VENOMOUS SNAKES
OF THE WORLD

VENOMOUS SNAKES
OF THE WORLD

A Manual for Use by U.S. Amphibious Forces

Based on *Poisonous Snakes of the World*
by the Department of the Navy,
Bureau of Medicine and Surgery

Revised and Updated by
Scott Shupe

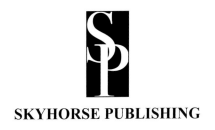

SKYHORSE PUBLISHING

All inquiries should be addressed to Skyhorse Publishing, 307 West 36th Street, 11th Floor, New York, NY 10018.

Skyhorse Publishing books may be purchased in bulk at special discounts for sales promotion, corporate gifts, fund-raising, or educational purposes. Special editions can also be created to specifications. For details, contact the Special Sales Department, Skyhorse Publishing, 307 West 36th Street, 11th Floor, New York, NY 10018 or info@skyhorsepublishing.com.

Skyhorse® and Skyhorse Publishing® are registered trademarks of Skyhorse Publishing, Inc.®, a Delaware corporation.

Visit our website at www.skyhorsepublishing.com.

10 9 8 7 6 5 4 3 2 1

Library of Congress Cataloging-in-Publication Data is available on file.

ISBN: 978-1-62087-623-7

Printed in China

CONTENTS

Introduction

Nearly half a century ago in 1965, three of the world's most noted herpetologists and medical professionals, in conjunction with the United States Navy's Bureau of Medicine and Surgery, cooperated to produce what at that time was perhaps the most comprehensive publication on the world's venomous snake species yet published. The book, *Poisonous Snakes of the World*, quickly became an important reference, not only for military personnel, but also medical professionals, herpetologists, and reptile keepers. Even today it remains a popular book among naturalists, book collectors, zoo personnel, and snake enthusiasts. In keeping with the current understanding of the terms "Poisonous" vs. "Venomous," the word poisonous has been changed to venomous in the title and throughout the text of this new manual.

This volume was inspired by the epic work *Poisonous Snakes of the World*, from nearly fifty years ago. Many reptile enthusiasts over the years have mused aloud about their yearnings for an updated version of that original publication, complete with color photos rather than black and white, and encompassing all the new species that were unknown or omitted from the 1965 edition. This project was conceived as a revised and updated version of *Poisonous Snakes of the World*. However, it soon became apparent to the author that the body of knowledge about venomous snakes has evolved enormously through the decades. In *Poisonous Snakes of the World,* there were less than 175 species of venomous snakes described. Today, the number of venomous snake species known to science exceeds 600. In addition to many new species having been described, many subspecies have been elevated to full species status, and in some instances there are species that are now assigned to entirely different genera. Even more dramatic, taxonomic changes have resulted in a few species being assigned to entirely different families.

In a classic example of how much the taxonomy of venomous snakes has changed since the publication of *Poisonous Snakes of the World* in 1965, the cobra species *Naja anchietae* (Ancheita's Cobra) was once considered to be a subspecies of *Naja annulifera* (Snouted Cobra). Meanwhile, the Snouted Cobra was formerly regarded as a subspecies of *Naja haje* (Egyptian Cobra). Thus, what was regarded in 1965 as a single species has now become three species in Africa with a fourth newly described species in the Arabian Peninsula. An even greater example are the Saw-scaled Vipers (*Echis*) which once consisted of only two species but now boast eleven recognized species and several subspecies within some of those eleven species. The North American rattlesnake species *Crotalus viridis* (Prairie Rattlesnake) was for many years regarded as a polymorphic species consisting of eight subspecies. It is now known that the complex formerly known as the "Prairie Rattlesnakes" contains six separate species (according to the Center for North American Herpetology). These are just a few examples of the extent of the changes that have occurred in the study of these animals over the last five decades.

While this book was inspired by the 1965 publication *Poisonous Snakes of the World*, this writer does not presume to possess the knowledge and expertise of the original authors. It is hoped by the revisionist author that this book will stand on its own merit and gain acceptance and use by both the U.S. military as well as the herpetological community.

In deference to the those early giants who produced *Poisonous Snakes of the World;* and upon whose shoulders this author and indeed all modern herpetologists stand, I have elected to include in this volume (where still appropriate) many excerpts and direct quotes from that 1965 book. The original authors were in a class far above this writer's status insofar as their scientific credentials and capabilities are concerned. Their work was peer reviewed and they themselves were selected for the task of writing the original book by the American Society of Icthyologists and Herpetologists.

Insofar as the taxonomic nomenclature used in this manual is concerned, this author found many diverse and varying views on the subject. It is in many ways heartening to see so much work being done on venomous snakes by researchers around the world, but also somewhat frustrating to be writing a book at a time when there is so much new and divergent research being conducted. The conclusions of the various researchers are often in conflict and as a result the current taxonomy of many species is controversial. Faced with these conflicting opinions (or as the researchers themselves would say "evidence"), the author was forced to make a choice regarding whose evidence was most acceptable.

In this case that difficult task was made easier due to the fact that this book is intended as a manual for U.S. military personnel. The Information Services Division of the Armed Forces Pest Management Board relies heavily upon the taxonomic classification used by the EMBL Reptile Database (personal communication, Harold Harlan). The Reptile Database is a website published by the European Molecular Biological Laboratory. While there are many within the professional herpetological community that do not follow completely everything contained in the Reptile Database, there are others who do accept its version of current reptile taxonomy. Moreover, as this book is intended mainly as a military manual, it seems logical to follow the same guidelines used by the Armed Forces Pest Management Board. For the most part that has been done in this manual. However, I have deviated at times from what is contained within the Reptile Database. For instance, in dealing with North American species, I have followed the classifications used by the Center for North American Herpetology, notably the publication *Standard Common and Current Scientific Names for North American Amphibians, Turtles, Reptiles & Crocodilians* (Collins & Taggart 2009). Likewise in chapter 14 (USPACOM-Part 2) which deals with mainly Australian species, I have at times deferred to the classification used by two Australian sources. One was the University of Adelaide's Clinical Toxinology Resources website (www.toxinology.com) and the other was a website known as the Australian Reptile Online Database (www.arod.com.au/).

Finally, it is important to note that many scholars in the science of herpetology will find much to criticize in this book. Among them will likely be many of those who generously contributed photographs, forwarded scientific papers, and generally tried to steer this author in the direction of scientific accuracy. Despite their efforts and my own, this volume remains an unscientific book. Experts in herpetology have not reviewed it for complete scientific accuracy, and it is a book written mostly for laypersons. *Its goal is to help lay military personnel deal with the small threat that venomous snakes pose to them and to their mission.* That said, it is hoped that the photos and information contained herein will also find acceptance and use by many others, especially by those who appreciate nature in general and snakes in particular.

Scott Shupe, 2012

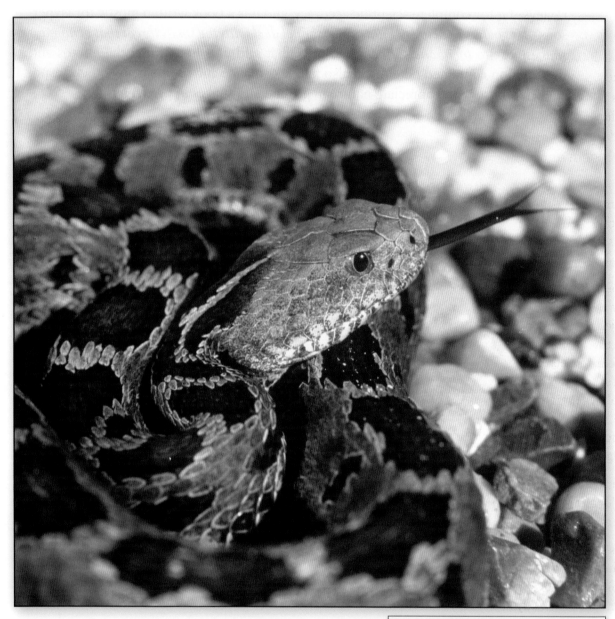

Mexican Pygmy Rattlesnake,
Crotalus ravus

CHAPTER 1
GENERAL INFORMATION

There may be as many as a half million bites and 20,000 deaths per year from snakebite worldwide (Kasturiratne et al. 2008). That figure is about half of the number of deaths attributed to venomous snakes worldwide when this book was originally published in 1965. In all probability, the death estimates are low, given that in many undeveloped regions of the world snakebite deaths often go unrecorded.

Personnel of the U.S. Navy and Marine Corps may find themselves stationed or visiting in many parts of the world, particularly the countries bordering the oceans. In some of these countries, snakebite is a significant public health hazard.

American military forces have never experienced casualty rates from snake envenomations sufficiently high as to jeopardize the outcome of an operation. However, the threat of snakebite may create a morale problem sufficient to delay an operation or cause unnecessary fear during its execution. While snakebite has been rare and fatalities therefrom have been even more uncommon in the military forces, it does constitute a medical emergency requiring immediate attention and considerable judgment in management.

This manual is designed to facilitate identification of the major groups (genera) of venomous snakes and to identify the most dangerous species.

It is not practical to by-pass the specialized terminology of herpetology completely, but herpetological terms are avoided whenever possible. Those that are used are defined in the glossary or are evident from examinations of the figures.

Geographic definitions of regions discussed are provided because of differences in the use of such words as Middle East, Southeast Asia, Near East, et cetera. Snakes found in more than one region are listed in each.

A second aim of the manual is to give suggestions for preventing snakebite, and a third aim is to indicate practical first aid measures should snakebite occur. Principals and procedures for medical managment of snake envenomation are discussed, but it is not a purpose of the manual to evaluate all the varied and sometimes conflicting therapeutic regimens that have appeared in the medical literature.

A list of specific references is included at the end of each chapter. There are two groups of references that are titled CURRENT REFERENCES and ORIGINAL REFERENCES. The list of current references contains all the specific references used in revising and updating this volume. The original references is a list of all the specific references used in the original (1965) text. The list of general references at the back of this manual is also from the original text. A space for notes will be found at the end of most chapters. This may be used for additional references and information gained under local circumstances.

CURRENT REFERENCES

Kasturiratne A, Wickremasinge AR, de Silva N, Gunwardena NA, Pathmeswaren A, et al. 2008. "Estimation of the Global Burden of Snakebite." PLoS Med., 5(11):e218 DOI 10.1371 /journal.pmed.0050218.

Swaroop, S. and B. Grab. 1954. *Snakebite Mortality in the World.* Bulletin of the World Health Organization, 10 35-76.

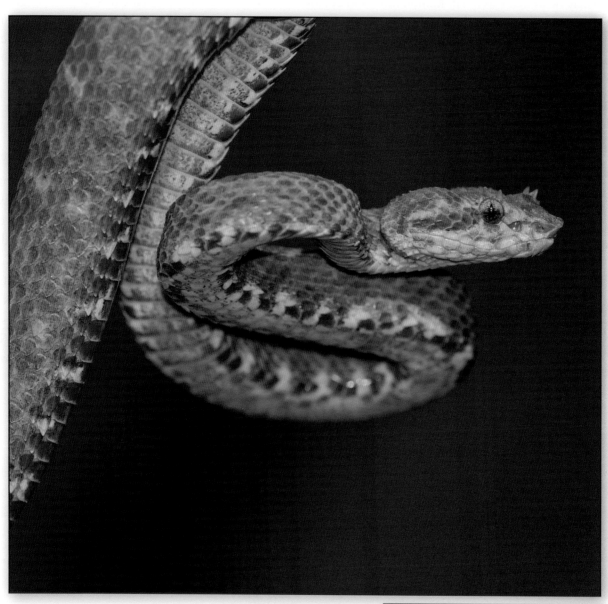

Eyelash Viper,
Bothriechis schlegeli, red phase

CHAPTER 2
PRECAUTIONS TO AVOID SNAKEBITE

The best way to keep from being bitten by snakes is to avoid them. However, since there is little choice in a duty assignment, there are certain precautions to be taken in "snake country."

When in a snake-infested country, it is important to:

1. **Remember that snakes are probably more afraid of humans than humans are of snakes.** Given the chance snakes will usually retreat to avoid an encounter.

2. **Learn to recognize the venomous snakes in the area of operation.** Avoid killing harmless snakes.

3. **Avoid walking around after dark.** Many venomous snakes are nocturnal and will travel at night far beyond the distances they may venture during the day. If you must walk at night be sure to wear boots.

4. **Remember that snakes in general avoid direct sunlight,** and that they are most active at moderate conditions.

5. **Avoid caves, open tombs, and known snake den areas.** Snakes live in areas which afford protection and which may be frequented by other small animals. They may be found in considerable numbers in caves and open tombs during the hibernation period which in most snakes extends from fall until early spring. They may also seek out these same areas during the summer months.

6. **Remember that venomous snakes may be found at high altitudes,** and that they can climb trees and fences.

7. **Walk on clear paths as much as possible.** Avoid tall grass and areas of heavy underbrush or ground covering. Always wear protective clothing in these areas.

8. **Avoid swimming in waters where snakes abound.** Most land species of venomous snakes swim well, and may, under unusual circumstances, bite while in the water. Sea snakes are not uncommon in the Indo-pacific area.

9. **Avoid sleeping on the ground whenever possible.**

10. **Avoid walking close to rocky ledges.** Give snakes a wide passage, just in case.

11. **Avoid hiking alone in snake-infested areas.**

12. **Avoid horse-play involving live or dead snakes.** Snakes should not be handled carelessly. Teasing people with snakes may have unexpected and unfortunate results.

Specific Precautions:

1. The following **DON'Ts** are suggested for those in snake country.

2. **DON'T** put your hands or feet in places you cannot look, and

3. **DON'T** put them in places without first looking.

4. **DON'T** turn or lift a rock or fallen tree with your hands. Move it with a stick, or with your foot if your ankle and leg are properly protected.

5. **DON'T** disturb snakes.

6. **DON'T** put your sleeping bag near rock piles or rubbish piles or near the entrance to a cave.

7. **DON'T** sit down without first looking around carefully.

8. **DON'T** gather firewood after dark.

9. **DON'T** step over a log if the other side is not visible. Step on it first.

10. **DON'T** enter snake-infested areas without adequate protective clothing.

11. **DON'T** handle freshly killed venomous snakes. Always carry them on a stick or in a bag if they must be returned to the command post.

12. **DON'T** crawl under a fence in high grass or in an uncleared area.

13. **DON'T** go out of your way to kill a snake. Thousands of people are bitten by snakes each year merely because they try to kill them withou tknowing anything about their habits or habitats.

14. Finally, **DON'T PANIC!**

Many military personnel may find reading the above list of precautions understandably disconcerting. Military missions in general and combat missions in particular often require doing some of the exact things cautioned against on the above list.

However even in circumstances where violating these precautions is necessary to the success of the mission, the actual threat posed by snakes is *proportionately* small. Venomous snakes evolved their venom primarily as a means of securing their food, (i.e., killing prey). Although most will bite in defense if threatened, they usually prefer to retreat or remain hidden. Only when hard pressed will most species inflict a bite.

Many defensive bites by snakes that have been approached too closely or trodden upon inadvertently, will not result in a life-threatening envenomation. Snakes control the amount of venom they inject, and usually the more frightened the snake the more dangerous the bite. Some defensive bites often result in only small doses of venom being injected and a small percentage of defensive bites may be "dry" bites, where no venom is injected at all.

On the other hand, when fighting for its life an enraged and terrified snake will often inject a larger dose of venom, thus increasing the likelihood of a life threatening bite. For this reason killing snakes is not recommended in instances where the option exists to simply move away from the snake.

Obviously, attempting to catch or handle snakes is a bad idea. As fundamental as that statement may sound to most people, the truth is that most venomous snakebites happen to people who are attempting to capture or handle the offending snake.

NOTES

CHAPTER 3

HOW TO RECOGNIZE SNAKE ENVENOMATION

INTRODUCTION

In most parts of the world, bites by nonvenomous snakes occur far more frequently than bites by venomous snakes. Since the differentiation is often difficult, all victims of snakebite should be brought under the care of a physician as quickly as possible.

In older texts, including the 1965 edition of this volume, the discussion of snakebite treatment and first aid usually included instructions such as "Whenever feasible the offending snake should be killed and brought with the victim to the physician." Although the identification of the offending snake has always been an important element in proper treatment, this advice is not without flaws. Attempting to kill a venomous snake can lead to additional bites, and even dead snakes have been known to reflexively envenomate careless handlers. In today's modern world a much safer tactic would be to take a picture of the snake and bring that to the physician. Almost everyone today has a cell phone or other device that can be used to accomplish this task. While a cell phone photo may not be as good a diagnostic tool as a dead snake, in most cases it should suffice for proper identification and it entails less risk. When possible to safely accomplish, a close up photo of the head along with a wide shot of the entire snake is most desirable for identification purposes.

While it is not always possible to identify the snake responsible for the bite by the tooth or fang marks found on the victim's skin, in some cases these may be of considerable value in differentiating between bites by venomous and nonvenomous species. Bites by the vipers (Old World vipers, pit vipers of Asia, eastern Europe, and the rattlesnakes and related species of the Americas) usually result in one or two relatively large puncture wounds of varying depth, depending on the size of the snake, the force of its strike, and other factors.

In most cases, additional tooth marks are not seen. Bites by the elapid snakes (cobras, mambas, tiger snake, taipan, coral snakes, and related species) usually produce one or two small puncture wounds, although occasionally there may be one or two additional punctures. Sea snake bites are characterized by multiple (2 to 20) pinhead-sized puncture wounds. In some cases the teeth may be broken off and remain in the wound.

Proper identification of fang or tooth marks may be complicated in those cases where skin tears result from jerking an extremity away during the biting act. This is a particular problem in viper bites where long scratches or even lacerations are inflicted by the fangs. In bites by elapid snakes there may be superficial scratches from the snake's mandibular and palatine teeth. Thus, it can be seen that while fang or tooth patterns may be of assistance in determining the identity of an offending snake, they should not be depended upon as the deciding factor in establishing the diagnosis.

It should be noted that one can be bitten by a venomous snake and not be envenomated. In 3 to 40 percent of the bites inflicted by venomous snakes, no signs or symptoms of envenomation develop. This may be due to the fact that the snake does not always inject venom, or if venom is ejected that it does not enter the wound, as can sometimes happen in very superficial bites. This important fact should always be considered before specific treatment is started.

Venom Apparatus

The venom apparatus of a snake consists of a gland, a duct, and one or more fangs located on each side of the head (fig. 1). The size of these structures depends on the size and species of the snake. Each venom gland is invested in a connective tissue sheath which is invaded by the muscles that contract it during discharge of the venom. The innervation of these muscles is different from that controlling the biting mechanisms: thus, the snake can control the amount of venom it ejects. It can discharge venom from either fang, from both, or from neither. Snakes rarely eject the full contents of their glands.

Most rattlesnakes probably discharge between 25 and 75 percent of their venom when they bite a human. The true vipers discharge about the same, perhaps slightly less. There appears to be a greater variation in the amount an elapid may discharge. Many victims of elapid envenomations have minimal signs and symptoms; others show evidence of severe envenomation.

The fangs of the vipers are two elongated, canaliculated teeth of the maxillary bones. These bones can be rotated so that the fangs can be moved from their resting positions against the upper jaw, to their biting positions, approximately perpendicular to the upper jaw. These snakes have full control over their fangs, raising or lowering them at will as when striking, biting, or yawning. The two functional fangs are shed periodically and are replaced by the first reserve fangs. The fangs of the elapid snakes are two enlarged anterior maxillary teeth. These teeth are hollow and are fixed in an erect position.

Snake Venoms

The venom of most snakes is a complex mixture, chiefly proteins, many of which have enzymatic activity. Some of the effects of snake venoms are due to the nonenzymatic protein portions of the venom, while others are due to the enzymes and enzymatic combinations. The symptoms and signs of snake envenomation may be complicated by the release of several substances from the victim's own tissues. These autopharmacologic substances sometimes render diagnosis and treatment more difficult.

The arbitrary division of venoms into such groups as neurotoxins, hemotoxins, and cardiotoxins, while having some useful purpose in classification, has led to much misunderstanding and a number of errors in treatment. In the years since the original publication of this volume the terms *cytotoxin, myotoxin, nephrotoxin,* and *necrotoxin,* have come into wide use in describing the physiological effects of snake venoms. Additionally, terms such as *procoagulant, haemorrhagic,* and *anticoagulant* are frequently used in discussions involving hemotoxins. It has become increasingly apparent that these divisions are over-simplified and misleading. Neurotoxins can, and often do have cardiotoxic or hemotoxic activity, or both; cardiotoxins may have neurotic or hemotoxic activity, or both; and hemotoxins may have the other activities. It is best to consider all snake venoms capable of producing several changes, sometimes concomitantly, in one or more of the organ systems of the body.

It is also apparent that quantitative and perhaps, qualitative differences in the chemistry of venoms may occur at the species level and may, in fact, be evident in snakes

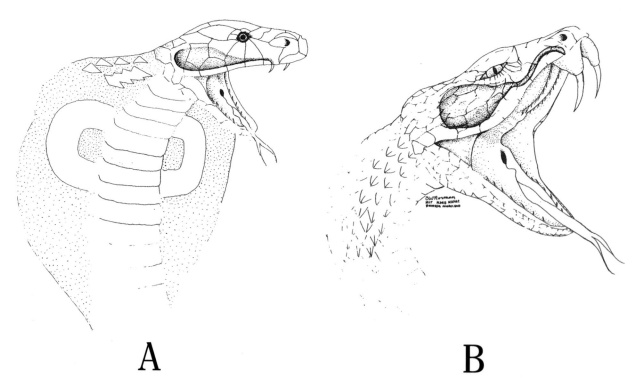

A   B

FIGURE 1. Figures of fangs, venom ducts, and venom glands of : A. Cobra (Elapidae), and B. Viper (Viperidae). The fangs of elapid snakes are much shorter than those of vipers and do not rotate. In each case the venom glands lie outside the main jaw muscles toward the back of the head. The venom ducts lead from the glands to the bases of the hollow fangs.

of the same species taken from different geographic areas. Thus, differences in the symptoms and signs of envenomation may occur even when similar snakes are involved in a series of accidents.

In Table 1 are given the names of some of the more important venomous snakes of the world, their adult average lengths, the approximate amount of dried venom contained within their venom glands (adult specimens), and the intraperitoneal and intravenous LD50 in mice, as expressed in milligrams of venom (on a dry weight basis) per kilogram of test animal body weight. The purpose of this table is to demonstrate the considerable differences that exist in the lethality of various snake venoms.

In general, the venoms of the vipers cause deleterious changes in the tissues both at the site of the bite and in its proximity, changes in the red blood cells, defects in coagulation, injury to the blood vessels; and, to a lesser extent, damage to the heart muscle, kidneys, and lungs. The venom of the tropical rattlesnake, Crotalus durissus, cause more severe changes in nerve conduction and neuromuscular transmission than do other crotalid venoms. The venoms of the elapid snakes cause lesser local tissue changes, but often cause serious alterations in sensory and motor function as well as cardiac and respiratory difficulties.

SYMPTOMS AND SIGNS

The symptoms, signs, and the gravity of snake venom poisoning are dependent upon a number of factors: the age and size of the victim, the nature, location, depth, and number of bites, the length of time the snake holds on, the extent of anger or fear that motivates the snake to strike, the amount of venom injected, the species and size of the snake involved, the condition of its fangs and venom glands, the victim's sensitivity to the venom, the pathogens present in the snake's mouth, and the degree and kind of first aid and subsequent medical care. It can be seen that snakebites may vary in severity from trivial to extremely grave.

The findings given in tables 2, 3, and 4 are those observed in what may be termed typical or moderately severe cases of snake envenomation. While they are not complete, they do provide a ready reference of the more commonly observed sequelae of bites by venomous snakes.

Diagnosis of crotalid envenomation is dependent upon the presence of one or more fang marks, and immediate and usually progressive swelling, edema, and pain. In most cases, swelling and edema are constant findings and are usually seen about the injured area within 10 minutes of the bite. In the absence of treatment, the swelling progresses rapidly and may involve the entire injured extremity within one hour. Generally, however, swelling and edema spread more slowly, and usually over period of 8-36 hours. Swelling and edema are most marked following bites by the North American Rattlesnakes (excluding the Mohave, Massassaugas, and pygmy rattlesnake) and the American lance head vipers (Bothrops, Rhinocerophis, and Bothropiodes). Swelling is slightly less marked following bites by the Malayan Pit Viper (Calloselasma rhodostoma) the Asian Pit Viper genus Trimeresurus, and the American moccasins (Agkistrodon). It is least acute following bites by the cascabel or South American Rattlesnake (Crotalus durussus terrificus).

In many cases, discoloration of the skin and ecchymosis appear in the area of the bite within several hours. The skin appears tense and shiny. Vesicles may form within 3 hours, and are generally present by the end of 24 hours. Hemorrhagic vesiculations and petechiae are common.

Pain immediately following the bite is a common complaint in most cases of crotalid envenomations. It is most severe following bites by the South American pit vipers (except for the cascabel, which is less severe); the eastern diamondback, western diamondback, and timber rattlesnakes of North America, and the Asian pit vipers.

Weakness, sweating, faintness, and nausea are commonly reported. Regional lymph nodes may be enlarged, painful, and tender. A very common complaint following bites by some rattlesnakes, and one sometimes reported following other pit viper bites, is tingling or numbness over the tongue and mouth or scalp. Paresthesia about the wound is sometimes reported. Viperid envenomation is characterized by burning pain of rapid onset, swelling and edema, and patch skin discoloration and ecchymosis in the area of the bite. Extravasation of blood from the wound site is common in Russell's and saw-scaled viper envenomations. The failure of the blood to clot is a valuable diagnostic finding. Bleeding from the gums, and the intestinal and urinary tracts is common in severe Russell's and saw-scaled viper bites.

Cobra envenomaton is characterized by pain usually within 10 minutes of the bite, and this is followed by localized swelling of slow onset, drowsiness, weakness, excessive salivation, and paresis of the facial muscles, lips, tongue, and larynx. The pulse is often weak, blood pressure is reduced, respirations are labored, and there may be generalized muscular weakness or paralysis. Ptosis, blurring of vision, and headache may be present. Contrary to popular opinion, necrosis is not an uncommon consequence of cobra envenomations. In bites by the kraits a similar clinical picture is usually seen, except that there is very little or no local swelling or severe pain. The systemic manifestations may often be more severe, and shock, marked respiratory depression, and coma may rapidly develop. Abdominal pain is often intense following envenomation by the kraits, mambas, and taipans. Envenomation by coral snakes may resemble krait bites. The bite is usually less painful, and there is occasionally a sensation of numbness about the wound. Chest pain, particularly on inspiration, is sometimes reported. Localized edema is minimal and necrosis is rare.

Mamba envenomation is characterized by weakness, nausea and vomiting, blurred vision, slurred speech, excessive salivation, headache, and abdominal pain. These findings are often followed by hypotension, respiratory distress, and shock.

Envenomation by most of the Australian-Papuan elapids produces drowsiness, visual disturbances, ptosis, nausea and vomiting, headache, abdominal pain, slurring of speech, respiratory distress, and generalized muscular weakness or paralysis. Hemoglobinuria may be found early in the course of the symptoms.

Sea snake envenomations are usually characterized by multiple pinhead-sized puncture wounds, little or no localized pain, oftentimes tenderness and some pain in the skeletal muscles and in particular, the larger muscle masses and the neck. This pain is increased with motion. The tongue feels thick and its motion may be restricted. There may be paresthesia about the mouth. Sweating and thirst are common complaints, and the patient may complain of pain on swallowing. Trismus, extraocular weakness or paralysis, dilation of the pupils, ptosis and generalized weakness may be present. Respiratory distress is common in severe cases. Myoglobinuria is diagnostic.

Little is known about the problem of envenomation by rear-fanged colubrid snakes. The African boomslang and bird snake are know to produce severe envenomations, which on rare occasions may be fatal. (These snakes are described on p. 202.) Other species of colubrids, some with enlarged grooved fangs and some with solid teeth, are know to bite and may be venomous. The manifestations of bites by known venomous colubrids, such as the mangrove snake (Boiga dendrophila) of southeast Asia, the "culebra de cola corta" (Tachymenis

peruviana) of western South America, the parrot snakes (Leptophis) of tropical America and several other species are known to cause local pain and swelling, sometimes accompanied by localized skin discoloration and ecchymosis; and in the more severe envenomation, increased swelling and edema which may involve the entire injured extremity, general malaise, and fever. The acute period may persist of 4 to 7 days. In the decades since the original publication of this volume a new family of mostly harmless snakes, the Lamprophiidae, has been described. Within this family is a single genus (*Malpolon*) of southern Europe and north Africa that is mildly venomous and has caused at least one death. It is important to differentiate envenomation by colubrids and others from that of more dangerous elapids and vipers.

In summary, any snakebite associated with immediate (and sometimes intense) pain, followed within several minutes by the appearance of swelling and subsequently edema is usually diagnostic of envenomation by a viper. Elapid envenomation, on the other hand, is not so easily diagnosed during the first 10 minutes following the bite. Pain, usually of minor intensity, may appear within the first 10 minutes, although in some cases it is not reported for 30 minutes or even longer. Swelling usually appears 2 or 3 hours following the bite and tends to be limited to the area of the wound. The first systemic sign of elapid envenomation is usually drowsiness. This is often apparent within 2 hours of the bite. Ptosis, blurring of vision, and difficulties in speech and swallowing may also appear within several hours of the bite. It can be seen how important it is in cobra, mamba, krait, taipan, tiger, and coral snake bites to determine the identity of the offending reptile as quickly as possible. A difference of 30 minutes to 1 hour in initiating treatment in elapid bites may make the difference between life and death.

TABLE 1. - Yield and lethality of venoms of important venomous snakes

Snake	Average length of adult (inches)	Approximate yield, dry venom (mg.)	Intraperitoneal LD$_{50}$ (mg./kg.)	Intravenous LD$_{50}$ (mg./kg.)
North America				
A. Rattlesnakes (*Crotalus*)				
Eastern diamondback (*C. adamanteus*)	33–65	370–720	1.89	1.68
Western diamondback (*C. atrox*)	30–65	175–325	3.71	4.20
Timber (*C. horridus horridus*)	32–54	95–150	2.91	2.63
Prairie (*C. viridis viridis*)	32–46	25–100	2.25	1.61
Great Basin (*C. v. lutosus*)	32–46	75–150	2.20	—
Southern Pacific (*C. v. helleri*)	30–48	75–160	1.60	1.29
Red diamond (*C. ruber ruber*)	30–52	125–400	6.69	3.70
Mojave (*C. scutulatus*)	22–40	50–90	0.23	0.21
Sidewinder (*C. cerastes*)	18–30	18–40	4.00	—
B. Moccasins (*Agkistrodon*)				
Cottonmouth (*A. piscivorus*)	30–50	90–148	5.11	4.00
Copperhead (*A. contortrix*)	24–36	40–72	10.50	10.92
Cantil (*A. bilineatus*)	30–42	50–95	—	2.40
C. Coral snakes (*Micrurus*)				
Eastern coral snake (*M. fulvius*)	16–28	2–6	0.97	—
Central and South America				
A. Rattlesnakes (*Crotalus*)				
Cascabel (*C. durissus terrificus*)	20–48	20–40	0.30	—
B. American lance-headed vipers (*Bothrops*)				
Barba amarilla (*B. atrox*)	46–80	70–160	3.80	4.27
C. Bushmaster (*Lachesis mutus*)	70–110	280–450	5.93	—
Asia				
A. Cobras (*Naja*)				
Asian cobra (*N. naja*)	45–65	170–325	0.40	0.40
B. Kraits (*Bungarus*)				
Indian krait (*B. caeruleus*)	36–48	8–20	—	0.09
C. Vipers (*Vipera*)				
Russell's viper (*V. russelii*)	40–50	130–250	—	0.08
D. Pit vipers (*Agkistrodon*)				
Malayan pit viper (*A. rhodostoma*)	25–35	40–60	—	6.20
Africa				
A. Vipers				
Puff adder (*Bitis arietans*)	30–48	130–200	3.68	—
Saw-scaled viper (*Echis carinatus*)	16–22	20–35	—	2.30
B. Mambas (*Dendroaspis*)				
Eastern green mamba (*D. angusticeps*)	50–72	60–95	—	0.45
Australia				
A. Tiger snake (*Notechis scutatus*)	30–56	30–70	0.04	—
Europe				
A. Vipers				
European viper (*Vipera berus*)	18–24	6–18	0.80	0.55
Indo-Pacific				
A. Sea snakes				
Beaked sea snake (*Enhydrina schistosa*)	30–48	7–20	—	0.01

TABLE 2. - Signs and symptoms of crotalid bites

Symptoms and Signs [1]	North American Rattlesnakes (Crotalus)	Central and South American Rattlesnakes (Crotalus)	North American Moccasins (Agkistrodon)	American Lance-headed Vipers (Bothrops)	Asian Lance-headed Vipers (Trimeresurus)	Malayan Pit Viper (Agkistrodon)
Swelling and edema	+++[5]	+	++	+++	+++	+++
Pain	++	++	+	+++	++	+++
Discoloration of skin	+++	+	+	+++	+++	+++
Vesicles	+++		+	+++	++	++
Ecchymosis	+++	+	++	+++	+++	+++
Superficial thrombosis	++		–	++	–	–
Necrosis	++		+	+++	+	+
Sloughing of tissue	++		–	+++	+	+
Weakness	++	+++	+	++	++	+++
Thirst	++	+++	+	++	+	++
Nausea or vomiting or both	++	+++	+	++	–	–
Diarrhea	+	+++	–		+	+++
Weak pulse and changes in rate	+++	+++	+	+++	+++	++
Hypotension or shock	+++	+	+	+++	++	++
Sphering or destruction of red blood cells	++		–		–	–
Increased bleeding time	++	+	–	+++	+	+
Increased clotting time	+++	++	+	+++	++	++
Hemorrhage [2]	+++		–	+++	++	++
Anemia	++		–	++	+	+
Blood platelet changes [3]	++		–	++	+	+
Glycosuria	++		+		–	–
Proteinuria	++	+	+	++	+	+
Tingling or numbness [4]	++	+++	–	++	+	–
Fasciculations	+	+++	–		–	–
Muscular weakness or paralysis	+	+++	–	+	–	–
Ptosis	+	+++	–	+	–	–
Blurring of vision	+		–	+	–	–
Respiratory distress	++	+++	+	++	–	–
Swelling regional lymph nodes	++	+	+	++	+	–
Abnormal ECG	+	++	–	+	++	++
Coma	+	++	–	+	+	+

[1] In the more severe cases the intensity of the symptoms and signs may be markedly increased. In addition, there may be severe respiratory distress, cyanosis, muscle spasms, and secondary shock leading to death.

[2] Bleeding may be from the gastrointestinal, urinary, or respiratory tracts, from the gums, or it may be subcutaneous. In *Trimeresurus* bites the hemorrhage is usually confined to the locus of the wound. Bleeding from the gums is common following *Bothrops* envenomation.

[3] Platelets may be increased in mild poisonings and markedly decreased in severe cases.

[4] Often confined to the tongue and mouth, but may involve the scalp and distal parts of the toes and fingers as well as the injured part.

[5] (+ to +++) = Grading of severity of symptom, sign or finding, (–) = Of lesser significance or absent, ( ) = Information lacking.

TABLE 3. - Symptoms and signs of viperide bites

Symptoms and Signs	Russell's Viper (*Vipera russelii*)	Saw-Scaled Viper (*Echis carinatus*)	Levantine Viper (*Vipera lebetina*) and related species	European Viper (*Vipera berus*)	Puff Adder (*Bitis arietans*)
Swelling and edema	+++	+++	++	++	++
Pain	+++	+++	++	++	+++
Discoloration of skin	+++	++	++	++	+++
Weakness	++	++	+	++	++
Nausea or vomiting or both	++	+	+++	++	++
Abdominal pain	++	+	+++	+	++
Diarrhea	++	+	+++	+	++
Thirst	++	+++	+	++	+
Chills or fever	++	++	++	-	+
Swelling regional lymph nodes	+	+	++	++	++
Facial edema	+	-	++	+	+
Dilatation of pupils	++	+	+	+	+
Weak pulse and changes in rate	++	+	++	+	+
Albuminuria	++	+	++	-	-
Proteinuria	++	++	++	-	-
Hypotension	++	++	++	+	++
Shock	++	++	++	+	++
Hemorrhage[1]	++	+++	++	+	++
Anemia	++	++	+	-	-
Vesicles	++	++	++	+	++
Ecchymosis	++	++	++	+	+++
Necrosis	++	+	+	-	++
Decreased platelets	+	+	+	-	+
Prolonged clotting time	+++	+++	++	-	+

[1] Usually limited to area of wound in puff adder and European viper bites. However, bleeding from the gums, intestine and urinary tract may occur, particularly in saw-scaled viper and Russell's viper envenomations.

TABLE 3. - Symptoms and signs of elapide bites (cont.)

Symptoms and Signs	Cobras (*Naja*)	Kraits (*Bungarus*)	Mambas (*Dendroaspis*)	Taipan (*Oxyuranus*)	Coral Snakes (*Micrurus*)
Pain	++	+	+	+	++
Localized edema	+	-	-	-	+
Drowsiness, weakness	+++	+++	++	+++	+++
Feeling of thickened tongue and throat, slurring of speech, difficulty in swallowing	+++	+++	+++	+++	++
Ptosis	+++	+++	++	+++	++
Changes in respiration	++	+++	++	+++	++
Headache	++	++	++	+++	++
Blurring of vision	++	++	+++	+++	++
Weak pulse and changes in rate	++	++	++	+	++
Hypotension	++	++	++	+	+
Excessive salivation	+++	+++	+++	+	++
Nausea and vomiting	+	++	+++	+++	+
Abdominal pain	+	+++	+++	+++	+
Pain in regional lymph nodes	+	++	+++	+++	+
Localized discoloration of skin	++	-	-	-	+
Localized vesicles	+	-	-	-	-
Localized necrosis	+	-	-	-	-
Muscle weakness, paresis or paralysis	++	++	++	+++	+
Muscle fasiculations	+	+	+	+	+
Numbness of affected area	++	+++	+	+	++
Shock	++	++	++	+	+
Convulsions	+	+	-	-	-

ORIGINAL REFERENCES

CAMPBELL, C.H. 1964. "Venomous Snake Bite inPapua and Its Treatment with Tracheotomy, Artificial Respiration and Antivenene". Trans. R. Soc. Trop. Med. Hyg. 58: 263-273.

CHRISTENSEN, P. A. 1955. South African Snake Venoms and Antivenoms. South African Institute Medical Research, Johannesburg, 142 p.

EFRATI, P. and REIF, L. 1953. "Clinical and Pathological Oservation of Sixty-five Cases of Viper Bite in Isreal". Amer. J. Tro. Med. Hyg. 2: 1085-1108.

GENNARO, J. F., JR. 1963. "Observations on the Treatment of Snakebite in North America", p. 427-446. In H.L. Keegan and W.W. Macfarlane, *Venomous and Poisonous Animals and Noxious Plants of the Pacific Region*. Pergamon, Oxford.

HEATWOLFE, H. and BANUCHI, I.B. 1966. "Envenomation by the Colubrid Snake, Alsophis portoricensis". Herpetological 22: 132-134.

KAISER, E. and MICHL, M. 1958. Die Biochemie der Tierischen Giftie. F. Deutticke, Wien, 258 p.

KLAUBER, L. M. 1956. *Rattlesnakes, Their Habits, Life Histories, and Influence on Mankind*. University California Press, Berkeley. 2 vol.

MOLE, R. H. and EVERARD, A. 1947. "Snakebite by Echis carinata". Quart. J. Med. 16: 291-303.

REID, H.A. 1961. "Myoglobinuria and Seasnake Bite Poisoning". Brit. Med. J. 1: 1284-1289.

REID, H.A., THEAN, P.C., CHAN, K. E. and BAHARAM, A. R. 1963. "Clinical Effectes of Bites by Malayan Viper (*Ancistrodon rhodostoma*)", Lancet 1:617-621.

RUSSELL, F.E. 1962. "Snake Venom Poisoning", Vol II, p. 197-210. In, G. M. Piersol, *Cyclopedia of Medicine, Surgerey and the Specialties*. F.A. Davos. Philadelphia.

SAWAI, Y., MAKINO, M., TATENO, L., OKONOGI, T. and MITSUHASHI, S. 1962. "Studies on the improvement of treatment of Habu Snake (*Trimeresurus flavoviridis*) Bite". 3. Clinical Analysis and Medical Treatment of Habu Snake Bite on the Amanmi Islands. Hap. H. Exp. Med. 32: 17-138.

SCHENONE, H. and REYES, H. 1965. "Animales ponzonosos de Chile". Bol. Chileno de Parasitol. 20: 104-108.

WALDER, C. W. 1945. "Notes on Adder Bite (England and Wales)". Brit Med J. 2:13-14.

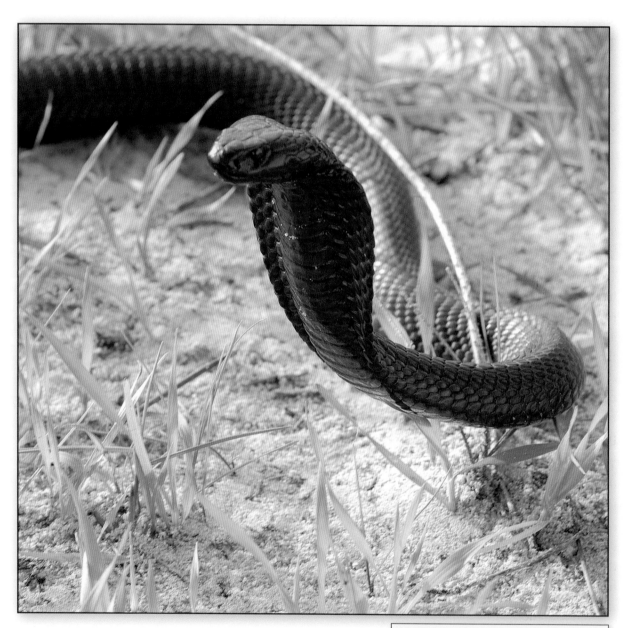

Western Barred Spitting Cobra,
Naja nigricincta, black phase

CHAPTER **4**
FIRST AID

INTRODUCTION

Since this volume was first published in 1965 understanding of snake venoms (and the way those venoms impact on living tissues) has expanded considerably. Likewise, the first aid and treatment of venomous snake bites has undergone significant change. So much so in fact, that the chapter written on this subject by the previous authors was so outdated that this author has elected to re-write this chapter completely.

Of course, some of the original advice for snakebite first aid remains valid. Such common sense things as getting the victim to a medical facility as soon as possible is perhaps even more imperative today than ever before. It has long been known that while there are some first aid measures that should be undertaken, the real treatment begins in the hospital; and it is now known that many of the accepted first practices from decades ago are a waste of time.

There has always been a "catch 22" involved in advice regarding snake bite first aid. The statement that the victim should "get to a medical facility as soon as possible, with the least amount of physical exertion as possible" leaves a real dilemma for a soldier or sailor who may be alone in the field and far from help.

Fortunately, most snakebite victims are not alone when these incidents occur, and in today's modern world rapid transport to a medical facility is nearly always possible.

GENERAL CONSIDERATIONS

The best advice in regards to snakebite first aid of course is to avoid being bitten in the first place! Obvious as this advice may seem, the truth is that most victims of venomous snakebites could have avoided being bitten. Snakes are retiring animals that usually try to avoid conflict. Most species bite only as a last resort. In general snakes, even venomous snakes, are afraid of people and if left alone they are not a threat. Thus, the easiest way to avoid being bitten is to avoid snakes.

Ironically, it is the snake's fear of man that leads the snake to bite. Venomous snakes have only one defense, and that is to bite. So, when trod upon by a giant, two-legged creature like a human, the snake's response is to bite. In truth, this is not how most human snakebites occur. The majority of bites are the result of people trying to kill, capture, or otherwise molest the offending snake (see page 3 chapter 2, Precautions to Avoid Snakebite.)

The first thing that should be discussed in regards to modern snakebite first aid is that nearly all the old methods recounted time and again through the years are *no longer regarded as valid and in fact are actually counter-productive.* These contraindicated tactics include topical applications of chemicals or ice, application of electrical current, and the famous "cut & suck" method of first aid. This latter tactic called for incisions made into the tissues and suction applied to the wound. This first aid method was discussed at length in the original publication of *Poisonous Snakes of the World* in 1965 and although it was long considered useful as a means of removing some of the venom from the victim, it is now known that this method is futile as a first aid measure.

One of the now disregarded actions discussed in the old "cut and suck" first aid method included instructions on the use of a constriction band around the bitten extremity above the bite. The idea was to retard the spread of venom through the body. Once again, the use of a constricting band (or a tourniquet) *is strongly contraindicated and should never be used in snakebite first aid.*

There is however a newer method whose aim is similar and that can be a useful first aid measure for some types of purely neurotoxic elapid snakes. That method, known as "pressure immobilization" or the "Sutherland technique," can help retard the spread of certain neurotoxic venoms and is a useful first aid method for the bites of coral snakes, kraits, sea snakes, many Australian elapids, and some cobra species. Also known as a "compression wrap" this technique involves firmly (but not too tightly) wrapping the bitten extremity *from distal to proximal* with a wide, elastic-type bandage in much the same way as one would wrap a sprained ankle.

CAUTION: **This method is for use only on snakes having purely neurotoxic venoms that do not have necrotic properties.** Nearly all vipers and many cobras (especially spitting cobras) have venoms that are strongly proteolytic and cause significant tissue damage. Applying a compression wrap to a bite by species such as these will increase the danger and severity associated with the necrotizing effect of the venom.

Insofar as first aid for vipers and other species whose venom precludes the use of the compression bandage, there is little that can be done to slow or prevent the absorption of the venom. One course of action that can be undertaken is to immobilize the bitten extremity to prevent movement of the limb. General restriction of movement and exertion by the patient is also important, as exerting movements may increase the spread of the venom through the body. Reassuring the victim and beginning arrangements for transport to a medical facility as soon as feasible are two other considerations that apply to any snakebite situation regardless of the species of snake involved. If trained to do so, starting an intravenous infusion of fluids can be useful in helping to delay or lessen the effect of one of snake envenomation's most deadly consequences, hypovolemic shock. In fact, it is useful for anyone administering first aid to regard a venomous snakebite as a form of trauma, where management of shock can be of paramount importance.

In the earlier (1965) edition of this book it was advised that medical corpsmen be trained in the use and administration of antivenom. This consideration today seems unnecessary as prompt transportation to medical facilities is normally possible, and antivenom treatment is not without some risk.

One factor that remains critical is in the making of a proper identification of the offending snake. In years past, including in this book's original edition, it was advised that the offending snake should be killed in order to facilitate proper identification. Certainly, having the dead snake on hand for examination is the ideal situation when attempting to make a proper identification. These actions however can entail some significant risks for personnel involved. Additional snakebites can easily occur to the personnel attempting to kill the snake. Even normally placid snakes when fighting for their life and escape is impossible, are capable of a spirited defense and even a dead snake can reflexively bite and inject venom. Thus, attempting to kill the snake and bring it to the hospital with the victim may not be the best solution to the need for proper identification. In today's world nearly everyone carries a cell phone with a camera function, or a small digital pocket camera of some variety. Most of these are capable of taking photographs that are of high enough quality to allow for proper identification of the offending snake by hospital personnel.

When taking photos of a snake for ID purposes, both a whole body photo and a close up photo of the head is most useful. Of course, care should be taken. Even dead snakes should not be handled and can be moved with a stick if necessary to reveal the animal for photography. A zoom feature is highly recommended, especially if the snake is still alive!

In such a case maintaining a safe distance of at least six feet is recommended when photographing a medium-sized (2 to 4 foot) snake. Smaller snakes can be more closely approached (3 feet), while larger snakes should be given correspondingly greater separation distances.

Finally, there may be rare circumstances where a soldier or sailor may find themselves in a situation where simply moving away from the snake is not an option, as for instance in the rare occurance of finding a snake in a bivouac (tent or shelter). In such circumstances killing a venomous snake may be necessary. If a snake must be killed to ensure the safety of nearby personnel it should be done as quickly and cleanly as possible. A wounded, enraged, and terrified snake is a much more dangerous animal than one that is casually encountered.

SIX STEPS IN SNAKEBITE FIRST AID *(all species)*

1. Immobilize bitten extremity and restrict overall movement.

2. Watch for signs of shock and react accordingly.

3. Reassure victim.

4. Arrange for transport to medical facility.

5. Photograph snake with cell phone or other device. If possible get a whole body shot then use zoom function if available to get a close up of the head. Keep a safe distance from the snake (see above).

OR IF THE SNAKE CAN BE KILLED AND COLLECTED; this method ensures that anyone familiar with the snakes of the region should be able to make a proper identification (see chapter 6, Recognition of Venomous Snakes.)

When collecting a dead snake for transport/identification, **DO NOT HANDLE THE SNAKE**, use a stick or tongs to lift the snake into a box or bag for transport.

EXTRA STEP FOR PURELY NEUROTOXIC ELAPIDS SNAKES

(including Coral Snakes, Kraits, King Cobra, Sea Snakes, and many Australian snakes.)

6. Apply compression bandage. **DO NOT USE COMPRESSION BANDAGE ON SNAKES THAT HAVE NECROTIZING COMPONENTS IN THEIR VENOM.**

Author's Note: *Much of the information contained in this chapter was supplied by Kristen Wiley and Jim Harrison of the Kentucky Reptile Zoo and Venom Laboratory.*

NOTES

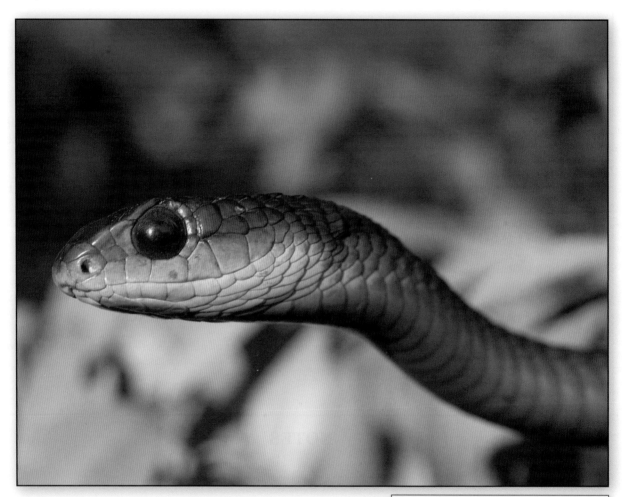

Boomslang (female),
Dispholidus typus

CHAPTER 5
MEDICAL TREATMENT

Author's Note:

Although the original authors of this chapter were medical profesionals and much of what was contained in the original edition regarding snakebite treatment remains relevant, it was written in 1965 and some of that material is now contraindicated.

The information for the outline for snakebite procedures that appears below was provided by Kristen Wiley and Jim Harrison of the Kentucky Reptile Zoo and Venom Laboratory. Though neither of these individuals are medical doctors, the procedures they have outlined have been developed over the last several decades in response to many venomous snakebites by a wide variety of species from around the globe.

These protocols are those that have been used successfully in treating the many bites experienced by both these individuals while working at their facility.

1. The proper identification of the offending snake is critical in determining the course of treatment.

Exact identification down to species level may not be as critical, but knowing whether the offending snake was a type of pit viper verses a species of krait or coral snake is *imperative*. First of all, identification is necessary to ascertain which type of antivenom should be used, but it can also be very important in regards to the methods of supportive therapy.

Therefore, it is highly recommended that some of the medical personnel within a deploying unit have some knowledge of the venomous snakes in the area to which the unit is deployed. This is especially true in regions of the world outside of the United States. The following recommendations assume some knowledge of the venomous snakes of the area by treating physicians.

Without this basic information, the snakebite scenario contains so many complicating factors and becomes so complex that it is impossible to give proper guidance.

The treatment regime and antivenom used (Coralmyn Antivenom) for treating North American coral snake bites is the same regardless of the species of coral snake involved. This also applies to all North American pit vipers, as the CroFAB Antivenom is effective against all pit vipers in the United States. However, there may be subtle differences in treatment regimes with certain pit vipers (copperhead bites and pygmy rattlesnake bites for instance very rarely warrant the use of antivenom). Thus exact identification down to species level is less critical in the United States, and the only really crucial information required is whether the offending snake was a venomous snake, and if so, was it a pit viper or a coral snake.

2. The primary treatment for snakebite is antivenom.

Although not all venomous snakebites will require antivenom, and its use does carry some risk of allergic reaction, if the need for antivenom therapy is apparent *it should begin immediately.* Unlike many types of trauma, where the stabilization of the patient is followed by surgery or other treatment, in the snakebite scenario, antivenom is crucial to both the initial stabilization as well as the treatment. Therefore the administration of antivenom should begin as soon as it becomes apparent that the patient has experienced a significant envenomation. The best results with antivenom use are achieved if it is administered within two hours of the bite. In some instances, however, it can still be used *with decreasing results* for up to 24 hours post bite.

Antivenom is administered intravenously by dilution (normally 1:10) in a saline drip (follow instructions contained in the antivenom package). The amount of antivenom needed to neutralize the venom will depend upon the amount of venom injected. Likewise the rate of infusion should depend upon the severity of symptoms weighed against the risk of allergic reaction. Infusion of a large amount of antivenom very rapidly may increase the risk of anaphylaxis. Since the amount of venom injected into the victim is impossible to determine, an initial dose of 10 vials is recommended. The protocol of the Kentucky Reptile Zoo regarding antivenom use is: *"If antivenom is needed, it is usually needed in larger rather than smaller amounts."* In the case of Australian species where the antivenoms are manufactured by Commonwealth Serum Laboratories (CSL), which come in much larger vials, 1 or 2 vials is adequate as an initial dosage.

Adequate antivenom supplies, *for each dangerous snake species found in the area of deployment*, is of paramount importance. Hours wasted trying to locate the correct antivenom can mean the difference between life and death for the snakebite victim. Again, it is important to note that in cases of severe envenomation by deadly species, antivenom therapy needs to begin at the earliest possible time. Although in almost every case it is impossible for treatment to be administered to personnel in remote locations, antivenom should be available at the first location to which injured personnel are evacuated.

Finally, as with any other type of trauma, a variety of supportive therapies may be needed. In the case of many neurotoxic species artificial ventilation may be necessary, sometimes for an extended period of several days. In these types of cases it is important to remember that the patient may be conscious, aware, and able to feel pain but unable to respond.

Bites by other mainly non-neurotoxic species such as the vipers also may require aggressive supportive therapy to combat hypovolemia, coagulopathy, etc.

3. Determination to give antivenom.

Antivenom should be given if any of the following symptoms appear in bites by vipers and other NON-NEU-ROTOXIC SPECIES.

Any symptoms of systemic poisoning (coagulopathy, hypovolemic shock, etc.). Local symptoms that can be signs of serious envenomation by non-neurotoxic venoms include swelling that progresses several inches or more beyond the site of the bite and significant discoloration (ecchymosis).

Antivenom should be given if any of the following symptoms appear in bites by NEUROTOXIC SPECIES. In bites by neurotoxic species antivenom is warranted in any bite by a snake having venom that is a *pre-synaptic neurotoxin.* Asian kraits and Australian taipans are a good example. In these species death occurs by respiratory paralysis. Once the symptoms of paralysis have progressed to the point of impairing normal respiration, antivenom will not be able to reverse this effect. Respiratory paralysis can last for several days, resulting in the need for artificial respiration. Any patient exhibiting signs of pre-synaptic poisoning (usually manifested as descending flaccid paralysis in which the first symptoms are paralysis of cranial nerves resulting in ptosis, loss of speech, confusion, etc.), should be treated with antivenom immediately. Even if administered prior to the onset (or at the earliest onset) of these symptoms, antivenom may not stop the progression of paralysis and aggressive supportive therapy (artificial respiration) may be necessary for up to several days.

Bites by neurotoxic snakes possessing *post-synaptic neurotoxins* usually respond to antivenom even after symptoms are well developed The American coral snakes, *Micrurus* are an exception, and reversal of respiratory paralysis in these snakes may not respond to antivenom once the symptoms have progressed to a point of respiratory failure. Thus, prophylactic antivenom therapy is recommended for treating all bites by members of this genus.

Snakebites by species possessing *post-synaptic neurotoxins* may also respond to treatment with anticholinesterase drugs.

Neurotoxic bites may present symptoms rapidly or very gradually, sometimes not manifesting for up to 12 hours. Victims of bites by neurotoxic species (even those showing no immediate signs of envenomation) should be observed closely for 24 hours.

4. Types of Antivenoms currently available.

Most antivenoms available today fall into one of two groups known as IgG and FAB'2. These antivenoms seem to have a longer half life in the body and therefore if the initial dose is sufficient to neutralize the amount of venom injected, they typically require only a single dosage.

CroFAB antivenom (used for treating bites of North American pit vipers) has a shorter half life and the venom-antivenom complex is more likely to dissociate. As a result, CroFAB typically requires repeated smaller doses over an approximately 72 hour period.

5. Potential complications.

When administering antivenoms, always be prepared for anaphylaxis. Have epinephrine available and be watchful for signs of allergic reaction.

Although many antivenom manufacturers advise the use of skin tests prior to the administration of antivenom, the protocol used by the Kentucky Reptile Zoo is that a skin test can increase the likelihood of, or initiate anaphylaxis, and skin tests are thus contraindicated.

6. Non-antivenom treatments.

There are a number of snake species throughout the world for which no antivenom is currently available. In such cases, supportive therapy is the physician's only option. Some widely used supportive therapies are listed below.

SUPPORTIVE THERAPY FOR NEUROTOXIC SNAKES:

*Anticholinesterase drugs may be beneficial in treating bites in which *post-synaptic neurotoxins* are the major source of pathology (American coral snakes and Australian death adders for instance).

*Snakebites that involve respiratory failure due to paralysis can be managed by artificial respiration.

SUPPORTIVE THERAPY FOR NON-NEUROTOXIC SNAKES:

*Treat coagulopathy. Fresh frozen plasma can replace depleted clotting factors but is usually not necessary and *is contraindicated if the effects of the venom have not yet been neutralized.*

*Most non-neurotoxic snakebites cause significant pain and pain management drugs may be important.

*Fasciotomy is rarely needed. Even though swelling may mimic superficial appearance of compartment pressure syndrome, this is actually very rare in snakebite. Fasciotomy procedure should ONLY be employed if doppler or intracompartmental pressure manometry indicates pressures are elevated, AND if venom has been neutralized to avoid bleeding risks. In the rare case where pressures are known to be elevated, more antivenom may lower pressures and should be the first treatment regime.

NOTES

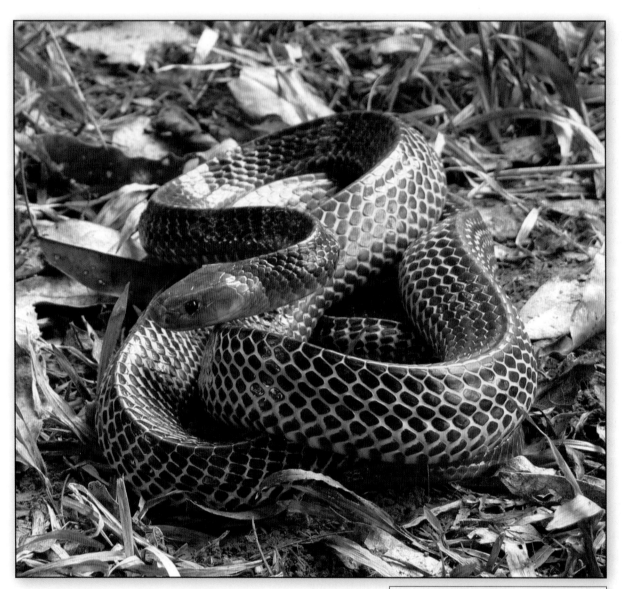

Red-headed Krait,
Bungarus flaviceps

INTRODUCTION

This chapter is designed primarily for identification of freshly killed snakes, not live snakes seen in the field, nor long preserved and faded museum specimens. Identification of live snakes in the field requires practice and experience, and the guidelines do not lend themselves to brief verbal descriptions, as a rule. It is to be hoped that the snakes submitted for identification will have their heads on and not be too badly smashed. Identification is considerably more complicated if the head is badly mutilated, and a decapitated body may be unidentifiable.

GENERAL PROCEDURES IN IDENTIFICATION

It is assumed that the user of this manual will have some knowledge of where the specimen he or she is trying to identify came from. For example, if a suspected coral snake is brought in for identification, there will be no reason to differentiate it from the 40 or so species of coral snakes found from Mexico southward if it is known that it was collected in North Carolina. Knowledge of the area of habitat narrows the field considerably. Identifying snakes from tropical areas often poses a problem in that tropical snake faunas are much richer in the numbers of species, and the distribution of some of these is poorly known. Nevertheless, if this manual is used correctly, and if there is an adequate specimen to work with, it should be possible to distinguish first between venomous and nonvenomous snakes, then, if venomous, to ascertain the correct generic identification in about 90 percent of the cases, and finally to arrive at the correct species in about 3 out of 4 cases.

First, if there is any doubt that the animal is a snake and a venomous one, or if the family of the snake is unknown, then Key to the Families of Snakes, page 29 this chapter, should be consulted. If the snake is known to be a ven-

omous land snake, then refer to the correct geographic section of chapter 7 and thence to the descriptions of the common species of the area; if a venomous marine snake, refer to Chapter 8.

If practicable every medical unit that enters an area where snakebite is a hazard should build up an identified collection of local venomous and nonvenomous snakes. Small individuals or just the heads of large snakes should be sufficient. Such collections are often essential for rapid identification of dangerous species.

If the specimen cannot be identified readily, it may be:

1. An aberrant individual or one from an atypical population;

2. An uncommon species listed in the regional table but not described in detail;

3. An unknown species or one not previously known from that geographic region;

4. A harmless species incorrectly identified as venomous. (To confirm the family, recheck characteristics using Key to the Families, this chapter.)

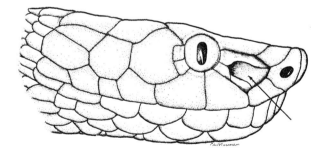

Figure 2. Drawing of head of pit viper, showing the position and appearance of the loreal pit. This heat sensitive structure is characteristic of the family Crotalidae.

In examining an unidentified snake look first at the head. In all pit vipers (family Crotalidae) there is a deep hollow between the eye and nostril and slightly below a line connecting the two (see Figure 2). The impression is one of an extra nostril. (A large pit viper, Bothrops atrox, is known in Mexico as cuatro narices or four nostrils.) These pits are actually sensitive heat receptors. They absolutely identify a snake as a pit viper, since they are not seen in any other type of snake. However, some pythons and boas do have pits on the upper lip. The pits may be difficult to recognize for they are often camouflaged by the head markings so that they are not visible except by close inspection; this offers another reason for bringing the intact snake in for identification.

DISTINGUISHING FEATURES IN IDENTIFICATION

Venom Apparatus

Fangs and venom glands are the only anatomic features that set venomous snakes apart from nonvenomous ones. Caution is demanded in examining the mouth of a freshly killed snake; the biting reflex may persist in a severed head for as long as 45 minutes. The long, moveable fangs of vipers, normally sheathed in whitish membrane and rotated parallel to the roof of the mouth, can be readily demonstrated and recognized. Fangs of elapid snakes (cobras, kraits, mambas, and related species) are smaller in size, located toward the front of the mouth, and fixed to the jaw (see Fig. 3). In cobras, mambas, and some other species they are large enough to be readily recognized, but in coral snakes and some other small elapids this is not the case. Enlarged anterior teeth are seen also in some nonvenomous snakes and can be confusing. Sea snake fangs are small and hard to distinguish. Rear fangs in colubrid snakes are rather difficult to see and extremely difficult to differentiate from nongrooved enlarged teeth found at the back of the jaw in many nonvenomous snakes. Fortunately, only a few rear-fanged snakes in Africa are sufficiently dangerous that their identification is important, and the fangs on these kinds are quite long.

Head Shields

The size and arrangement of shields on the top and sides of the head are most helpful in snake identification. In the great majority of snakes the top of the head is covered by large symmetrical shields, typically 9 in num-

ber (see Fig. 4). More or less division of these shields into small scales is seen in many kinds of vipers, many boas and pythons, and in a few other kinds of snakes. Reduction of the number through fusion of shields is seen mostly in small burrowing snakes.

If there are typical large shields on the crown and no pit between the eye and nostril, look at the side of the head in front of the eye. The loreal shield (see Fig. 4) is absent in nearly all venomous snakes of the Elapidae as well as the African mole vipers (Viperidae). This shield is also lacking in a good many nonvenomous snakes, but many of these are small burrowers or strictly aquatic snakes which may be eliminated on other grounds. The size of the eye may be important (see GLOSSARY).

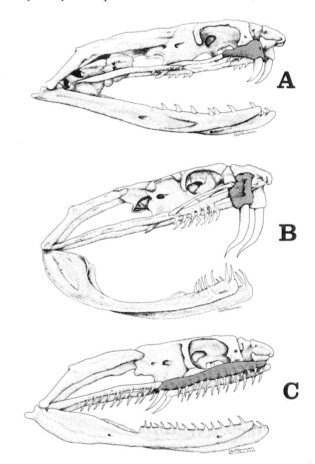

Figure 3. Skulls representative of various families of venomous snakes, showing lengths of maxillary bones (shaded) and positions and lengths of fangs. A. Cobra (Elapidae), showing short fang in front part of maxillary bone; B. Pit viper (Crotalidae), showing long fang on short maxillary bone; C. Rearfanged snake (Colubridae), showing short fang on rear part of long maxillary bone (other parts of skull diagrammatic only).

Eye Characteristics

The shape of the pupil of the eye should be noted in live or freshly killed snakes. Most snakes have round pupils, some have vertically elliptical pupils, and a few have horizontally elliptical pupils. Vertically elliptical pupils are characteristic of most vipers but some nonvenomous snakes also have this type. Most venomous elapids have round pupils.

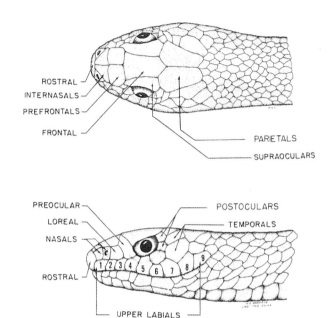

Figure 4. Head of typical colubrid snake, illustrating arrangement of scales from dorsal and lateral views. Any of these scales may be modified in shape or absent in various groups of venomous snakes.

Dorsal Scale Characteristics

The number of dorsal scale rows is sometimes important in snake identification. The method of counting is shown in Figure 5. While it is quite possible to make this count on a snake "in the round" so to speak, the inexperienced individual may obtain better results by skinning out a section of the body and flattening the skin. It is seldom possible to take a satisfactory scale count of a live snake. It is often desirable to note if the dorsal scales have a longitudinal raised ridge, keeled, or if they lack such ridges, smooth (see Fig. 6).

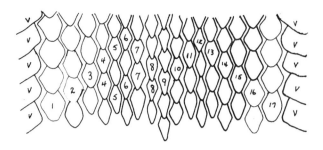

Figure 5. Method of counting dorsal scale rows. Figure drawn as though skin has been slit down belly and spread flat (V = ventral plates).

Ventral Scutes

In the vast majority of snakes, large transverse scutes extend the full width of the belly. These are considerably reduced in size in boas and pythons, some freshwater and burrowing snakes, and in many sea snakes (see Figure 7). They are completely absent in the burrowing blind snakes, and in some sea snakes. A complete count of the ventrals is routine procedure in systematic herpetology. It is easily done, but rather tedious, and is not required for most of the species identifications in this manual.

Tail

The tail of a snake begins at the anal plate which covers the opening of the cloaca. The form of the tail is often important in identification and virtually diagnostic in sea snakes and rattlesnakes. The subcaudal scutes are usually in a double row (paired); however, in some species, all or most may be in a single row (see Figure 8). A count of the subcaudals is routine.

Sex

Sex of a snake can sometimes be determined readily by observing eggs or developing young in the oviducts. Pressure by fingers or injection of liquid at the base of the tail will usually evert the copulatory organs or hemipenes of a male snake. The morphology of these organs is important in snake taxonomy. Usually they are rather large fleshy structures bearing spines or other ornamentation, but they may be quite smooth, small, and slender.

Color and Pattern

Color and pattern are the most widely used but, unfortunately, are the most deceptive criteria for snake identification. Color and patterns in snakes have evolved primarily for purpose of concealment and, as a result, totally unrelated snakes may appear very much alike. Many tree snakes, for example, are green with a light line on the flank, and many snakes that live in the crevices of rock or under bark have dark heads with a light collar at the nape. Real or apparent mimicry of venomous snakes by harmless species is very widespread and may involve similarities in behavior as well as appearance. Color and pattern vary greatly even within a species. In snakes of semiarid lands, it has been observed for centuries that there is often correspondence of general body color with the color of the soil. Abnormal increases of dark pigment (melanism) or its complete absence (albinism) can in rare cases give rise to black coral snakes or white rattlesnakes. Pattern is generally more constant than color, but several kinds of snakes may show both ringed and striped types of pattern. Pattern and colors of young snakes may be totally different from those of the adult. Sex differences in color and pattern are also seen.

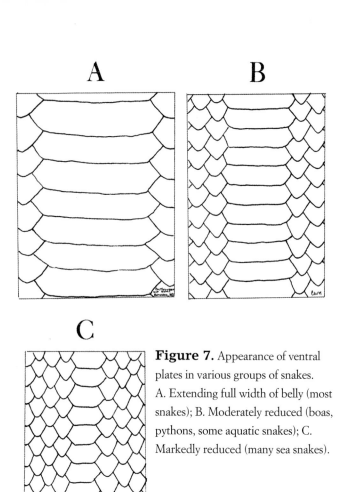

Figure 7. Appearance of ventral plates in various groups of snakes. A. Extending full width of belly (most snakes); B. Moderately reduced (boas, pythons, some aquatic snakes); C. Markedly reduced (many sea snakes).

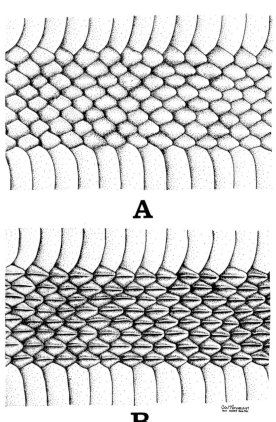

Figure 6. Figures of dorsal scales showing major types of scale ornamentation : A. smooth scales. B. keeled scales.

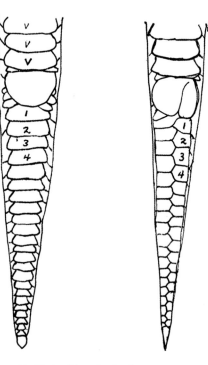

Figure 8. Undersides of tails of representative snakes. Snake with ENTIRE anal plate and a SINGLE row of subcaudal scutes; snake with DIVIDED anal plate and PAIRED rows of subcaudal scutes (V = ventral plates).

THE FAMILIES OF SNAKES

The keys given in Chapter 7 distinguish the various kinds of venomous land snakes from one another; Chapter 7 distinguishes the venomous sea snakes. Often, however, there are basic questions as to whether or not a snake is venomous, and to what family it belongs. Sometimes a family allocation will act as a double check on a tentative identification and also, occasionally, a family designation will be all that is possible because of the condition of the snake.

To identify an animal by use of this key, the reader must begin with the first couplet (pair of statements), decide which one describes the animal at hand, and then proceed to the couplet indicated at the end of the proper descriptive phrase. This procedure is followed with the next couplet and so on. Thus, an alternative decision is offered with each couplet until the reader finally determines the proper category for the animal. The animal must possess all of the characteristics mentioned in the proper line of couplets, not just the final characteristic. Therefore, it is always necessary to start at the beginning of the key.

The following key has been designed to sort out many kinds of nonvenomous snakes and snakelike animals before finally distinguishing between typical harmless snakes and venomous ones by the only positive means of identification of a venomous kind, the presence of fangs in the upper jaw. The following key should always be used if there is any question as to whether or not the animal at hand is a venomous snake:

KEY TO THE FAMILIES OF SNAKES

1. A. Body elongate, but legs or fins present on front and/or rear parts of body _____ NOT A SNAKE
   B. Body elongate, no legs or fins _____ 2

2. A. Skin slimy, with or without bony (fish-like) scales _____ NOT A SNAKE
   B. Skin dry, with thin horny scales _____ 3

3. A. Skin formed into distinct broad rings that extend around body _____ NOT A SNAKE
   B. Skin formed into small overlapping or juxtaposed scales (not in rings), at least on back _____ 4

4. A. Eye with a movable lid _____ NOT A SNAKE
   B. No movable lid _____ 5

5. A. Tail round in cross-section; not oar-shaped _____ 7
   B. Tail compressed into an oar-like blade _____ 6

6. A. Head covered with small granular scales; no large shields on crown; watersnakes of Southeast Asia _____ COLUBRIDAE
   B. Some crown shields present; see fig. 6; seasnakes, Chapter VIII _____ HYDROPHIDAE ☠

7. A. A row of enlarged, transverse scutes (ventrals) down the belly _____ 11
   B. Body scales uniform above and below _____ 8

8. A. Tail with an enlarged and ornamented scute or with several spiny scales near tip (SE Asia only); Indian rough-scaled snakes _____ UROPELTIDAE
   B. No such specialized tail, a single spine or none on tip _____ 9

9. A. Eye under a distinct round scale; most of head covered with small granular scales_____ 16

   B. Eye under irregularly-shaped head plate; head covered with enlarged scutes_____ 10

10. A. Scute containing nostril forms border of lip, 14 rows of scales around body; slender blindsnakes_____LEPTOTYPHLOPIDAE

    B. Scute containing nostril separated from lip by surrounding scales; more than 14 scale rows; typical blindsnakes_____ TYPHLOPIDAE

11. A. Ventral scutes extend full width of belly_____ 15

    B. Ventral scutes narrow, not extending width of belly_____ 12

12. A. Ventrals scarcely twice size of dorsals, or less_____ 13

    B. Ventrals distinctly enlarged, more than 3 times width of dorsals; boas and pythons_____ BOIDAE

13. A. Head mainly covered with small scales_____ 16

    B. Head covered with large scutes, though not in "typical" pattern (see fig. 6)_____ 14

14. A. A large median shield behind frontal; 15 scale rows (SE Asia only); sunbeam snake_____ XENOPELTIDAE

    B. No large median scute behind frontal; 17 scale rows or more (SE Asia and northern South America). Pipe snakes_____ ANILIDAE

15. A. A spur-like hook on either side of vent (often hidden in small depressions)_____ 12

    B. No indication of spurs_____ 16

16. A. One or two large fangs near front of upper jaw on each side_____ 17

    B. No sign of fangs at front of upper jaw. Typical harmless snakes; about 2,000 species, only 2 in C. and S. Africa are dangerous_____COLUBRIDAE

17. A. Long fangs on short maxillary bone which can rotate to erect them; no other teeth on maxillary_____ 18

    B. Short fangs on long maxillary bone which cannot rotate; usually teeth on maxillary bone behind fang; cobras and relatives_____ ELAPIDAE ☠

18. A. A loreal pit, see fig. 4; (SE Europe, Asia, and Americans only); pit vipers_____ CROTALIDAE ☠

    B. No loreal pit (Europe, Asia, and Africa only); Old World vipers_____VIPERIDAE ☠

☠ = Families of dangerously poisonous species.

PRESERVATION AND DISPOSITION OF UNIDENTIFIED SNAKES

Snakes that cannot be identified should be preserved in the manner given in the next paragraph and submitted to the nearest U.S. Naval Preventive Medicine Unit. Such units will provide identification service. If delivery to such a unit is not practicable, then contact the nearest natural history museum or other institution which might have a staff herpetologist and request help in identification. The two best preservatives to prepare a specimen for shipment or delivery to a herpetologist are:

1. Commercial formaldehyde diluted with 5 to 9 parts of water;
2. Grain alcohol diluted to 75 percent.

However, animals as large as most snakes will decay if placed in a preservative without some prior preparation. An ideal specimen and one which will remain in a state of minimum decay may be prepared by thoroughly injecting the body cavity and base of the tail with the preservative. A large syringe is the best means to inject the fluid, but if one is not available, multiple slits should be cut into the belly and the base of the tail and this will enable the preservative to reach the deep tissues.

Then put a wad of cotton or gauze into its mouth to hold it open. The specimen should then be neatly coiled, belly side up, in a container sufficiently large to cover the snake with the preservative. Do not crowd several specimens in a single container.

Large snakes of 5 feet or more in length should be eviscerated or skinned out leaving only the head and tail intact before placing them in a container of preservative. An intact head will be sufficient to differentiate between venomous and nonvenomous species.

After the specimen has hardened (5 to 7 days is usually required), it may be removed from the liquid, wrapped in damp rags, put in a plastic bag, and shipped to the herpetologist for identification. A tag should always be included which gives the location where the specimen was collected in enough detail so that it can be located on a map in an ordinary atlas. If the name of a small native village is used then the name of the district, department, county, or other political subdivision must be added. Other information to put on the tag which will greatly increase the scientific value of a specimen includes date of collection of specimen, approximate altitude, habitat, and the name and address of the collector. Use waterproof ink or a pencil in filling out the tag.

NOTES

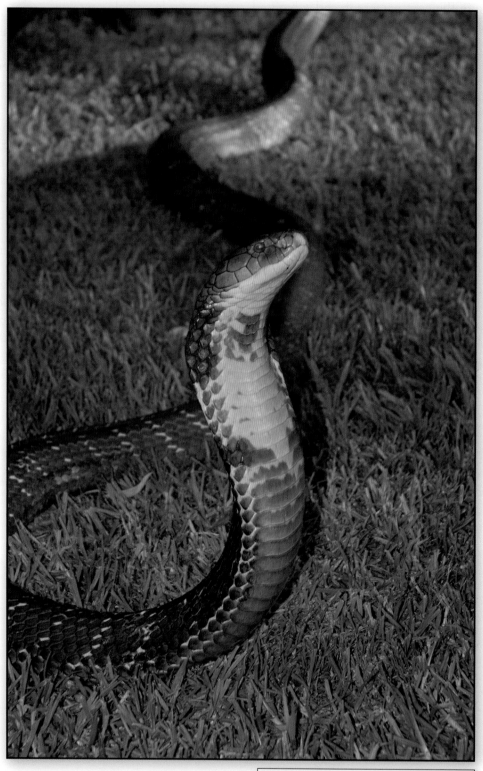

King Cobra,
Ophiophagus hannah

CHAPTER 7

INTRODUCTION

To facilitate the identification of many the of world's nearly 700 species of venomous snakes, the land areas of the globe have been divided into 6 regions (see map 1 page 33). The 6 divisions correspond to the world's 6 regions of command designated and used by the U.S. military. The following seven chapters correspond to these six regions (*Note*: *region six has two chapters*). In each chapter has been included a definition of the region with a map of the land area covered by that chapter and a list of the venomous snakes which occur in it and their distribution within the region. The main body of the text of each of the following chapters is divided into generic divisions and each division is headed by a description of the genus. Following thereafter are individual descriptions of the venomous species which are responsible for the largest numbers of bites within the area, or are believed to be of serious danger to any adult human inhabiting or entering the region.

The maps depicting the range of individual species were drawn by the author after viewing a variety of different publications and/or websites. At best, the range maps should be construed as being close approximations rather than exact descriptions of species distribution.

Likewise, the species descriptions are derived from previously published materials. There is a list of references at the end of each chapter listing the sources used in writing that specific chapter.

Except for those species within the United States the basis for the nomenclature used in this manual is derived mainly from the website *www.reptiledatabase.org*. For species found within the United

States the basis for nomenclature used was the publication *Standard Current and Scientific Names for North American Amphibians, Turtles, Reptiles, and Crocodilians* (2009) published by the Center For North American Herpetology (CNAH).

It should be noted that this arrangement may not be followed exactly by many experts around the globe. In fact, the classification of the world's venomous snake species has experienced some tumultuous changes in recent years. The advent of new technologies to analyze DNA, along with continued field and museum research turning up new information results in a huge number of publications in scientific journals around the world. Keeping track of all these changes is a formidable task, and disagreement regarding the conclusions of different researchers leads to contentious issues among scientists regarding the currently accepted taxonomic status of these animals. The most difficult task for this author was settling on which interpretation of the evidence should be used in the nomenclature of the snakes described in this book.

In the end, I elected to follow (generally) the same source(s) used by the Armed Forces Pest Management Board. Not all will be in agreement with this decision, and the author must take full responsibility for any errors and misinterpretations in regards to the scientific accuracy of this publication.

In the individual species accounts are headings titled *Description and Identification:, Distribution, Habitat, and Biology:,* and *Venom and Bite:*. Under the *Venom and Bite* section of each species account is a list of antivenoms for that particular species. Also within that section there may be a listing of the types of toxins known (or suspected) to occur within the venom of that species. The information regarding the types of toxins is taken from the Clinical Toxinology Resources website (www.toxinology.com)

The list of references appended to the end of each of the following chapters is not intended to be comprehensive, but indicates the main sources of information utilized in preparing the accounts and may serve as an introduction to the literature and authoritative websites available on the venomous snakes of each region (chapter).

The first set of references following each chapter appears under the heading CURRENT REFERENCES and those are the references used in the revision of this manual. The second group of references is under the heading ORIGINAL REFERENCES and consists of those references that were used by the original authors of this manual back in 1965.

Color photographs are provided for most of the dangerously venomous species described in this book. In some cases more than one photograph may be used to depict the different color morphs that often occur within a single species. It is important to note that some species can exhibit a very significant variety of colors or patterns, some of which may not be depicted with a photograph. In most cases where significant variation in color or pattern occurs within a single species, those variations are noted within the text section describing that species.

Finally, the reader should be aware that not every species of dangerously venomous snake is depicted in this book. There are over 70 species of Coral Snakes (*Micrurus*) alone found in Central and South America. Rather than treat each individual species to its own written account the author has chosen to depict those species that are the most significant clinically; the species that are most common; those that are most widespread; or those that are responsible for the most snakebite incidents and/or deaths have been chosen as representative examples of these diverse genera.

Finally, the original manual included a list of antivenom sources arranged by country. In this revised edition the author has elected to include antivenom information with each individual species account under the heading *Venom and Bite.*

NOTES

Map 1. Geographic divisions used in this book.

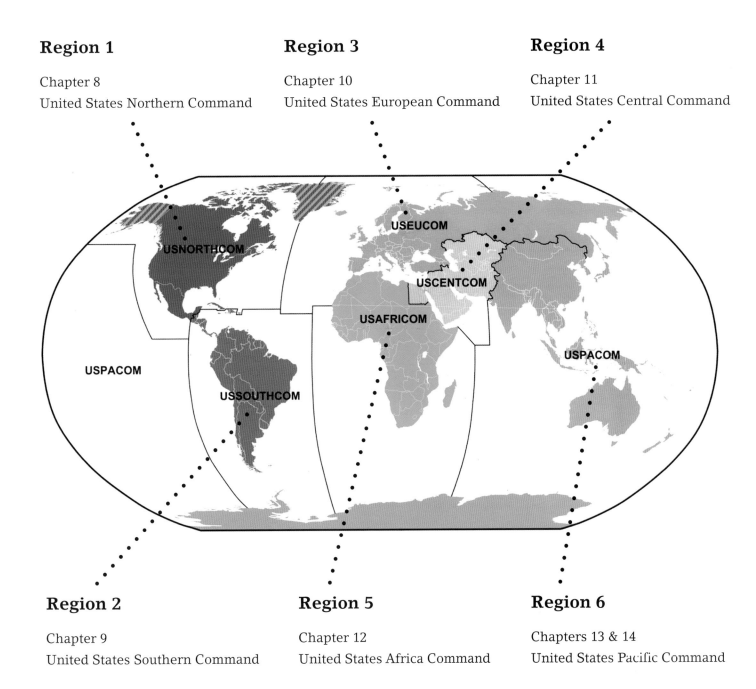

Region 1

Chapter 8
United States Northern Command

Region 3

Chapter 10
United States European Command

Region 4

Chapter 11
United States Central Command

USEUCOM

USNORTHCOM

USCENTCOM

USAFRICOM

USPACOM

USSOUTHCOM

USPACOM

Region 2

Chapter 9
United States Southern Command

Region 5

Chapter 12
United States Africa Command

Region 6

Chapters 13 & 14
United States Pacific Command

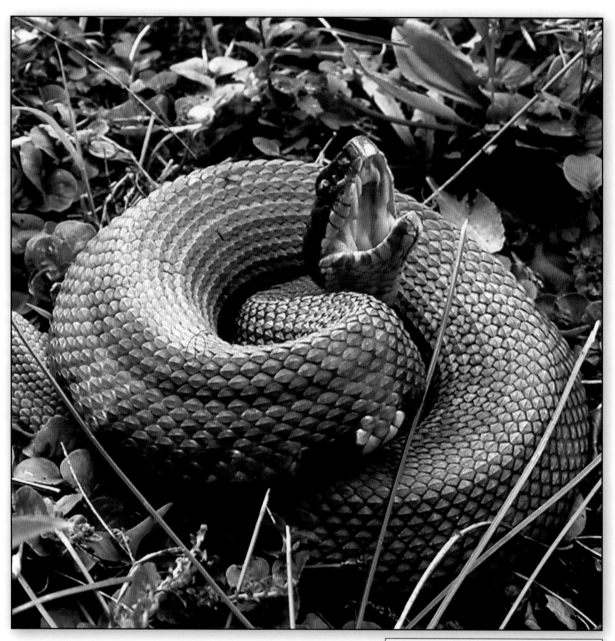

Cottonmouth,
Agkistrodon piscivorous

CHAPTER **8**

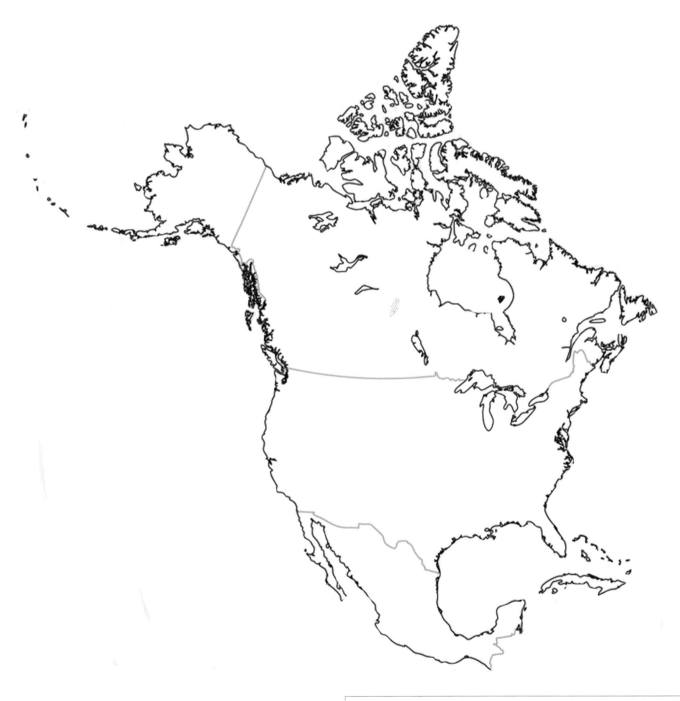

Map 2. Definition of region one: United States Northern Command. Canada, United States, and Mexico.

Introduction

The venomous snake fauna of the United States and Canada is well known and highly studied. Species native to Mexico however are less well known, and the exact range of many Mexican species remains unclear. Within the region covered by this section there are a total of 78 venomous snake species divided into two large families; the Viperidae (vipers) and the Elapidae (cobra family). In the USNORTHCOM region all vipers are members of the subfamily Crotalinae, or "pit viper" group. This group includes the moccasins, the rattlesnakes, and a large and diverse group of tropical pit vipers usually referred to collectively as the "Lancehead Vipers." Altogether there are 8 genera of pit vipers in this region, totaling 62 species. The region's other group of venomous snakes are members of the family Elapidae, often called the "cobra family," and this group consists of two genera of Coral Snakes with a total of 16 species.

Perhaps the best-known group of venomous snakes within this region are the rattlesnakes (genera *Crotalus* and *Sistrurus*). Rattlesnakes are one of the most numerous and diverse types of venomous snake within the region and many species are extremely dangerous. Mexico boasts the most rattlesnake species in the region (30), 12 of which also occur in the United States. A further 9 species are endemic to the United States and two of these extend their range northward into parts of southern Canada.

In southernmost Mexico there are several species of tropical pit vipers belonging to 6 genera. Most of these genera are represented by dangerous snakes capable of inflicting a fatal bite. These tropical pit vipers include the Mountain Pit Vipers (*Cerrophidian*), the Jumping Vipers (*Atripoides*), the Horned Vipers (*Ophyracus*), the Palm Pit Vipers (*Bothriechis)*, the Hognosed Vipers (*Porthidium*), and the Lance-headed Vipers (*Bothrops*). The latter genus, though represented in the region by a single species (*B. asper),* is responsible for a disproportionate number of deaths in southern Mexico.

The region's other pit viper group, the moccasins, genus *Agkistrodon,* are represented by 3 species, all of which have caused human deaths.

Micrurus and *Microides* make up the two genera of the Elapidae family found in the region. Of these, the *Microides* genus contains but a single species, while *Micrurus* is represented in the region by a total of 15 species,

only two of which range north of the Mexican border into the United States. All should be considered dangerous to man and several species are known to have killed humans.

The venomous snakes in this section occur from sea level to over 11,000 feet in elevation, and occupy nearly every habitat except for the boreal forests and tundra of Canada and Alaska. Venomous snakes occur in every state in Mexico and every state in the United States except Maine. In Canada, rattlesnakes occur in the southern portions Ontario, Saskatchewan, Alberta, and British Columbia.

Venomous snakebite is by no means a rare occurrence in this region. Of the several thousand venomous snakebites that occur in the United States each year, only a half dozen or so result in death. In Mexico, where the greatest number of venomous snake species occurs (67), and much of the population lives in rural areas, as many as 28,000 bites are recorded annually with up to 150 deaths per year (Gomez and Dart, 1995).

The map below shows the area covered by this chapter.

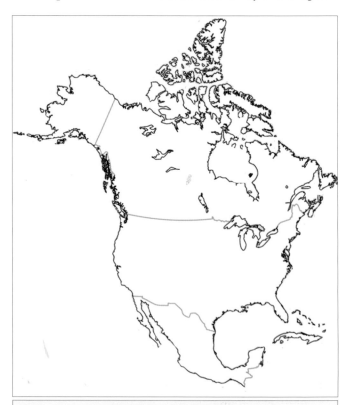

MAP 3. Region 1, United States Northern Command. Canada, United States, and Mexico.

Generic And Species Descriptions

Family - Elapidae

Genus - Micruroides

Sonoran Coral Snake

A single species, M. euryxanthus (Sonora Coral Snake), is recognized. It is found in the southwestern United States and in northwestern Mexico. It is a small snake but is considered dangerous.

Definition: Head small, not distinct from neck; snout rounded, no distinct canthus. Body slender and elongate, not tapered; tail short. Eyes small; pupils round.

Head scales: The usual 9 on the crown. Laterally, nasal scale is in contact with a single preocular scale (no loreal scale). Ventrally, mental scale separated from anterior chin shields by first infralabials.

Body scales: Dorsal scales smooth, in 15 oblique rows throughout body. Ventral scales 206-242; anal plated divided; subcaudals paired, 19-32.

Maxillary teeth: Two relatively large tubular fangs followed, after an interspace, by 1-2 small teeth.

Remarks: Differs from nonvenomous snakes as Micrurus does; differs from Micrurus of this region in the solid black head color which ends in a straight line across the parietals, and in the teeth behind the fangs. Oviparous.

Sonoran Coral Snake,
Micruroides euryxanthus

Description & Identification: The elongate body, unmodified rostral scale and black snout distinguish this species from the similarly-colored nonvenomous sand snakes (*Chilomeniscus*) and Shovel-nosed Snakes (*Chionactis*) that inhabit the same region.

The yellow or white-bordered red bands distinguish it from the king snakes (*Lampropeltis*) which have black-bordered red bands. Adults average 12 to 16 inches in length; occasional individuals attain a length of 20 inches, with a maximum of 24 inches. Snout and anterior part of head black, ending in a straight line across posterior tips of parietals. A light (yellowish or whitish) band on neck, followed by a red ring; remainder of body with alternating rings of black and red, each separated by light rings.

Tail bands alternating black and light.

Distribution, Habitat, and Biology: Found in most of Southern Arizona and extreme southeastern New Mexico southward through Sonora and southwestern Chihuahua to southern Sinaloa. Also found on Tiburon Island in the Gulf of California. Found from low desert to at least 5,000 feet. Sonora desert, mesquite grassland, and pine/oak woodlands are inhabited in the northern portions of its range as well as in thorn forests farther south.

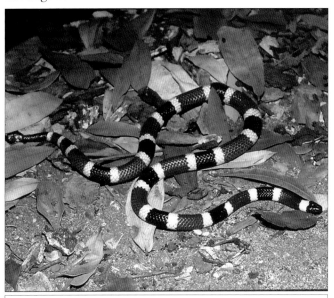

PHOTO 1. Sonoran Coral Snake, *Micruroides euryxanthus.*

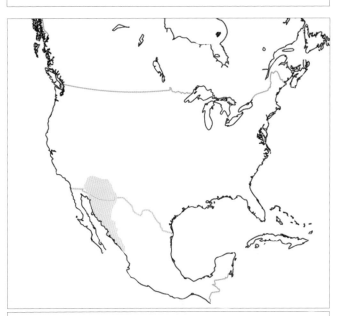

MAP 4. Range of the Sonoran Coral Snake, *Micruroides euryxanthus.*

Venom and Bite: Post-synaptic neurotoxins and systemic myotoxins possibly present. This small and secretive snake is inoffensive and very few bites have been reported. No deaths have been recorded from its bite. However, its venom is highly toxic and it should not be treated carelessly.

Family - Elapidae

Genus - Micrurus

American Coral Snakes

When the book *Poisonous Snakes of the World* was published in 1965 there were about 40 species of *Micrurus* known to science. Today, that number has nearly doubled (some sources list up to 78 species) and new species are still being discovered. Some species boast several subspecies and many exhibit significant variation both geographically and within specific populations. To further complicate identification, there are numerous nonvenomous snake species that mimic the coral snakes in color and pattern. To say that this genus presents an identification problem for the lay individual is an understatement, but from a practical standpoint of snakebite treatment, one need only be concerned with identifying an offending snake as a member of the *Micrurus* genus. This task is best accomplished by noting the *absence of a loreal scale and the 15 rows of smooth scales at midbody.*

This genus is contained entirely in the western hemisphere and most species occur in Central and South America. *Micrurus* is found from the Coastal Plain of the southeastern United States (two species) through much of Mexico (15 total species), all the way to central Argentina in South America.

Definition: Head small, not distinct from neck; snout rounded, no distinct canthus. Body elongate, slender, not tapered; tail short. Eyes small; pupils round.

Head scales: The usual 9 on the crown. Laterally, nasal scale in contact with single preocular (no loreal scale). Ventrally, mental scale separated from anterior chin shields by first infralabials.

Body scales: Dorsals smooth in 15 rows throughout body. Ventral scales 177-412, anal plate divided or entire; subcaudals 16-62, usually paired but more than 50 percent single in some species.

Maxillary teeth: Two relatively large tubular fangs with indistinct grooves; no other teeth on bone.

Most coral snakes have color patterns made up of complete rings of yellow (or white), black, and red. In some species however, the typical triad pattern is replaced by black and red rings, black and white rings, black and orange, or black and yellow. Still others can have the red

or black rings greatly expanded with only a few rings at either the head, the tail, or both; producing a nearly all red or all black snake. When threatened many species elevate the curled tip of the tail, presumably to fool a predator into thinking the snakes tail is the head. Coral snakes are inoffensive animals that do not coil and strike in the manner of the vipers or cobras. Bites from coral snakes invariably occur from the victim handling the snake, stepping on it barefoot, or carelessly placing a bare hand onto the snakes body. However, their venom is highly toxic and all species should be considered potentially deadly.

Antivenom for coral snakes in this region (Coralmyn) is produced by Instiudo Bioclon in Mexico. Although many coral snake bites will not result in envenomation, a lethal envenomation may not produce significant symptoms for several hours. Thus, persons bitten by coral snakes must always seek immediate medical attention and administration of antivenin is advised even in asymptomatic patients.

Eastern Coral Snake,
Micrurus fulvius

Description and Identification: Head small; body slender with little taper; tail short; scales smooth with high gloss. End of snout black followed by a broad yellow band across the base of the head and a wide black neck ring. Body completely circled by black, red, and yellow rings - red and yellow rings touching. If the red and black rings touch each other, if the end of the snout is red, whitish, or speckled, and if the colors fail to encircle the body, the snake is not a North American Coral Snake. These rules apply only in the United States and are not true in tropical America. The average length is 23 to 32 inches, but specimens of 4 feet in length have been recorded.

Distribution, Habitat, and Biology: Found in the coastal plain of the southeastern United States from southeastern North Carolina to southern Mississippi, including all of Florida. Inhabits nearly all biomes within its range except permanent wetlands. Most common in areas with sandy soils. Both nocturnal and diurnal in habits, and frequently forages actively in the morning. Fairly secretive, spending much of its time hidden beneath leaf litter, logs, etc., on the forest floor. Feeds on lizards and smaller snakes. All coral snakes are oviparous and this species typically lays 6 to 12 eggs.

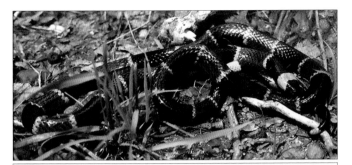

Photo 2. Eastern Coral Snake, *Micrurus fulvius*.

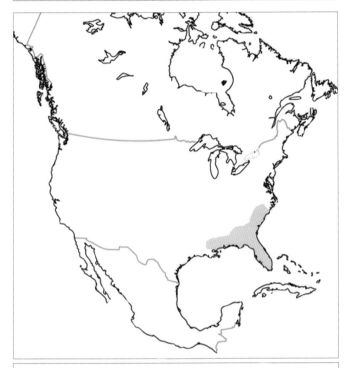

Map 5. Range of the Eastern Coral Snake, *Micrurus fulvius*.

Texas Coral Snake,
Micrurus tener

Description and Identification: All the descriptive characters for the previous species (*M. fulvius,* Eastern Coral Snake) are applicable to this very similar species. In this snake, however, the red rings contain larger black spots and the yellow ring on the head does not extend to the end of the parietal scales.

Distribution, Habitat, and Biology: Found from Louisiana and southern Arkansas west through the eastern half of Texas and south to northern Veracruz and parts of central Mexico. In habits, feeding and reproduction similar to the Eastern Coral Snake (*M. fulvius*). While it also occupies many of the same types of habitats including southern evergreen woodlands and deciduous woodlands, it's range encompasses a wide variety of other habitats including mesquite grassland, upland oak woodlands, rocky canyons, dry forest and scrub, and thorn forest. There are very four similar subspecies of this snake, three of which are endemic to Mexico. In size it is also similar to the previous species averaging 24 to 30 inches with an absolute maximum of 4 feet.

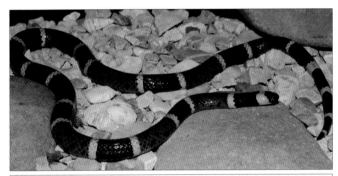

Photo 3. Texas Coral Snake, *Micrurus tener*.

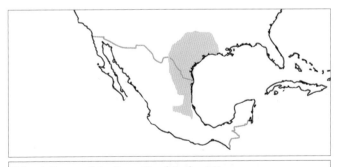

Map 6. Range of the Texas Coral Snake, *Micrurus tener*.

Venom and Bite: Post-synaptic neurotoxins and systemic myotoxins. Although this is a usually docile species that has at times been handled freely by unknowing children without incident, some individuals are very quick to bite at the slightest provocation. Their venom is highly toxic and they can attain a large size for a coral snake. The venom kills by paralyzing the diaphragm, and the victim dies of suffocation. Numerous deaths from this snake have been recorded over the years. Although many bites will not result in envenomation, a lethal envenomation may not produce significant symptoms for several hours. Thus, persons bitten by coral snakes must always seek immediate medical attention and administration of antivenin is advised even in asymptomatic patients. "Coralmyn" antivenom is produced in Mexico by Instituto Bioclon.

Venom and Bite: Post-synaptic neurotoxins and systemic myotoxins. Presumably very similar to that of the Eastern Coral Snake. Thus capable of inflicting a very dangerous bite. Antivenom for the Texas Coral Snake (Coralmyn) is produced in Mexico by Instituto Bioclone.

Variable Coral Snake,
Micrurus diastema

Description and Identification: Previously known as the Atlantic Coral Snake, there are seven subspecies of this highly variable coral snake. Many exhibit a typical coral snake pattern of triad rings, but in others the light rings may be greatly reduced or lacking. Some have black pigment heavily diffused in the red rings, or in both the red and yellow rings. These are medium sized coral snakes that rarely reach three feet in length.

Ventral scales 188-228, subcaudals 38-47. 15 scale rows at midbody, no loreal scale, anal plate divided.

As with other coral snake species, identification of *M. diastema* is complicated by the presence of nonvenomous look alike species which occur within its range. Most notable among these mimics are *Lampropeltis triangulum* and *Urotheca elapoides*.

Distribution, Habitat, and Biology: Ranges from southern Veracruz to western Honduras on the Atlantic slope including all of the Yucatan Peninsula. In addition to its range in Mexico this species can also be found throughout Belize, northern Guatemala, and western Honduras in Central America (USSOUTHCOM). All habitats of the lower to middle elevations of the Atlantic slope are utilized. Secretive and terrestrial, its habits, food preferences, and reproduction are similar to other members of its genus (see Eastern Coral Snake on page 38).

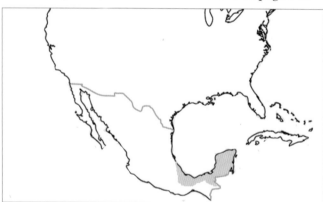

Map 7. Range of the Variable Coral Snake, *Micrurus diastema*, in the USNORTHCOM region.

Venom and Bite: Post-synaptic neurotoxins and systemic myotoxins present. There is little information on the effects of its bite on humans. It is likely a very dangerous snake that is capable of killing. Coralmyn antivenom is listed by the manufacturer (Institudo Bioclone of Mexico) to be effective in treating bites by *M. diastema*.

West Mexican Coral Snake,
Micrurus distans

Description and Identification: A coral snake in which the red bands are significantly wider than the yellow and black bands, producing a snake whose body color is mostly red. Adults average 2-3 feet with a maximum of 42 inches. The crown of the head is black and black extends to behind the eye on the top of the head. The yellow nape band extends forward under the eye and may encompass the upper labial scales; and there may be light pigment on the snout as well.

Previously called Broad-banded Coral Snake.

Distribution, Habitat and Biology: Found in western Mexico from southern Sonora to Guerrero. This coral snake has a remarkable harmless mimic which inhabits the same region. The neotropical milksnake *Lampropeltis triangulum nelsoni* has the same broad red bands and narrow black bands. However, as in most coral snake mimics, the black bands occur in pairs; and occurrence never found in coral snakes.

This species inhabits the tropical deciduous forests and thorn forest of the pacific slope from sea level to nearly 4,000 feet.

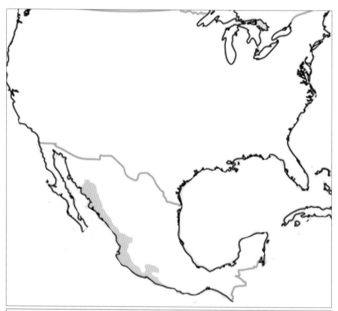

Map 8. Range of the West Mexican Coral Snake, *Micrurus distans*.

Venom and Bite: Post-synaptic neurotoxins and systemic myotoxins present. At least one death has been recorded from the bite of this snake. Coralmyn antivenom by Bioclone of Mexico is recommended for treating bites.

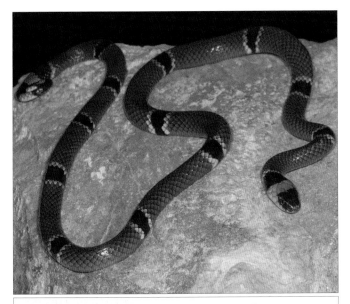

PHOTO 4. West Mexican Coral Snake, *Micrurus distans*

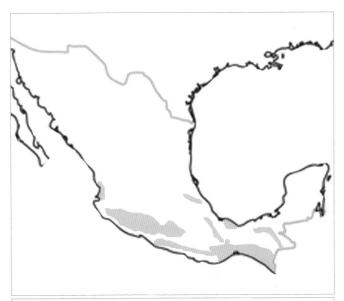

MAP 9. Combined ranges of all of other coral snake species found within the USNORTHCOM region.

Additional Species: In addition to the four species of *Micrurus* coral snakes described already, there are another 12 species that occur in the USNORTHCOM region. All have relatively restricted ranges in southernmost Mexico. Most exhibit either the classic red, black and yellow ringed pattern or are red with black rings. All should be considered dangerous to man.

These other 12 species are listed below:
Brown's Coral Snake, *Micrurus browni*
Balsan Coral Snake, *Micrurus laticollaris*
Blotched Coral Snake, *Micrurus bernardi*
Bogart's Coral Snake, *Micrurus bogerti*
Elegant Coral Snake, *Micrurus elegans*
Oaxacan Coral Snake, *Micrurus ephippifer*
Tuxtlan Coral Snake, *Micrurus limbatus*
Long ringed Coral Snake, *Micrurus latifasciatus*
Ixtlan Coral Snake, *Micrurus nebularis*
Zapotilan Coral Snake, *Micrurus pachecogili*
Nayarit Coral Snake, *Micrurus proximans*
Tamaulipen Coral Snake, *Micrurus tamaulipensis*

Finally, one other coral snake species ranges into the southern tip of Mexico from Central America. Information on that species, the Central American Coral Snake, *Micrurus nigrocinctus,* is available in Chapter 9 covering the USSOUTHCOM region (see page 75).

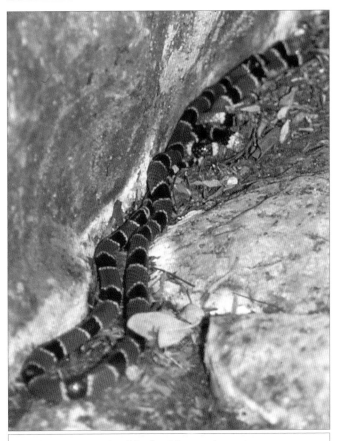

PHOTO 5. Brown's Coral Snake, *Micrurus browni*

Family - Viperidae

Subfamily - Crotalinae - Pit Vipers

Genus - Agkistrodon

American Moccasins

Four species are recognized. All are found in the US-NORTHCOM region. One species (the Cottonmouth) is endemic to the United States, one is endemic to Mexico (Taylor's Cantil); a third (Copperhead) exists in both countries, and the fourth (Common Cantil) is a primarily Mexican species that also ranges into Central America. All have been responsible for human fatalities. The Copperhead is the least dangerous and most survive its bite. The Cottonmouth, Taylor's Cantil, and Common Cantil however are all dangerous species.

Definition: Head broad, flattened, very distinct from narrow neck; a sharply distinguished canthus. Body cylindrical or depressed, tapered, moderately stout to stout; tail short to moderately long. Eyes moderate in size, pupils vertically elliptical.

Head scales: The usual nine on the crown.

Laterally, loreal pit separated from labials or its anterior border formed by second supralabial. Loreal scale present or absent.

Body scales: Dorsals keeled, with apical pits, in 23 to 27 rows. Ventrals 127-157, subcaudals single anteriorly, 19-71.

Copperhead,
Agkistrodon contortrix

Description and Identification: Head triangular; body moderately stout; facial pit present; pupil elliptical; most of subcaudals undivided.

There are five subspecies of copperheads, thus this species does show some variation in color. However, the basic pattern is constant among all specimens of copperhead. The ground color is some shade of brown (dark brown, tan, reddish-brown, orange-brown, or pinkish buff) with darker brown, hourglass shaped bands across the body. Belly is pinkish white with large dark spots or mottling; top of head yellowish to coppery red; sides paler; end of tail yellow in young, black to dark greenish or brown in adult. The cross bands are narrow in the center of the back and wide on the sides in eastern specimens, only slightly narrowed at the top of the back in western specimens.

Averages 2-3 feet in length; maximum slightly over 4 feet; males larger than females. There is an unofficial record of 58 inches from a captive specimen (personal observation).

Distribution, Habitat, & Biology: Ranges across most of the eastern United States except for northern New England and the Great Lakes region; south to the Atlantic and Gulf Coasts (exclusive of peninsular Florida); west to the Big Bend region of western Texas. It is most common in the deciduous forests of the east, the southern evergreen forests of the coastal plain, and the hemlock-hardwood forests in the Appalachian plateau. It also may be found in wooded regions within the southern plains as well as mountain habitats in the Chihuahua Desert. Frequents wooded, hilly country in the north and west; lowland woods in the south; sometimes plentiful in populated areas. In mountainous areas it frequently hibernates in rocky ledges with rattlesnakes and various nonvenomous species. Feeds on a variety of

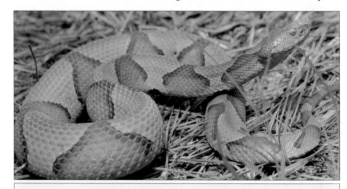

Photo 6. Southern Copperhead, *Agkistrodon contortrix*

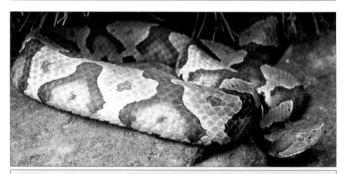

Photo 7. Northern Copperhead, *Agkistrodon contortrix mokasen*

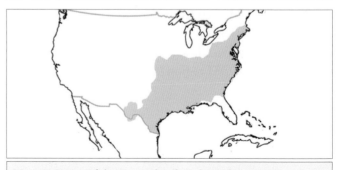

Map 10. Range of the Copperhead, *Agkistrodon controtix.*

small mammals and amphibians as an adult, insects and other invertebrates when very young.

Venom and Bite: Procoagulants and myotoxins possibly present. The Copperhead ranges throughout much of the highly populated eastern United States. Although secretive and normally inoffensive, it is a common snake in many areas of its range and in the eastern United States it is responsible for more venomous snakebites than any other snake. Fortunately, the venom is not highly toxic and although fatalities have been recorded, deaths from copperhead bites are extremely rare. The venom can be highly destructive to local tissues and can lead to permanent crippling of an extremity or loss of digits.

Antivenin is usually unwarranted in treating copperhead bites, but if needed Cro-fab Antivenom (Ovine) produced by Protherics, Inc., is listed as having cross reactivity in treating Copperhead bites. Also available is Bioclon Antivipmyn (Equine) and Tri-Antivipmyn (Equine) from Instituto Bioclon both of which are listed as having possible cross reactivity to Copperhead venom.

Cottonmouth,
Agkistrodon piscivorous

Description & Identification: A pit viper related to the copperhead but very widely confused with the harmless water snakes of the genus *Nerodia*. For identification of dead specimens, note presence of facial pit, elliptical pupil, and undivided subcaudals; all features lacking in nonvenomous water snakes within the range of the cottonmouth. For field identification, the head of the cottonmouth is decidedly heavier and eyes less prominent than in the harmless water snakes. A chunky, heavy-bodied snake. Adults are usually a uniform brown, dark brown to nearly black above. Some specimens will have darker, hourglass shaped bands across the back, especially on freshly molted individuals. These freshly molted snakes may be olive in color between the cross bands. Young and immatures exhibit a banded pattern that is quite distinct at birth and which gradually fades with age (see inset photo). Most are full grown at about 4 feet, but cottonmouths can reach 6 feet.

Distribution, Habitat, & Biology: Found throughout the coastal plain of the southeastern United States from southeast Virginia to Texas. Ranges up the Mississippi Valley to southern Illinois and west to extreme southeastern Kansas and eastern Oklahoma. Absent from the Appalachian Plateau and Interior Highlands. They are primarily aquatic animals usually found in close proximity to water.

However, on rare occasions they may wander far from water. Their primary habitat is swamps, marshes, creeks, oxbows, and other aquatic situations in the lowlands of the Coastal Plain of the southeastern United States, but they can also be found within mountain streams high into the Ozark Plateau and their range sometimes follows river valleys well into the southern plains of Texas and Oklahoma.

Baby Cottonmouths possess a bright yellow tail tip that is wriggled to imitate a grub or worm and lure small animals to within striking distance. This yellow tail fades with age. This species name comes from it's peculiar behavior whenever threatened . If under threat, a Cottonmouth will open it's mouth and show the fangs, revealing the white "cotton" membrane inside of the mouth (see photo 9 below). If this threat display fails to ward off a potential attacker, these snakes will often strike savagely, but usually only as a last resort and their reputation for being aggressive is exaggerated. Although these snakes are highly aquatic, they may leave their wetland environment in the fall to hibernated on higher ground, and at this time they can be seen far from water. The belief that a Cottonmouth cannot bite underwater is erroneous, as is the old wives' tale about "balls" of large numbers of snakes being encountered.

Cottonmouths will eat almost any animal small enough to swallow, including other snakes. Their primary food is fish and amphibians.

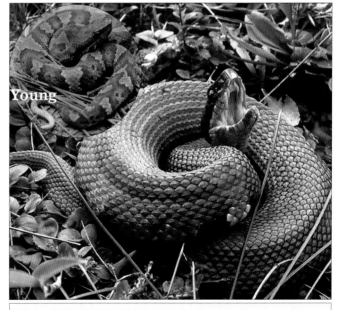

PHOTOS 8 & 9. Cottonmouth, *Agkistrodon piscivorous.*

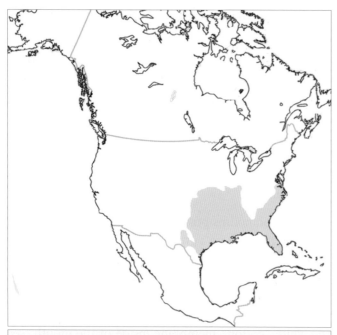

MAP 11. Range of the Cottonmouth, *Agkistrodon piscivorous.*

Venom and Bite: Systemic myotoxins and procoagulants present. Although most experts agree that the Cottonmouth fails to live up to its reputation as an aggressive animal, these snakes do tend to hold their ground when approached rather than flee in the manner of harmless water snakes. Bites by this snake are fairly frequent in the lower Mississippi Valley and along the Gulf Coast. Although fatalities are rare, the Cottonmouth is a snake that is capable of killing a human. They can attain a large size and their venom is fairly toxic. The venom has strong proteolytic activity. Tissue destruction may be severe. In addition, these snakes often feed on carrion and their mouths can harbor pathogenic bacteria which can lead to serious infections, deep tissue abscesses, and life threatening septicemia.

"Crofab" Antivenin (Ovine) is produced by Protherics, Inc., (USA) and the venom of the Cottonmouth is used in the production of this product. Thus "Crofab" antivenom is the antivenin of choice in treating Cottonmouth bites. Also available is Bioclone "Antivipmyn" (Equine) and "Tri-Antivipmyn" (Equine) from Instituto Bioclon (Mexico) both of which are listed as having possible cross reactivity to Cottonmouth venom.

Taylor's Cantil,
Agkistrodon taylori

Description and Identification: Also known as Mexican Moccasin. A chocolate brown, reddish brown, or nearly black pit viper with dark transverse bands which alternate with lighter bands of white, yellowish, or orange pigment. Some individuals are nearly solid black with flecks of yellow or white. There are two distinct light lines on the face, one runs from the snout along the top of the canthus through the eye to the back of the jaw, and another runs from the snout along the upper labials for the entire length of the mouth. Young snakes are more distinctly patterned and have the bright yellow tail characteristic of the young of all *Agkistrodon* species. Old adults can be quite dark, nearly solid black, but most show at least some light flecking.

The top of the head is covered by 9 large plates and there are 23 rows of heavily keeled scales at mid body. Ventrals 127-138; subcaudals 40-56, divided anteriorly.

Can reach a length of 3 feet.

Distribution, Habitat, & Biology: This species has a restricted range in northeastern Mexico that includes the south half of Tamaulipas and small portions of the states of Neuvo Leon, San Luis Potosi, Veracruz, and Hildalgo. Mesquite-grasslands, thorn forest, and tropical deciduous forest are all listed as habitats (Campbell and Lamar, 2004). Apparently this species is more like the copperhead in habitat preference, showing a liking for dryer, upland habitats.

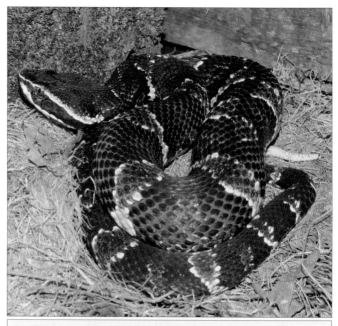

PHOTO 10. Taylor's Cantil, *Agkistrodon taylori*

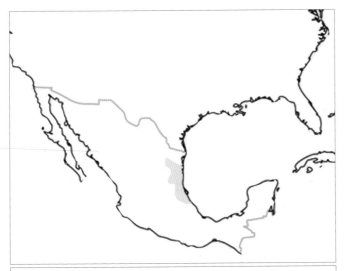

MAP 12. Range of the Taylor's Cantil, *Agkistrodon taylori.*

Venom and Bite: There appears to be little information regarding this species venom and its effects on humans. Systemic myotoxins, procoagulants, and haemorragins are possibly present in the venom. The very similar *A. bilineatus* is known to be capable of killing, and there is no reason to assume that the Taylor's Cantil is not a deadly species as well. Bioclon's "Antivipmyn" is the Anitivenom of choice for treating bites by this species.

Common Cantil,

Agkistrodon bilineatus

Description and Identification: Very similar to the preceding species. The two snakes were formally considered to be the same species. Common Cantils can vary in color from nearly black to reddish, or gray-brown. Like the preceding species they always show a pattern of transverse bands alternating between dark and lighter colors, and the light lines on the face are a consistent marker of both snakes. The Common Cantil may be distinguished by the fact that the light line running along the top of the mouth does not encompass the lower part of the supralabial scales (as in *A. taylori*). Instead, the lower part of the supralabials in this species are a dark color.

Scalation is similar to the preceding species.

Reaches a length of 55 inches.

Distribution, Habitat, and Biology: The lower and moderate elevations along the pacific coast of Mexico and Central America from southern Sonora south to Costa Rica. Within its range in the USNORTHCOM region this species is found in dryer habitats including dry forests and savannas. There are three subspecies of this snake, and it is also found in USSOUTHCOM region.

Venom and Bite: Venom toxins are presumed to be the same as for the previous species. *A. bilineatus* has proportionately longer fangs than *controtrix* or *piscivorous* and its venom is apparently quite potent. A number of deaths have been recorded. Severe tissue damage is said to frequently occur in victims which may sometimes lead to amputations. Bioclon's "Antivipmyn" and "Tri-Antivipmyn" (country of origin, Mexico) are both listed by the manufacturer as effective antivenoms for treating Cantil bites.

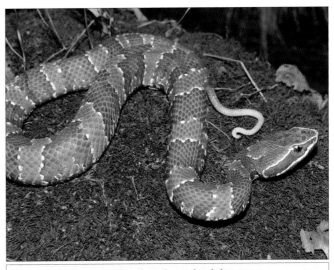

PHOTO 11. Common Cantil, *Agkistrodon bilineatus*

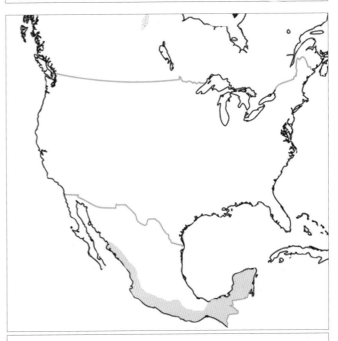

MAP 13. Range of Common Cantil, *Agkistrodon bilineatus* in the USNORTHCOM region.

Family - Viperidae

Subfamily - Crotalinae - Pit Vipers

Genus - Atropoides

Jumping Vipers

There are five species in this genus, four of which occur in the USNORTHCOM region, and two of those are also found in the USSOUHTHCOM region. The other two species in this region are endemic.

Definition: All are readily identified by their exceedingly stocky body shape. These are short, very thick bodied snakes with a series of dark, saddle shaped blotches down the back. The head is quite large with a broad snout and a prominent dark postocular stripe. These are short snakes, reaching a maximum length of only about 2 feet, but a large specimen may have a girth as big as a man's wrist. They have the ability to strike for an abnormally long distance, hence the name "Jumping Viper."

Dorsal scales heavily keeled in 21-29 rows; rostral scale concave and broader than high; ventrals 114-155; subcaudals undivided, 22-40.

Eyes comparatively small and separated from labials by several rows of small scales. Pupils elliptical.

Jumping Vipers

Atripoides nummifer (Mexican Jumping Viper), *Atripoides mexicanus* (Central American Jumping Viper), *Atripoides olmec* (Tuxtlan Jumping Viper), *and Atripoides occidus* (Guatemalan Jumping Viper)

Description and Identification: All four Jumping Viper species found within the USNORTHCOM region are for the most part indistinguishable to the lay observer. In fact, until recently they were all considered to be a single species. Thus, the author has elected to treat all four of these similar snakes together in this account.

All are short, thick-bodied pit vipers with dark saddle-shaped blotches on a tan or gray background.

Adults average 18 to 24 inches in length.

Ground color tan, light brown or gray with about 20 dark brown or black rhomboid blotches down the back, these are often connected with lateral spots to form narrow cross bands. Top of head dark with oblique post orbital band forming upper limit of light color on sides

of head. Ventral color whitish, sometimes blotched with dark brown. Snout rounded, canthus sharp. Body exceedingly stout; tail short.

Dorsal scales strongly keeled, tubercular in large individuals, in 23-27 rows at mid-body; fewer (19) posteriorly. Ventrals 125-135; subcaudals 26-36; all or mostly single. Eye separated from labials by 3-4 rows of small scales.

Distribution, Habitat, and Biology: The name Jumping Viper is appropriate for this species, as its stout body can strike for a distance greater than its length. Ranging from southern Mexico to Panama, Jumping Vipers are rain forest animals and occur in a wide variety of elevations throughout their range. As with many other pit viper species, the young have bright yellow tail tips. Immature snakes are reported to feed heavily on grasshoppers, while mice appear to constitute the mainstay of the diet for adults.

Venom and Bite: Myotoxins and haemorragins possibly present. The venom of jumping vipers is apparently not highly toxic, and they appear not to be deadly to humans. However, the venom is known to vary widely among snakes from different regions, and some may be more dangerous than others. These snakes also have a tendency to hang on after striking, a habit that can increase the amount of venom injected and thus increase the severity of the bite.

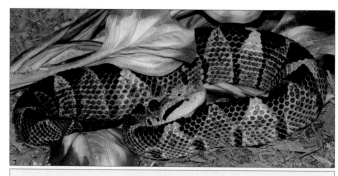

PHOTO 12. Mexican Jumping Viper, *Atripoides nummifer*

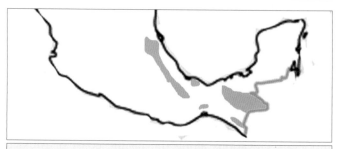

MAP 14. Range of Jumping Vipers in the USNORTHCOM region.

Family - Viperidae

Subfamily - Crotalinae - Pit Vipers

Genus - Bothriechis

Palm Vipers

These snakes are found mostly in the USOUTHCOM region. There are a total of nine species and all are decidedly arboreal in habits. Three species can be found in the southernmost tip of the USNORTHCOM region in the Mexican states of Chiapas and extreme southeast Oaxaca.

Definition: Average length about 2 feet but may reach 3 feet. Body moderate to slender. Tail moderate in length and prehensile. Head very distinct from neck with a sharply defined canthus.

Eyes moderate size with elliptical pupil.

Head Scales: Highly variable, some species have numerous small scales on top of the head while others have large, platelike scales. Two species have raised, spine-like scales above the eye.

Body Scales: Scale rows at midbody 17-25. Ventrals 134-175. Subcaudals 42-75, undivided.

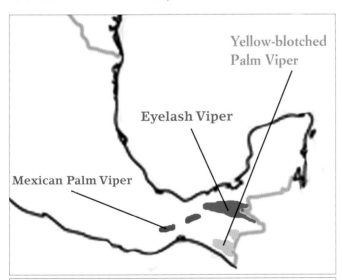

MAP 15. Range map for the three species of *Bothriechis* found in the USNORTHCOM region.

Yellow-blotched Palm Viper,
Bothriechis aurifer

Description and Identification: Average length about 2.5 feet. May rarely reach 3 feet. Ground color is green with a series of black bordered pale blotches down the center of the back and extending onto the tail. A broad, dark postocular stripe is usually present. Immature specimens are greenish yellow. Scales on top of the head anterior of the eyes are large and plate-like. Keeled scales in 18 to 21 scale rows at midbody. Ventrals 148-167, 48-64 subcaudals, mostly undivided. The iris of the eye in this species is greenish yellow and heavily diffused with darks specks.

Distribution, Habitat, and Biology: A primarily arboreal snake that hunts by day in trees and bushes in mountain cloud forests. Campbell and Lamar (2004) report treefrogs and rodents as prey, but small birds and lizards are probably also consumed.

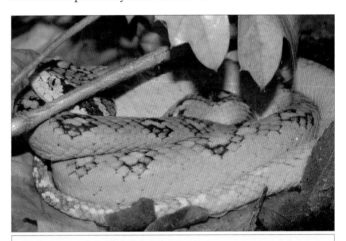

PHOTO 13. Yellow-blotched Palm Viper, *Bothriechis aurifer* (immature)

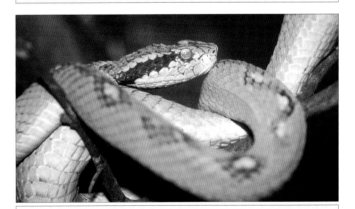

PHOTO 14. Yellow-blotched Palm Viper, *Bothriechis aurifer* (adult)

Venom and Bite: Procoagulants and haemorragins possibly present. Deaths from the bite of this species have been recorded. Instiudo Bioclon's "Tri-Antivipmyn" antivenom (manufactured in Mexico) is listed as having protective substances capable of neutralizing the toxic effects of the venom of *Bothriechis* species.

Mexican Palm Viper,

Bothriechis rowleyi

Description and Identification: Reaches a maximum length of just over 3 feet. Color is uniformly green or green with pale blue spots. There is no postocular stripe and the iris of the eye is yellow.

Young are yellowish green and have dark blotches. The head scales on top of the snout and anterior to the eyes are large and plate-like, and the head scales posterior to the eye are also relatively large in size compared to most other members of the genus.

Typically 19 scale rows at midbody (keeled), ventrals 154-166, subcaudals 53-66 and undivided.

Distribution, Habitat, and Biology: This species is found on forested slopes between 3,000 and 6,000 feet in elevation. Its range is quite small (see range map), and there is little information available on the natural history of the species. As with other members of this genus, these are primarily arboreal snakes that are mainly diurnal in habits. Tree frogs, lizards and birds are likely its diet.

Venom and Bite: Haemorragins present, procoagulants possibly present. The potency of this snake's venom is unknown. However, other closely related members of this genus have killed humans and this snake should be treated as highly dangerous. Antivipmyn antivenom by Bioclon of Mexico is the antivenom listed for treating bites by this genus. Tri-Antivipmyn antivenom can also be used to treat its bite.

Similar Species: There is one other similar *Bothriechis* species that also occurs in this region. The Eyelash Viper (*B. schlegelii*) can be told from the preceding species by the presence of raised, spine-like scales above the eye. This species is also widely found in the USSOUTH-COM region. For information see page 93, chapter 9 (USSOUTHCOM region).

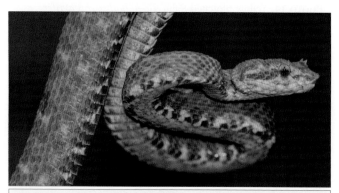

Photo 15. Eyelash Viper (red phase), *Bothriechis schlegelii*

Family - Viperidae

Subfamily - Crotalinae - Pit Vipers

Genus - Ophryacus

Horned Pit Vipers

There are only two species in this unusual genus and both are found in tropical Mexico, where they have a rather restricted range. They are superficially similar to the preceding genus (*Bothriechis*) from which they can be distinguished by the lack of a prehensile tail. They are also much less arboreal in habits, and one species is apparently entirely terrestrial. The name Horned Pit Viper comes from the fact that both species have raised, hornlike scales above the eye.

Definition: These are moderately stout snakes that reach a maximum length of just over two feet. The head is very distinct from the neck and rounded distally when viewed from above. Pupil elliptical.

Head Scales: Top of head covered with small scales with tubercular keels. Raised, hornlike projection above the eye.

Body Scales: 21 midbody scale rows (keeled). Ventrals 141-178. Subcaudals 36-57 (divided or undivided).

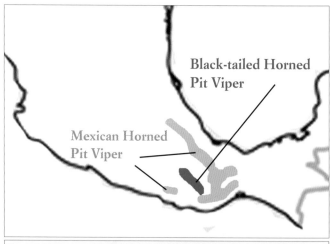

Map 16. Range map for the Horned Pit Vipers.

Mexican Horned Pit Viper,

Ophryacus undulatus

Description and Identification: The head viewed from above is ovoid in shape and quite distinct from the neck. The superocular scales above the eye are also distinctive, forming raised spine-like projections. The body is moderately stout. Eyes moderate, pupils elliptical. Scale rows at midbody 21. Ventrals 157-178. Subcaudals

37-57 (divided). The color is variable and may be gray, greenish brown, or greenish yellow. The ground color is sometimes diffused with dark speckling. A series of vertebral blotches running the entire length of the body are usually connected to form an irregular zig-zag pattern.

Distribution, Habitat, and Biology: This species occurs at intermediate elevations in the mountains of Hildago, Guerrero, Oaxaca, and Veracruz. Lamar and Campbell (2004) list as habitat "pine-oak and cloud forest." Despite it's superficial resemblance to the arboreal Palm Vipers, this genus is much more terrestrial in habits. As with many mountain species, these snakes appear to be primarily diurnal or crepuscular in habits. Rodents and lizards are reported as prey.

Venom and Bite: Nothing is known about the venom of this snake or the effects of its bite on humans. Tri-Antivipmyn antivenom is listed by Biolcon of Mexico as a treatment for bites by this genus.

Similar Species: The similar Black-tailed Horned Pit Viper (*O. melanurus*) can be found in a small area of southern Mexico in parts of the states of Pueblo and Oaxaca (see map 16 on page 48).

Family - Viperidae

Subfamily - Crotalinae - Pit Vipers

Genus - Cerrophidion and Mixcoatlus

Neotropical Mountain Pit Vipers

These two genera are so similar that they are being treated here together as a single genus. Indeed, all 8 species of the two genera are remarkably similar in morphology and biology. They owe their diversity to the fact that they are mountaintop animals that are genetically isolated from other populations.

There are five species of *Cerrophidion*, two of which are quite rare and have very restricted ranges in southern Mexico. One species, *C. godmani* (Godman's Mountain Viper) is fairly common and ranges from southern Mexico into the USSOUTHCOM region in Guatemala. Two more species *C. sasai* (Costa Rican Mountain Viper) and *C. wilsoni* (Honduran Mountain Viper) are endemic to the USSOUTHCOM region in Central America. The similar genus *Mixcoatlus* contains three species total and all are endemic to the mountains of southwest Mexico. In fact, all species of both genera are mountaintop snakes and all are primarily diurnal in habits.

Definition: These are small to medium sized snakes with a maximum length of about 30 inches. The head is large with a distinct neck. Body is only moderately stout and the tail is short.

Eyes moderate in size, pupils elliptical.

Head Scales: Variable. Some exhibit a few large plates similar to *Agkistrodon* (moccasins) while others have many small head scales reminiscent of *Crotalus* (rattlesnakes).

Body scales: There are 17-21 scale rows at midbody. Dorsal scales are moderately keeled. Ventrals 120-150, subcaudals 22-36 (undivided).

Mountain Pit Vipers
(genus *Cerrophidion*), C. godmani (Godman's) C. petlacalensis (Petlacala), and C. tzotzilorum (Tzotzil). (genus *Mixcoatlus*) M. melanurus (Black-tailed) M.barbouri (Barbour's), and M. browni (Brown's).

Description and Identification: The three species of *Cerrophidion* and three species of *Mixoatlus* found in the USNORTHCOM region are all variable in color and pattern, but all are similar in general appearance and in natural history. Most are quite rare and have very restricted ranges, thus the author has decided it expedient to treat all species in this single account.

These snakes vary considerably in color even among members of the same species, but they always show a dorsal pattern of dark vertebral blotches on a lighter ground color. The dorsal blotches are sometimes connected to form a zigzag pattern (especially anteriorly), and there are a series of corresponding small dark blotches laterally. The ground color may be reddish, brown, or gray. A dark post-ocular stripe is always evident. These are small to medium sized pit vipers with a proportionately large head.

Distribution, Habitat, and Biology: As their name implies these snakes are found only in mountainous habitats. Many are found only in very small areas consisting of individual mountain ranges in southern Mexico. One species (*C. godmani*) is fairly common and can be found from southern Mexico into Guatemala but even its range is disjunct and restricted to a series of highlands. These unusual pit vipers feed on a wide variety of prey including small mammals, birds, lizards, amphibians and large numbers of insects. Litters number from

2 to 12 with larger females producing the higher number of young. Unlike many pit vipers, the Mountain Pit Vipers are apparently strictly diurnal in habits. This may be a response to the cooler temperatures which prevail at the higher elevations where these snakes live.

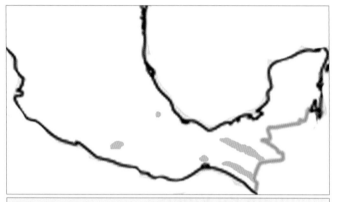

Map 17. Range of the Mountain Pit Vipers in the USNORTHCOM region.

Venom and Bite: Venom toxins that may be present include procoagulants and haemorragins. Although there are no known fatalities from the bite of any of these snakes, several accounts by Campell & Lamar (2004) cite significant localized symptoms (pain, swelling, discoloration) seen in a number of snakebite cases. Polyvalent Antivenom by Institute Clodomiro Picado (Costa Rica) is one of several antivenoms listed by www.toxinology.com (2012). Bioclon's Tri-Antivipmyn manufactured in Mexico is also a choice for treating bites.

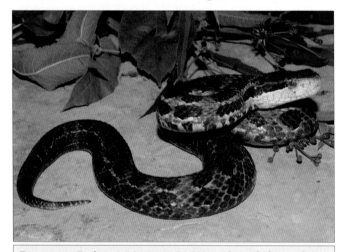

Photo 16. Godman's Mountain Pit Viper, *Cerrophidion godmani*

Lancehead Vipers

There are 23 species of Lancehead Vipers (some experts recognize more). All are dangerous snakes and several species rank among the most deadly snakes in the western hemisphere. They range from tropical regions of southern Mexico throughout Central America to southern South America. Most are snakes of lowland regions that are primarily nocturnal in habits. A few species range high into mountains where they may be more diurnal in movements.

Most average 3 to 4 feet in length but several species can exceed 6 feet.

Definition: Head broad, flattened, very distinct from narrow neck. Body slender to moderately stout. Tail moderately long, non-prehensile.

Scales on top of head small and keeled.

Eyes moderate in size, elliptical pupil.

Loreal pit present.

Dorsal scales keeled, 21-33 rows at midbody.

Ventrals 141-240. Subcaudals (divided) 33-95.

A single species, the Terciopelo (*B. asper*) can be found in the USNORTHCOM region.

Terciopelo,
Bothrops asper

Description and Identification: Head triangular and distinct from the neck. Body moderately slender. Eyes moderately large, pupils elliptical. Scale rows at midbody 25-29, heavily keeled. Subcaudals 56-70, mostly undivided. Ventrals 185-220. Adults average about 4 feet but can reach a length in excess of 7 feet. The color of these snakes is confusingly variable, and they may be brown, gray, yellowish, reddish, olive, or very dark charcoal. The dorsal pattern varies somewhat in discernability, however it is consistently a pattern of dark triangles on each side of the body which meet at the top of the back. These dark markings are edged in a lighter pigment that also highlights the center of each triangle. This pattern runs the entire length of the body and onto the tail. A narrow, dark postocular stripe is nearly always present from the eye to the angle of the jaw. Young snakes may have a yellow tail tip.

Distribution, Habitat, and Biology: The Terciopelo is mostly a lowland animal, found in rain forest from sea level to moderate elevations of up to 3,600 feet. It is most often found in the vicinity of rivers and streams. These are ground dwelling snakes and the color and pattern of the Terciopelo is highly cryptic. They are nearly invisible when coiled atop the leaf litter on the forest floor. They are ambush predators that as adults feed mostly on small mammals and birds. Young snakes will eat invertebrates, frogs, and lizards. These snakes are often referred to as "Fer-de-lance," but that name should be reserved for the Martinique Lancehead *Bothrops lanceolatus*.

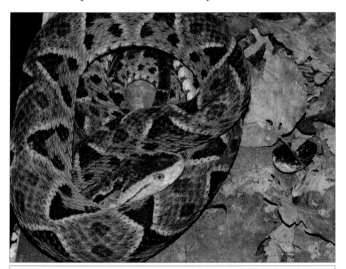

Photo 17. Terciopelo, *Bothrops asper*

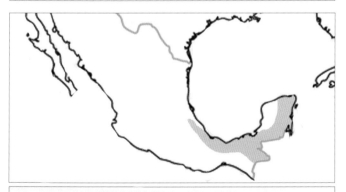

Map 18. Range of the Terciopelo, *Bothrops asper* in the USNORTHCOM region.

Venom and Bite: Venom contains procoagulants, haemorragins, and systemic myotoxins. Its large size, long fangs, extended reach when striking and its propensity to defend itself at the slightest provocation make this one of the most dangerous snakes in the western hemisphere. In addition, it possesses a highly toxic venom and can deliver large doses deep into tissues. The venom can cause severe necrosis (hemorrhage is often cause of death) and inhibits the clotting factor of the blood. Severe envenomations that do not receive prompt and proper medical attention often result in death. The Terciopelo is a fairly common snake throughout its range and it sometimes occurs around human habitations. It is thus responsible for a significant number of snakebite deaths. Two antivenoms of choice for treating bites from this snake are "Tri-Antivipmyn" (Mexico) and "Antiofidico Bothropico Polivalente" (Ecuador).

Family - Viperidae

Subfamily - Crotalinae - Pit Vipers

Genus - Porthidium

Hognosed Pit Vipers

Most of the nine species of these small to medium sized pit vipers have a distinctive upturned snout. This character is more apparent in some species than others, but all have some degree of "hognosed" appearance. There are four species found within the USNORTCHCOM region, three of which are endemic and one that ranges farther south into the USSOUTHCOM region where the other five species are also found.

Definition: Triangular head very distinct from neck. Body slender to moderately stout. Canthus sharply defined. Rostral scale always higher than wide.

Eyes moderately large, pupil elliptical.

Dorsal scales heavily keeled in 21- 27 rows at midbody. Ventrals 136-176, subcaudals 25-44.

Adult range from about 20 inches to 2.5 feet in length.

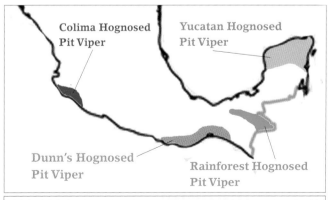

Map 19. Range of the Hognosed Pit Vipers in the USNORTHCOM region.

The World Health Organization's Venomous Snake Antivenom Database (www.int/bloodproducts/snakeantivenoms/database - 2012) lists the following antivenoms for treating bites by *Porthidium* species.

Product: Polyvalent Antivenom ICP
Manufacturer: Instituto Clodomiro Picado
Country of Origin: Costa Rica
Product: Antivipmyn
Manufacturer: Instituto Bioclon
Country of Origin: Mexico

Hognosed Pit Vipers

P. nasutum (Rainforest Hognosed Pit Viper),
P. dunni (Dunn's Hognosed Pit Viper),
P. yucatanicum (Yucatan Hognosed Pit Viper),
P. hespere (Colima Hognosed Pit Viper).

Description and Identification: All four species of Hognosed Pit Vipers found in the USNORTHCOM region are fairly similar in appearance and biology and are thus treated together in this account. When the head is viewed in profile there is a distinct upturn of the snout and on some the snout is elevated enough to create a "rhinoceros" like appearance (*P. nasutum and P. dunni*). All are moderately stout snakes. The ground color is brown, tan, gray, or reddish brown. There is a series of dark vertebral blotches down the back that sometimes form a zigzag pattern, or the blotches may appear squarish and be paired of slightly offset on each side of the spine. A vertebral stripe is sometimes present. Immature snakes have a bright yellow tail tip.

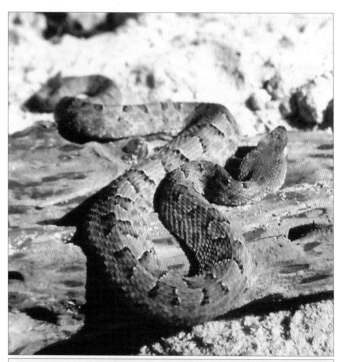

PHOTO 19. Yucatan Hognosed Pit Viper, *Porthidium yucatanicum*

Distribution, Habitat, and Biology: These are mostly lowland animals in this region. They inhabit both tropical rainforest and drier deciduous woodlands. Primarily nocturnal and crepuscular in habits they feed on a variety of small vertebrates. Lizards are reportedly a main source of food but their diet also includes frogs, mice, and birds. Invertebrates are also eaten.

Venom and Bite: Though dangerous, these snakes are not generally regarded as being deadly to humans. However one species, *P. nasutum,* the Rainforest Hognosed Pit Viper, has caused human deaths. Its venom contains procoagulants and possibly haemorragins.

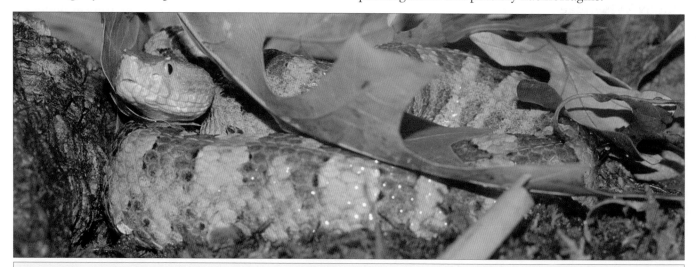

PHOTO 18. Dunn's Hognosed Pit Viper, *Porthidium dunni*

Rattlesnakes

Rattlesnakes are distinctively American serpents that can be almost always identified by the jointed rattle at the tip of the tail. The rattle is vestigial in a single rare species found on an island off the Mexican coast. It is too small to be a good filed identification characteristic in the pygmy rattlesnake (Sistrurus miliarius) and in the young of some other small rattlesnakes. Although most of the rattle can easily be pulled or broken off, the base or matrix usually remains. Rarely the entire tail tip including the rattle matrix may be missing as a result of injury. Nine large crown shields are seen in rattlesnakes of the genus *Sistrurus*. In the genus *Crotalus* the crown shields are more or less extensively fragmented. The facial pit is present in all rattlesnakes. Scales are keeled and the subcaudals are undivided.

Species identification among rattlesnakes may be difficult, but it is often important. The venoms show significant differences that can influence treatment and prognosis. "Cro-fab" Ovine Antivenom by Protherics, Inc. is recommended for most North American rattlesnake species. "Antivipmyn" (Equine) and "Tri-Antivipmyn" (Equine) antivenoms by Institudo Bioclone are most useful in treating bites by Mexican, Central American, and South American rattlesnakes and likely have some degree of effectiveness against all rattlesnake venoms.

The larger species of rattlesnakes feed principally upon small mammals; the smaller species mostly upon lizards. All rattlesnakes are live-bearing.

Family - Viperidae

Subfamily - Crotalinae - Pit Vipers

Genus - Crotalus

Rattlesnakes

About 37 species of rattlesnakes are currently recognized (some say 35, others 39). All but one species can be found in the USNORTHCOM region. Most species are in the southwestern United States and northern Mexico. One species, (C. durissus) ranges as far south as southern South America, two are found east of the Mississippi River, and two as far north as Canada. A few of the very small species, and small individuals of large species (less than 2 feet) may offer little danger, but most species do; some are highly dangerous.

Crofab antivenin by Protherics, Inc. is recommended in treating most North American rattlesnake bites, while Antivipmyn Tri manufactured by Bioclon of Mexico is effective for South American Rattlesnakes.

Definition: Head broad, very distinct from narrow neck, canthus distinct to absent. Body cylindrical, depressed, or slightly compressed, moderately slender to stout; tail short with a horny segmented rattle.

Eyes small, pupils vertically elliptical.

Head scales: Supraoculars present, a pair of internasals often distinct, occasionally a pair of prefrontals; enlarged canthal scales often present; other parts of crown covered with small scales. Laterally , eye separated from supralabials by 1-5 rows of small scales.

Body scales: Dorsals keeled, with apical pits. in 19-33 non oblique rows at midbody. Ventrals 132-206, subcaudals 13-45, all single or with some terminal ones paired.

Eastern Diamondback Rattlesnake,
Crotalus adamanteus

Description and Identification: Within its range the only large rattlesnake with distinct, diagonal, whitish stripes on side of head; tail more or less indistinctly ringed.

Olive green to dark brown with central series of darker diamond shaped blotches each with a somewhat lighter center and a distinct cream or yellow edge; belly cream heavily clouded with gray.

Average 3.5 to 5.5 feet; maximum nearly 8 feet.

Distribution, Habitat, and Biology: Coastal lowlands from North Carolina through Florida to extreme south-

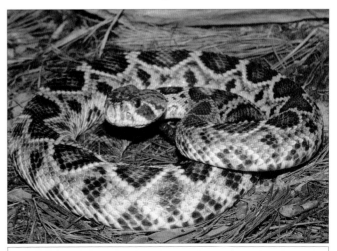

Photo 20. Eastern Diamondback Rattlesnake, *Crotalus adamanteus*

west Mississippi. Found in dry pine woods, palmetto thickets, old fields, and coastal dunes.

These snakes are good swimmers and may enter both fresh or salt water and can be found on many offshore islands. They avoid permanent wetlands. Primary prey of adults is rabbits, both cottontails and marsh rabbits. Also eaten are rice rats, squirrels and other rodents, and some ground nesting birds.

These snakes are famous among ecologists for their association with the Gopher Tortoise, a burrowing land turtle whose range closely parallels that of the Eastern Diamondback. The tortoises share their burrow home with these large rattlesnakes and provide the bulky serpents with rare access to underground shelter in extreme weather.

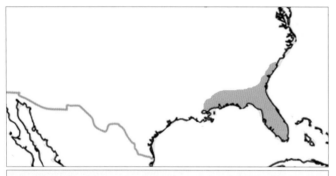

MAP 20. Range of the Eastern Diamondback, Rattlesnake, *Crotalus adamanteus.*

This species has experienced a severe decline in numbers since the publication of *Poisonous Snakes of the World* back in 1965. Today, Eastern Diamondback populations are fragmented and in serious trouble throughout their range. Habitat loss is the main culprit in this decline but a pervasive image of rattlesnakes as vermin exacerbates the problem .

Venom and Bite: The Eastern Diamondback has long fangs, large venom glands, and a highly toxic venom. It is thus one of the more dangerous members of the rattlesnake clan. A maximum envenomation by a large specimen would almost certainly be fatal without treatment, and this species has killed many humans. Bites from this species probably produce the highest mortality rate of any rattlesnake in the United States. "Cro-fab" (Ovine) antivenom manufactured in the U.S. by Protherics, Inc. is an effective agent for neutralizing the effects of this species venom. This snake's venom contains myotoxins, procoagulants, anticoagulants, haemorragins, and seconday nephrotoxins and necrotoxins. The venom gland capacity of 500 mg. or more (dry weight) is the highest of any rattlesnake.

Western Diamondback Rattlesnake,
Crotalus atrox

Description and Identification: Two light, diagonal stripes on side of head, posterior one extending to angle of mouth; tail distinctly ringed with black and gray or white, the black rings as wide as or wider than the pale ones; scales between supraoculars small; two scales between nasals and in contact with rostral.

General coloration buff, gray, brown, or reddish with diamonds that are less clear cut , often appearing dusty with indistinct light edges; belly cream to pinkish buff sometimes clouded with gray.

Average length 3 to 5.5 feet. Maximum 7 feet. Captive specimens in excess of 7 feet are known.

Distribution, Habitat, and Biology: Central Arkansas to southeastern California southward through most of Texas into Mexico to northern Veracruz and southern Sonora with an isolated population in Oaxaca. Inhabits many types of terrain from dry, sparsely wooded rocky hills to flat desert and coastal sand dunes. Often found in agricultural land and near towns. Generally avoids dense forest, swamps, and elevations above 5,000 feet in the United States, but may be found up to 8,000 feet in Mexico.

As with most large rattlesnakes, small mammals make up the bulk of the diet for adult snakes. Unlike many North American Rattlesnake species that are in a steep decline, populations of *C. atrox*, remain fairly healthy in much of their range.

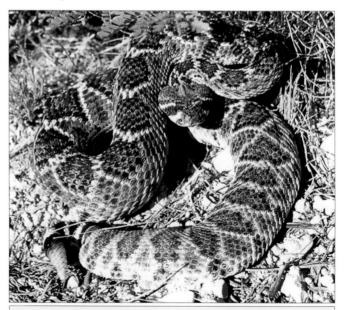

PHOTO 21 Western Diamondback Rattlesnake, *Crotalus atrox*

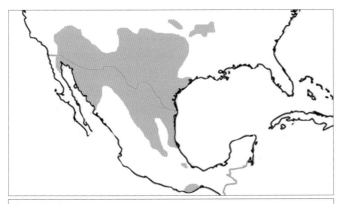

MAP 21. Range of the Western Diamondback Rattlesnake, *Crotalus atrox.*

Venom and Bite: The Western Diamondback has a reputation for having an irascible disposition and it is quick to strike. It's venom is less toxic than that of many other rattlesnakes, but it has large venom glands and yields more venom per bite than any other rattlesnake. It's fangs may exceed an inch in length, and venom may be injected deep into tissue.

To say that this is a potentially deadly species is an understatement, and in fact it is credited with causing more deaths in the United States than any other snake. "Crofab" (Ovine) antivenom is reportedly effective in treating bites by this species. "Tri-Antivipmyn" by Bioclon of Mexico has also been used to successfully treat bites by this species (personal communication - Jim Harrison). Venom contains procoagulants, haemorragins and secondary necotoxins.

Red Diamond Rattlesnake,
Crotalus ruber

Description and Identification: Separated from the Western Diamondback only by its more reddish color and minor details of scalation (usually 29 rather than 25 scale rows at midbody; first lower labial usually divided in ruber, undivided in atrox).

Average length 40 to 50 inches; maximum about five feet.

Distribution, Habitat, and Biology: Found in Baja California and southwestern California; this species and *C. atrox* meet only in a narrow zone in extreme northeastern Baja Norte and adjacent California. Red Diamond Rattlesnakes are largely confined to rocky hillsides with scrubby vegetation but at no great elevation.

The three large rattlesnakes, the Red Diamond, the Eastern Diamondback, and the Western Diamondback, are quite similar in appearance but differ somewhat in

behavior. The Red Diamond is the most diurnal of the group, although all may be active by day during cooler times of the year. Western Diamondbacks in the northern part of their range aggregate in large numbers to hibernate-a trait seen in some other species of rattlesnakes as well.

Temperament in the group shows much individual variation. Generally the Red Diamond Rattler is the mildest mannered and the Western Diamondback the most irritable. All may defend themselves with great vigor. They sometimes raise the head and a loop of the neck well above their coils to gain elevation in striking. All may occasionally strike without rattling. The Red Diamond Rattlesnake often hisses loudly.

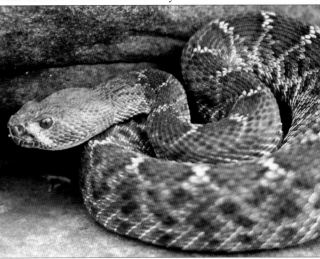

PHOTO 22. Red Diamond Rattlesnake, *Crotalus ruber*

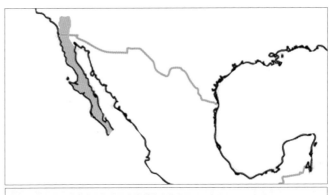

MAP 22. Range of the Red Diamond Rattlesnake, *Crotalus ruber.*

Venom and Bite: Procoagulants and haemorragins. The venom of the Red Diamond Rattlesnake is definitely less toxic than that of other large American Rattlesnakes and fatalities from its bite are rare. The Western and Eastern Diamondbacks cause most of the snakebite fatalities in the United States. However, this is a large species capable of delivering a large dose of venom, and its bite can sometimes kill.

Mohave Rattlesnake,
Crotalus scutulatus

Description and Identification: Very similar to the Western Diamondback and Prairie Rattlesnake in appearance. Scales on top of head between and anterior to the eyes large, resembling shields of most snakes; dark rings on tail much narrower than light spaces between them; general color often greenish, olive, or tan.

Average length 30 to 40 inches; maximum about 4 feet.

Proper identification of the Mohave Rattlesnake is important in the event of a snakebite, as this species has a neurotoxic element to the venom that has a marked effect on respiration. To distinguish from the Western Diamondback note that on the Mohave the *white bands on the tail are wider than the black bands*, opposite is true for the Western Diamondback. Differentiation from the Prairie Rattlesnake is best accomplished by noting the scales on the top of the head between the eye, which in the Mohave *consist of large shields* but in the Prairie Rattlesnake appear as numerous small scales.

Distribution, Habitat, and Biology: The Mohave Rattlesnake is a decidedly desert animal. In the southwestern United States this snake is common in Creosote Bush flatlands, upland desert scrub, and mesquite-grassland. Farther south in Mexico it may be found in pine-oak woodlands. While this snake does range throughout the Mohave Desert region, it also ranges across the Sonora and Chihuahua Deserts from southern California to western Texas and south to southern Mexico. It may be found in a wide variety of habitats within its range but never ascends to the higher elevations, preferring broad valleys, flatlands, or plains.

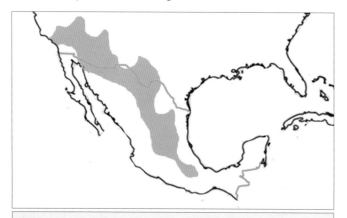

MAP 23. Range of the Mohave Rattlesnake, *Crotalus scutulatus.*

Venom and Bite: This species boasts one of the most toxic venoms of any rattlesnake. Powerful pre-synaptic neurotoxins, known as "mohave toxins" interfere with breathing. The insidious aspect of the venom is manifested in the fact that potentially lethal envenomations may not show the significant localized symptomology common to most pit viper bites. This can lead to a false sense of security in both victims and medical personnel unfamiliar with the species. "Crofab" (Ovine) antivenin by Protherics, Inc. is recommended for treating bites, and "Tri-Antivipmyn" by Bioclone of Mexico has also been used successfully (personal communication - Jim Harrison).

A professional American herpetologist was among the many deaths resulting from the bite of this highly dangerous species.

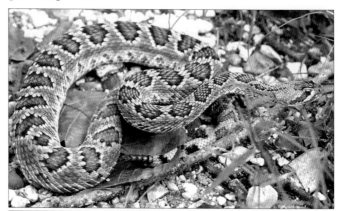

PHOTO 23. Mohave Rattlesnake, *Crotalus scutulatus*

The Western Rattlesnake Group

The next 7 species were once all considered to be subspecies of *Crotalus viridis*. Their biology is similar and although they vary considerably in color, the basic pattern of a series of rhomboid shaped dorsal blotches is common to all. The exact taxonomy of this group is disputed. Here the author has followed the sixth edition of *Standard Common and Current Scientific Names for North American Amphibians, Turtles, Reptiles and Crocodilians* published by The Center for North American Herpetology in 2009.

The rattlesnakes of this group are largely diurnal, although they avoid intense light and heat and may become nocturnal during the hottest parts of the summer. In the northern part to their range they assemble in great numbers to hibernate.

In disposition these snakes are, on average, less irritable than diamondbacks and less likely to make a determined defense. A characteristic defensive gesture is to protrude the tongue as far as possible and wave it slowly up and down.

Bites from rattlesnakes in this group are relatively common. There is evidence that venom of the Pacific species *C. oreganus* and *C. helleri* is more toxic than that of the eastern species *C. viridis*, and it is a highly dangerous snake. The species with the most toxic venom in the group however is the diminutive Midget Faded Rattlesnake *C. concolor.*

Prairie Rattlesnake,
Crotalus viridis

Description and Identification: Light diagonal line behind the eye narrow; body blotches rectangular, usually with narrow light edges; ground color often greenish gray or olive brown.

Average length 3 to 4 feet; record 5 feet. Males are larger than females.

Light Diagonal lines on the side of the head extend behind angle of the mouth. The light rings on the tail are the same color as the body, not white as in *C. atrox* and *C. scutulatus*. Dorsal blotches rhomboid rather than diamond shaped.

Distribution, Habitat, and Biology: Found throughout the great expanse of the North American prairie from the high northern plains of southern Alberta and Saskatchewan in Canada to the desert grasslands of northern Coahuila, Mexico. In the United States its range includes parts of North Dakota, South Dakota, Wyoming, Montana, Idaho, Colorado, Nebraska, Kansas, Oklahoma, Texas, New Mexico, and Arizona as well as a tiny portion of southwestern Minnesota and western Iowa. Native mixed grass prairies and short grass prairies are its primary habitat, but it also ascends into mountains as high as 10,000 feet where it may be found in meadows, forests, or most commonly talus slopes and rocky canyons. In the southern portions of its range it lives in mesquite-grassland and desert grasslands. Avoids low, hot desert.

Some populations in the far north may migrate several miles between summer feeding grounds and winter hibernacula. Large, communal hibernating dens are common on the northern plains where suitable hibernacula is rare. Small mammals, birds, and lizards are the preferred prey.

Venom and Bite: The venom of the Prairie Rattlesnake ranks fairly high in toxicity, and deaths from the bite of this snake are not rare. Researchers have noted two distinct venom types in this species. Specimens from farther north possess a venom that is high in muscle destroying properties (myotoxins), while snakes in the southern portions of this species range may contain some amount of neurotoxins. Procoagulants and haemorragins are also present. The Ovine antivenin "Crofab" is reportedly polyvalent against most North American Rattlesnake species and is likely the best choice of antivenom for treating bites by this species. Antivipmyn antivenom and Tri-Antivipmyn by Bioclon of Mexico is also effective.

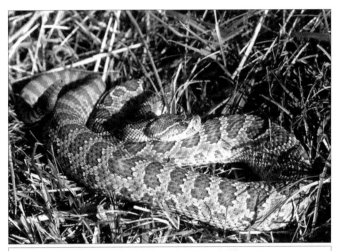

PHOTO 24. Prairie Rattlesnake, *Crotalus viridis viridis*

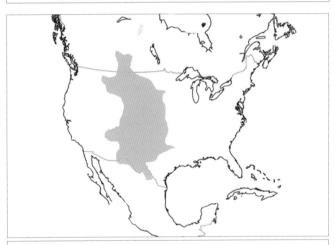

MAP 24. Range of the Prairie Rattlesnake, *Crotalus viridis.*

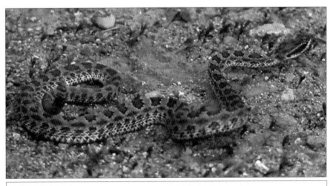

PHOTO 25. Hopi Rattlesnake, *Crotalus viridis nuntius*

Great Basin Rattlesnake,
Crotalus lutosus

Description and Identification: Light stripe behind eye wide; dorsal blotches usually without light edges; ground color buff or drab yellow. Ground color between dorsal blotches about as wide as the blotches.

Average length 24-35 inches; maximum 50 inches.

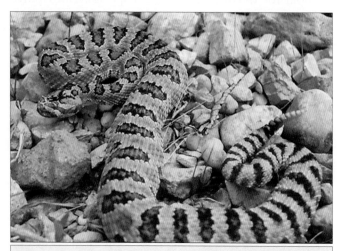

PHOTO 26. Great Basin Rattlesnake, *Crotalus lutosus.*

Distribution, Habitat, and Biology: Inhabits the Great Basin region of western Utah, southern Idaho, southeastern Oregon, and most of Nevada. Sagebrush desert, arid and semi-arid rocky areas.

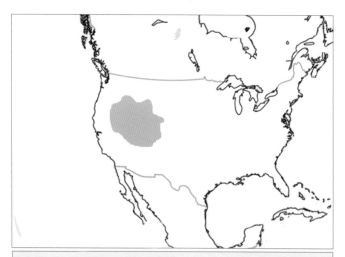

MAP 25. Range of the Great Basin Rattlesnake, *Crotalus lutosus.*

Venom and Bite: As with other members of the Western Rattlesnake group, the Great Basin Rattler is capable of inflicting a fatal bite. Crofab antivenom by Protherics, Inc. is recommended for treating bites of North American Rattlesnakes. Myotoxins and haemorragins are known to be present in venom.

Northern Pacific Rattlesnake,
Crotalus oreganus

Description and Identification: In this species the dorsal blotches are wider than the spaces between them and the tail rings are well defined and quite uniform in width. The ground color ranges from brown or reddish brown to buff. Length 3 to 4 feet.

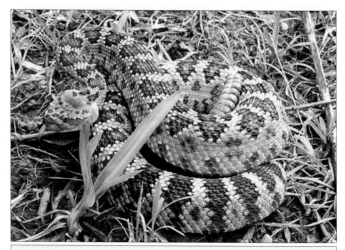

PHOTO 27. Northern Pacific Rattlesnake, *Crotalus oreganus*

Distribution, Habitat, and Biology: Ranges from southern British Columbia in Canada southward through the pacific northwest to south central California. Inhabits grasslands, sagebrush desert, and rocky canyons and talus slopes in mountains.

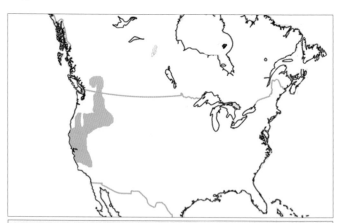

MAP 26. Range of the Northern Pacific Rattlesnake, *Crotalus oreganus.*

Venom and Bite: Myotoxins, procoagulants, and haemorragins present. As with other members of the Western Rattlesnake group, the Northern Pacific Rattlesnake is capable of inflicting a fatal bite.

Southern Pacific Rattlesnake,
Crotalus helleri

Description and Identification: May be tan or olive but usually very dark in color, being gray to almost black. Dark dorsal saddles usually readily discernible even in the darkest of specimens. Averages 3 to 4 feet in length.

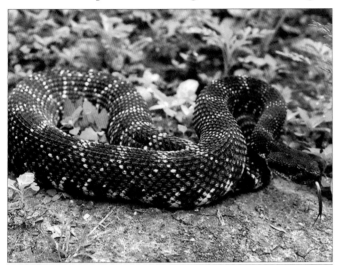

Photo 28. Southern Pacific Rattlesnake, *Crotalus helleri*

Distribution, Habitat, and Biology: Ranges from the southern third of California south to the northern tip of Baja Sur in Mexico. It shuns desert areas in preference for foothills and in southern California it is found from the pacific coast eastward into the coastal ranges, avoiding the deserts of southeast California.

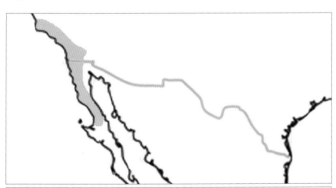

Map 27. Range of the Southern Pacific Rattlesnake, *Crotalus helleri.*

Venom and Bite: Myotoxins, procoagulants, and haemorragins present. The venom of this species is quite toxic and bites from this snake often result in fatalities unless treated with antivenom therapy. Crofab (Ovine) antivenom is listed as being effective against this species.

Arizona Black Rattlesnake,
Crotalus cerberus

Description and Identification: Very similar to the preceding species, but sometimes nearly solid black. On the darkest specimens the dorsal blotches may be obscured. The easiest way to distinguish between these two very similar species is by geography, as their ranges are separated by several hundred miles (see range maps).

Distribution, Habitat, and Biology: The Arizona Black Rattlesnake inhabits the mountains and foothills of the Mogollon Rim region of Arizona and New Mexico.

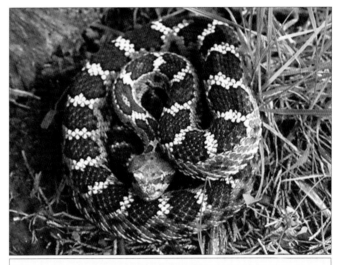

Photo 29. Arizona Black Rattlesnake, *Crotalus cerberus*

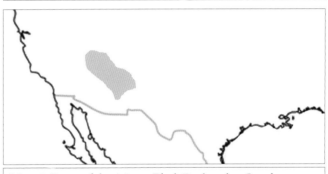

Map 29. Range of the Arizona Black Rattlesnake, *Crotalus cerberus.*

Venom and Bite: As with other members of the Western Rattlesnake group, the Arizona Black Rattlesnake is presumed to be capable of inflicting a fatal bite.

Grand Canyon Rattlesnake,
Crotalus abyssus

Description and Identification: This species is characterized by its yellowish, reddish, or pinkish coloration and by the fact that the dorsal blotches are faded or absent.

Distribution, Habitat, and Biology: This species range is restricted to the immediate vicinity of the Grand Canyon in northeastern Arizona and southern Utah. Occurs both in the canyon and along the rim where it often intergrades with *C. lutosus.*

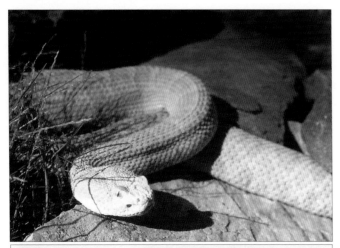

Photo 30. Grand Canyon Rattlesnake, *Crotalus abyssus*

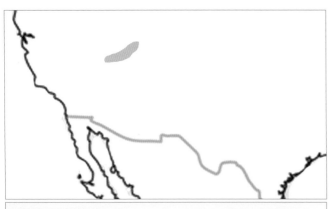

Map 30. Range of the Grand Canyon Rattlesnake, *Crotalus abyssus.*

Venom and Bite: Little is known about the venom of this rare snake, but it is most likely a dangerous species. Myotoxins, procoagulants, and haemorragins are presumed present.

Midget Faded Rattlesnake,
Crotalus concolor

Description and Identification: This is the smallest of the western rattlesnake group and adults rarely exceed two feet (record 3 feet). In coloration these snakes may be creamy yellow, tan, or rarely pinkish.

The dorsal blotches are only slightly darker than the ground color, producing a faded effect.

Distribution, Habitat, and Biology: This snake occurs only to the west of the continental divide. throughout western Colorado and eastern Utah. It may also be found well in a small area of southwest Wyoming along the Green River.

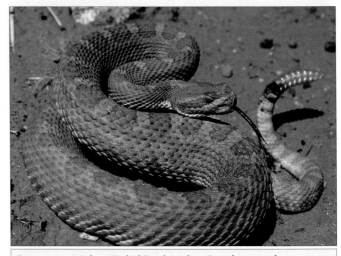

Photo 31. Midget Faded Rattlesnake, *Crotalus concolor*

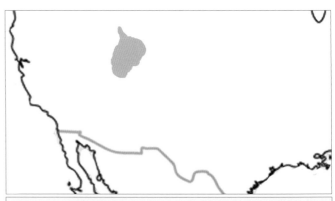

Map 31. Range of the Midget Faded Rattlesnake, *Crotalus concolor.*

Venom and Bite: Studies of the venom of the Midget Faded Rattlesnake have shown it to be as much as 10 to 30 times as toxic as that of the Prairie Rattlesnake. Despite its small size, this species should be considered as very dangerous. Myotoxins, procoagulants, and haemorragins.

Timber Rattlesnake,
Crotalus horridus

Description and Identification: The only rattlesnake in the eastern United States showing the combination of small scales between the eyes, no prominent light stripes on the side of the head, and in adult snakes, a black tail.

Yellow, gray, buff or pale brown with sooty black cross-bands or chevrons narrowly edged with pale yellow or white; often an amber, pinkish or rusty stripe down the middle of the back; belly cream to pinkish white more or less suffused with dark gray.

Specimens from upland areas of the eastern United States are sometimes almost uniformly black above.

Snakes from the lowlands of the coastal plain regions (often called Canebrake Rattlesnake) may be pinkish or purplish between the dark chevrons.

Average length 3 to 4 feet; maximum a little over 6 feet. The largest specimens tend to come from the more southerly areas of its range.

Distribution, Habitat, and Biology: New England to the Florida panhandle, west to central Texas, north in the Mississippi Valley to southeastern Minnesota. Found in wooded rocky hills in the northern part of the range (Timber Rattlesnake), swamps and lowland forest in the south (Canebrake Rattlesnake).

As their name implies, this is a woodland species, and their range closely approximates that of the eastern deciduous forests. In the northern part of their range Timber Rattlesnakes congregate in numbers to bask and hibernate in rocky bluffs and ledges; a habit which has greatly facilitated their extermination in populous areas. This species is now considered to be threatened or endangered in many northeastern states, though their numbers remain fairly healthy in the southern regions.

Adult Timber Rattlesnakes feed on a wide variety of small mammals and birds. Squirrels and Chipmunks are a favored prey. Though mainly terrestrial, they have been know to climb into low bushes and trees.

Venom and Bite: Rather mild tempered, they often do a good deal of preliminary rattling and feinting before striking. This rattlesnake and the Copperhead are used in religious rituals by snake handling cults in the southern Appalachian Mountains. Bites among cultists are fairly frequent, and no medical care is immediately given as a rule. Dozens of fatalities have occurred among these snake handlers. Myotoxins, mixture of procoagulants,

and haemorragins present. Some specimens from the coastal plain possess a neurotoxic component to their venom (Canebrake Toxin) and are thus more dangerous than specimens found farther north.

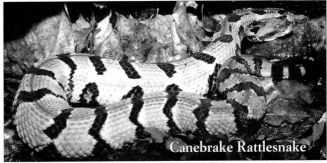

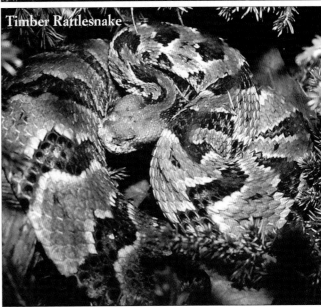

PHOTOS 32 & 33. Timber Rattlesnakes, *Crotalus horridus*

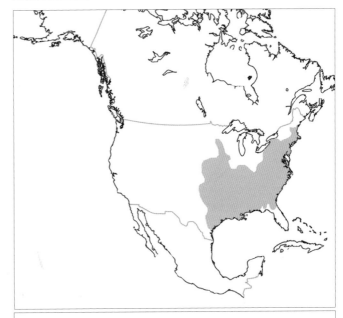

MAP 32. Range of the Timber Rattlesnake, *Crotalus horridus.*

Panamint Rattlesnake,
Crotalus stephensi

Description and Identification: Tan or gray, often has a reddish or purplish hue in the ground color. Markings on back consist of dorsal blotches anteriorly which connect with side blotches to form distinct crossbands beginning about 1/3 of the way back from the head. Tail distinctly banded.

Distribution, Habitat, and Biology: Named for the Panamint Mountains of California's Death Valley, which is the heart of this species' range. These snakes can tolerate exceedingly high temperatures and though mainly nocturnal during summer months they may be seen abroad in late afternoon when temperatures are still quite high.

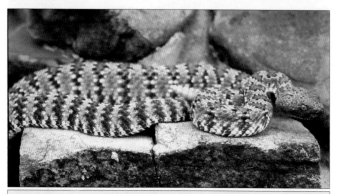

Photo 34. Panamint Rattlesnake, *Crotalus stephansi.*

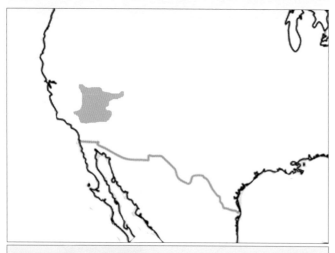

Map 33. Range of the Panamint Rattlesnake, *Crotalus stephensi.*

Venom and Bite: There is little information on the potency of this snake's venom but Campbell and Lamar (2004) report a maximum venom yield of 129 mg., which is probably a lethal dose for a human.

Speckled Rattlesnake,
Crotalus mitchelli

Description and Identification: An extremely variable species in color and pattern. Ground color may be gray, blueish, creamy yellow, tan, or pink. Area between bands heavily diffused with dark speckling. Specimens colors always tend to match the color of the rocks or gravel of their environment, and individuals occurring in areas of lava flows are black. Dorsal markings usually consist of bands but may be blotches, especially anteriorly. Tail is distinctly ringed. Maximum length abut 40 inches.

Distribution, Habitat, and Biology: Extreme south east Nevada, eastern Arizona, and s.w. California south throughout the Baja Peninsula of Mexico. Arid, rocky, desert terrain is the primary habitat, but is also found in chaparral and juniper/pine woodlands.

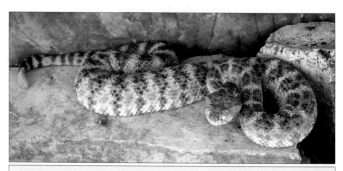

Photo 35. Speckled Rattlesnake, *Crotalus mitchelli*

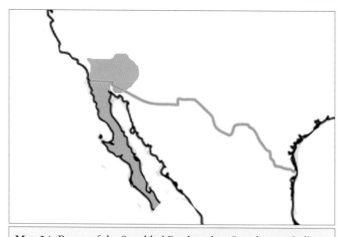

Map 34. Range of the Speckled Rattlesnake, *Crotalus mitchelli.*

Venom and Bite: As with many venomous snakes, this species' venom varies considerably in potency from one geographic region to another. Some specimens are quite dangerous to man.

Sidewinder Rattlesnake,
Crotalus cerastes

Description and Identification: Presence of a horn-like scale above the eye identifies this rattlesnake.

Cream, tan, gray, light brown or pinkish with rows of darker spots; tail ringed.

Average length 18 to 25 inches; maximum about 30 inches; females slightly larger than males.

Distribution, Habitat, and Biology: Deserts of southeastern California and southern Nevada southward through western Arizona into adjacent Sonora and Baja Norte, Mexico. Most common in sandy flats and dunes with sparse vegetation; sometimes on arid, rocky hillsides.

Sidewinders often rest during the day with part of their body buried under sand and they are usually active at night. The sidewinding type of motion, difficult to describe but unmistakable when seen, is characteristic of this snake and some heavy-bodied sand vipers of Africa and Asia. It is used occasionally by some other desert snakes including a few other species or rattlesnakes. The name sidewinder is also applied incorrectly to other kinds or small rattlesnakes in the southwestern United States.

The disposition of the sidewinder is about the same as that of the western rattlesnake group. Bites, formerly quite unusual, have become more frequent with the growing use of desert areas for residential and recreational purposes.

Three subspecies of this snake are currently recognized and all three are very similar in appearance. Each occupies a different desert region and the common name indicates the specific desert where they are found, the Mohave Desert, the Sonoran Desert, and the Colorado Desert.

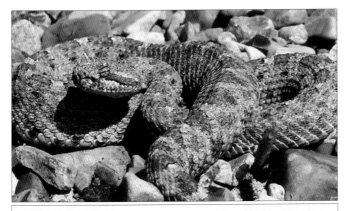

PHOTO 36. Colorado Sidewinder, *Crotalus cerastes laterorepens*

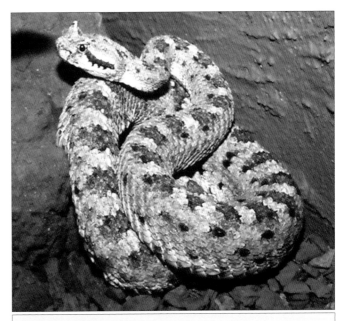

PHOTO 37. Mojave Sidewinder Rattlesnake, *Crotalus cerastes cerastes*

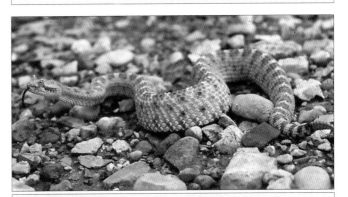

PHOTO 38. Sonoran Sidewinder Rattlesnake, *Crotalus cerastes cercobombas*

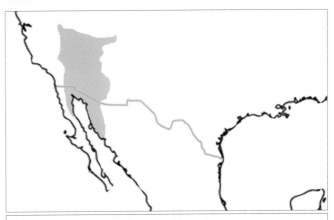

MAP 35. Range of the Sidewinder Rattlesnake, *Crotalus cerastes.*

Venom and Bite: These small snakes have a limited amount of relatively weak venom and this is probably not a deadly species.

Mexican West Coast Rattlesnake,
Crotalus basiliscus

Description and Identification: The only rattlesnake within its range with diamond shaped dorsal markings. Body moderately stout and rather triangular in cross section. Adults average 4 to 5 feet. Maximum length of wild specimens is just under seven feet, but some captive reared individuals have exceeded the 7 foot mark (personal observation, Scott Shupe).

Head uniform grayish brown or olive green except for dark post orbital bar and lighter labials; no distinct markings on crown or neck. Body brown or grayish olive with 26-41 dark, light edged, rhomboid shape (diamond) blotches. Tail gray, darker-banded or almost unicolor without distinct markings. White or cream colored below.

Dorsals strongly keeled, in 25-29 rows at midbody, fewer posteriorly. Ventrals 174-206; subcaudals 18-36.

Distribution, Habitat, and Biology: The coastal plain and mountain slopes of western Mexico from southern Sonora to central Oaxaca. Mainly an inhabitant of thorn forest, but ranges upward into tropical rain forest in the south.

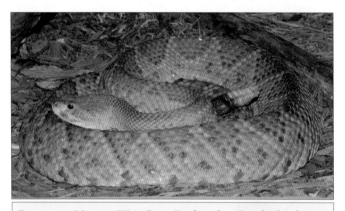

Photo 39. Mexican West Coast Rattlesnake, *Crotalus basiliscus*

Venom and Bite: This snake is equal in size to both the Eastern and Western Diamondbacks and like those two species it is a highly dangerous snake capable of injecting large doses of virulent venom deep into tissues. "Antivipmym" and "Tri-Antivipmyn" antivenoms by Bioclon of Mexico are listed as being effective in treating bites by this species. The venom is known to contain a mixture of procoagulants and haemorragins. Mytoxins are probably present along with secondary neprotoxic and necrotoxic activity. The venom yield of up to 350 mg. (dry weight) is second only to the Eastern Diamondback (Minton 1974).

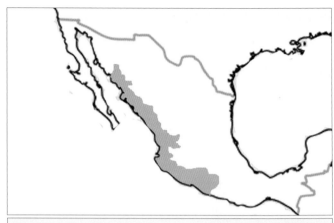

MAP 36. Range of the Mexican West Coast Rattlesnake, *Crotalus basiliscus.*

Similar Species: There are three other very similar rattlesnake species native to southern Mexico. *C. culminatus,* the Northwestern Neotropical Rattlesnake, *C. tzabcan,* the Yucatan Neotropical Rattlesnake, and *C. totonacus,* the Totonacan Rattlesnake. Range map 37 below shows the geographic distribution of these other three similar species.

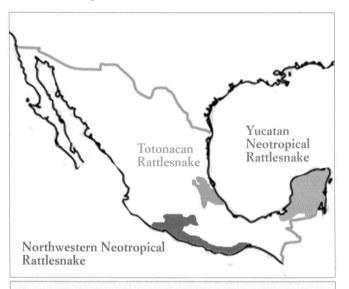

MAP 37. Range of the Totonacan Rattlesnake, *Crotalus totonacus,* the Yucatan Neotropical Rattlesnake, *Crotalus tzabcan,* and the Northwestern Neotropical Rattlesnake, *Crotalus culminatus.*

Middle American Rattlesnake,
Crotalus simus

Much of this species range is in the USSOUTHCOM region, although it does range into the USNORTH-COM region in southernmost Mexico and the Yucatan Peninsula. For information on this species see chapter 9, USSOUTHCOM region, page 117.

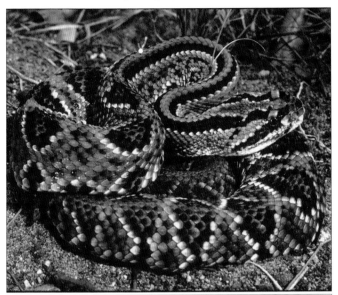

Photo 40. Middle American Rattlesnake, *Crotalus simus*

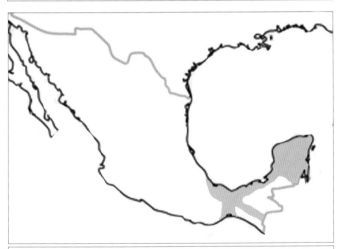

Map 38. Range of the Middle American Rattlesnake, *Crotalus simus* in the USNORTHCOM region.

Tiger Rattlesnake,
Crotalus tigris

Description and Identification: Highly variable in color, gray, blueish, or reddish to pink, being the most common color schemes. This snake has proportionately the smallest head of any rattlesnake, despite having a rather stout body. This rattlesnake has a distinctly banded pattern which, along with its exceptionally small head makes identification rather easy.

Distribution, Habitat, and Biology: Found from south central Arizona southward throughout most of Sonora, Mexico. The small head is an adaptation for pulling lizard prey out of rock crevices. Also eats mice. Maximum length about 3 feet.

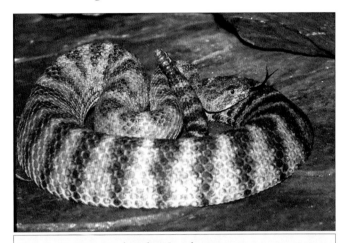

Photo 41. Tiger Rattlesnake, *Crotalus tigris*

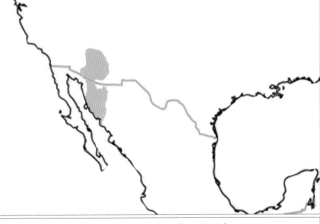

Map 39. Range of the Tiger Rattlesnake, *Crotalus tigris.*

Venom and Bite: Due to its small head, the Tiger Rattlesnake has a limited amount of venom. However, its venom is known to be highly toxic (containing pre-synaptic neurotoxins) and any bite by this species should be treated as life threatening.

Black-tailed Rattlesnake,
Crotalus molossus

Description and Identification: Ground color yellow gold, greenish gray, olive, or dingy brown. Specimens living in areas of lava flows may be solid black. The top of the head from the eyes forward is black, and the tail is solid black. Maximum length is just over four feet but most adults are around 3 feet.

Distribution, Habitat, and Biology: This wide-ranging snake is found from northern Arizona and New Mexico eastward to central Texas and southward throughout most of Mexico. Lives both in high mountains and low deserts.

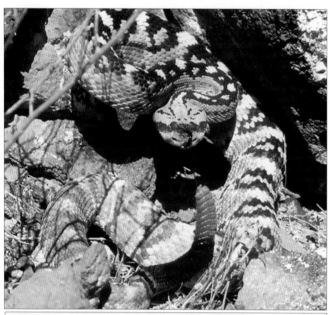

Photo 42. Black-tailed Rattlesnake, *Crotalus molossus*

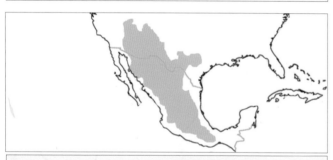

Map 40. Range of the Black-tailed Rattlesnake, *Crotalus molossus.*

Venom and Bite: Venom toxicity reportedly about the same as the Western Diamondback, thus a dangerous snake capable of killing a human. Haemorragins are known to be present in the venom. Procoagulants possibly present.

Mexican Lance-headed Rattlesnake,
Crotalus polystictus

Description and Identification: This distinctive rattlesnake can often be identified by the shape of the head alone. In this species the head is long and slender, an exceptional condition among rattlesnakes.

The pattern is also rather disinctive, consisting of a double row of oval blotches along the center of the back, with numerous more or less rounded blotches along the sides of the body. The ground color is usually light brown or tan, and the blotches are dark brown and narrowly edged in black. Average length 2-3 feet. Maximum 3.5 feet.

Distribution, Habitat, and Biology: This snake is restricted to central Mexico, where it lives in the highlands of the Mexican Plateau.

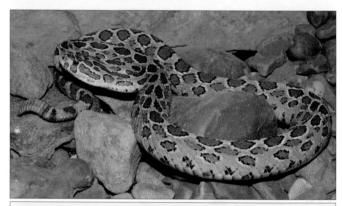

Photo 43. Mexican Lance-headed Rattlesnake, *Crotalus polystictus*

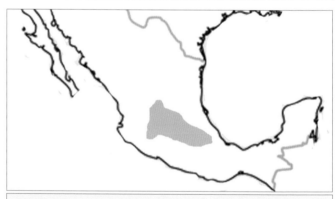

Map 41. Range of the Mexican Lance-headed Rattlesnake, *Crotalus polystictus.*

Venom and Bite: Unknown. The exceptionally long head of this rattlesnake accommodates long fangs and large venom glands. It should be considered a dangerous animal.

Baja California Rattlesnake,
Crotalus enyo

Description and Identification: Head narrow, eyes large. Dorsal scales 25-27, keeled. Anal scute undivided. Ground color brownish. Dorsal pattern of reddish or yellowish brown blotches that become more or less crossbanded posteriorly. Maximum recorded length 3 feet.

Distribution, Habitat, and Biology: Range restricted to the Baja Peninsula, encompassing the southern half of Baja Norte and all of Baja Sur.

"Frequents arid thornscrub, mainly in rocky canyons and mesas. Eats small rodents, lizards, and centipeds" (Stebbins 2003). Also found in desert, chaparral, tropical deciduous forest, and pine-oak forest (Campbell and Lamar 2004).

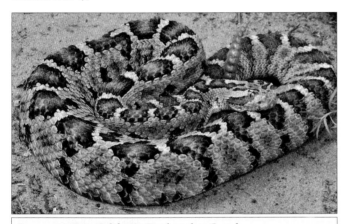

Photo 44. Baja California Rattlesnake, *Crotalus enyo*

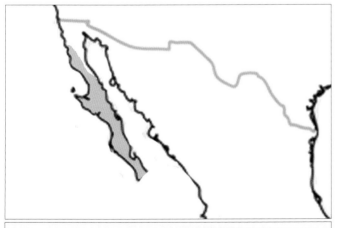

Map 42. Range of the Baja California Rattlesnake, *Crotalus enyo.*

Venom and Bite: Unknown. Should be considered potentially deadly.

Rock Rattlesnake,
Crotalus lepidus

Description and Identification: Averages about 2 feet with a record length of 33 inches. This species varies in color to match the color of the rocks where it lives. There are a total of four subspecies, and there is great variation even among the races. Many specimens present a pattern of distinct dark bars across the back contrasting sharply with a lighter background. In others the dark bars are faded but still distinct, and there is a profusion of dark stippling between the bars, with the stippling matching the colors of the dark bars. The ground color between the bars and/or stippling may be gray, greenish, purplish, or pinkish.

Distribution, Habitat, and Biology: The Rock Rattlesnake is usually found in association with rocky places such as canyons or talus slopes. They can also be found sometimes in lower desert areas, but they are more common on mountain slopes and canyons. They feed mostly on lizards, which is the most common vertebrate prey in the arid, rocky habitats where this species is found.

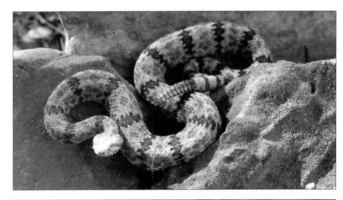

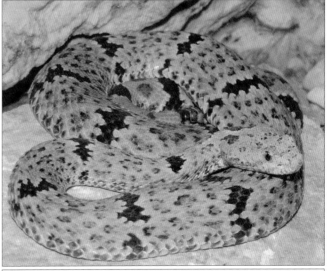

Photos 45 & 46. Rock Rattlesnakes, *Crotalus lepidus.*

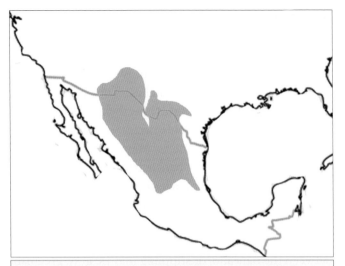

MAP 43. Range of the Rock Rattlesnake, *Crotalus lepidus.*

Mexican Pygmy Rattlesnake,
Crotalus ravus

Description and Identification: A small brownish rattlesnake with 9 plates on the crown. This is the only member of the Crotalus genus that exhibits this pattern of head scalation. Body moderately stout; head oval. Adults average about 20 inches in length; a large individual is 24 inches.

Ground color brown or gray with 25-35 small irregular blotches down the back, small lateral spots may fuse with the dorsal row to form irregular crossbands; 6-8 dark bands on tail. Head unicolor brown or with an arrow shaped median dark marking. Ventral surface yellowish, blotched with brown.

Dorsals moderately keeled, in 21-23 rows at midbody, fewer posteriorly. Ventrals 138-152; subcaudals 20-30.

In spite of the common name this species is not a true Pygmy Rattlesnake. That distinction belongs to the members of the genus *Sistrurus.*

Venom and Bite: These are small snakes with a low venom yield. Although no deaths have been recorded their venom is more toxic than that of many large rattlesnakes. Potential for a lethal bite cannot be excluded.

Similar Species: There are a number of other small, montane rattlesnake species that occur in isolated pockets on the Mexican Plateau. *C. aquilus,* the Queretaro Dusky Rattlesnake and *C. triseriatus,* the Mexican Dusky Rattlesnake are found in south central Mexico and both have significant ranges (see map below). *C. pusillus,* the Tancitaran Dusky Rattlesnake has a much more restricted range. Both *C. transversus,* the Cross Banded Mountain Rattlesnake and *C. stegnegeri,* the Sonaloan Long-tailed Rattlesnake are also quite rare and the latter is known from only about a dozen specimens.

Distribution, Habitat, and Biology: Found in the southern portion of the Mexican Plateau. Lives in a variety of forested habitats from medium to high elevations.

This snake was once considered to be a member of the *Sistrurus* genus because of the scales it has on the top of its head (nine plates instead of numerous small scales typical of most *Crotalus).*

Venom and Bite: This small species is not considered deadly to man.

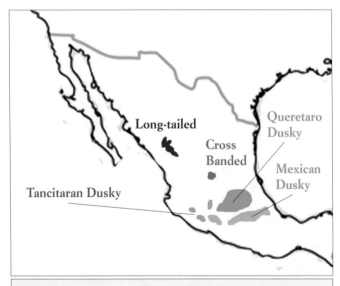

MAP 44. Range for miscellaneous Mexican mountain rattlesnakes.

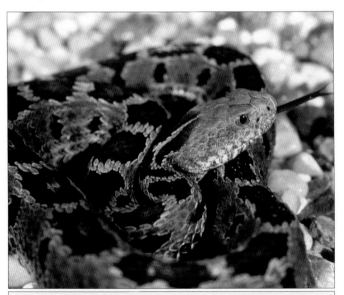

PHOTO 47. Mexican Pygmy Rattlesnake, *Crotalus ravus*

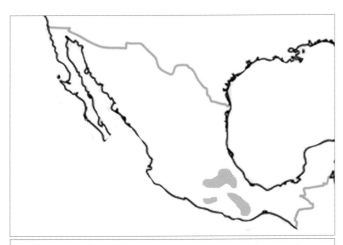

Map 45. Range of the Mexican Pygmy Rattlesnake, *Crotalus ravus*.

Twin-spotted Rattlesnake,
Crotalus pricei

Description and Identification: A small, grayish snake with a double row of dark gray to black vertebral blotches. Rarely exceeds 2 feet in length.

Distribution, Habitat, and Biology: Occurs in the United States only in a few mountain ranges in southeastern Arizona. More widespread in Mexico where it ranges through the Sierra Madre Occidental south to southwest Zacatecas, northern Jalisco and eastern Nayarit. A subspecies also occurs in the Sierra Madre Oriental in parts of San Luis Potosi, Tamaulipas, and Neuvo Leon.

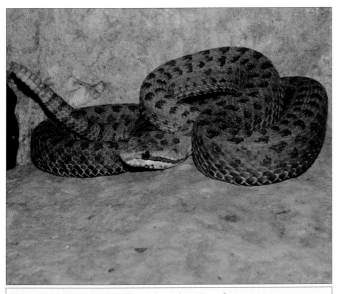

Photo 48. Twin-spotted Rattlesnake, *Crotalus pricei*

Venom and Bite: This is a small snake with correspondingly small fangs and small venom glands. Its habitat on the highest mountain slopes in remote areas means that it possess little threat to humans. However its venom is quite toxic and bites by this snake should be treated with caution.

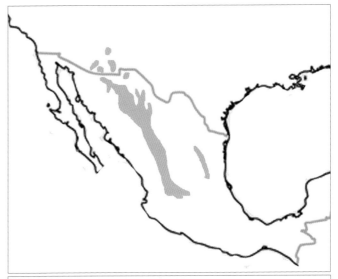

Map 46. Range of the Twin-spotted Rattlesnake, *Crotalus pricei.*

Similar Species: *Crotalus intermedius,* the Mexican Small-headed Rattlesnake is found in three disjunct localities in the southern highlands of Mexico. It is similar in many respects to the more northerly occuring Twin-spotted Rattlesnake.

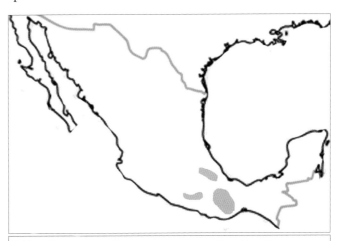

Map 47. Range of the Mexican Small-headed Rattlesnake, *Crotalus intermedius.*

Additonal Species: In addition to the previously described mainland species of the genus *Crotalus*, there are two other species endemic to offshore islands. *Crotalus catalinensis,* the Santa Catalina Rattlesnake found on Santa Catalina Island and *Crotalus tortugensis* Tortuga Island Rattlesnake on the island of Tortuga. Both these islands are in the Sea of Cortez (Mexico).

A unique feature of the Santa Catalina Rattlesnake is the absence of a fully developed rattle. Note the lack of a rattle on the specimen shown below.

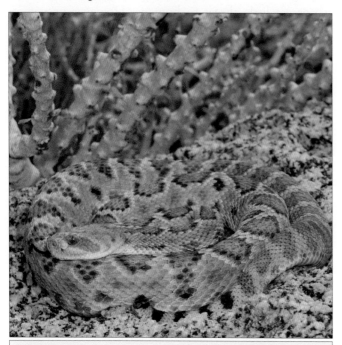

PHOTO 49. Santa Catalina Rattlesnake, *Crotalus catalinensis*

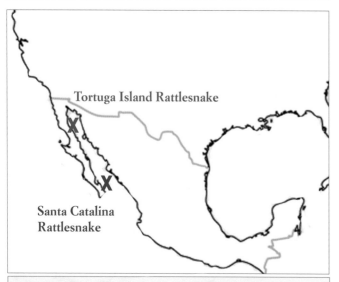

Tortuga Island Rattlesnake

Santa Catalina Rattlesnake

MAP 48. Range of the Santa Catalina Rattlesnake and the Tortugua Island Rattlesnake, *Crotalus catalinensis* and *Crotalus tortugensis*.

Family - Viperidae

Subfamily - Crotalinae - Pit Vipers

Genus - Sistrurus

Pygmy Rattlesnakes

Two species are recognized; formerly there were three but the Mexican Pygmy Rattlesnake has now been assigned to the genus *Crotalus*. Both species are found in the United States and one is found in disjunct, isolated populations in northern Mexico. Neither species is considered especially dnagerous, although S. catenatus is reported to sometimes cause deaths, especially in children.

Definition: Head broad, very distinct from narrow neck; canthus obtuse to acute. Body cylindrical, tapered, slender to moderately stout; tail short, terminating in a relatively small horny, segmented rattle.

Eyes small to moderate in size; pupils vertically elliptical.

Head scales: The 9 typical scales on the crown similar to that seen in *Agkistrodon*. Laterally, nasal in contact with upper preocular or separated from it by loreal scale; eye separated from supralabials by 1-3 rows of small scales.

Body scales: Dorsals strongly keeled, with apical pits, in 19-27 oblique rows at midbody, fewer anteriorly and posteriorly. Ventrals 122-160; subcaudals 19-39; all entire or a few posterior ones paired.

Massassauga Rattlesnake,
Sistrurus catenatus

Description and Identification: The large shields of the crown distinguish this species from all other United States rattlesnakes except the Pygmy Rattlesnake (S. miliarius). It is best differentiated from that species by the shorter tail and well developed rattle. Ranges of the two overlap only in small areas of Texas and Oklahoma.

Ground color gray, tan, buff, or yellowish with rows of dark gray, brown, or black spots often with narrow light edges; belly marbled with dark gray, black and white; tail barred. Specimens form the northeastern part of the range sometimes are uniformly black when adult.

Average length 18-29 inches; maximum 40 inches; males larger than females.

Distribution, Habitat, and Biology: This snake once ranged in a broad band from the Great Lakes region southwestward to extreme southeastern Arizona and southern Texas; also being found in two isolated, disjunct populations in northern Mexico. With changes wrought by man on its prairie habitat the species has disappeared from many areas formerly inhabited, and its range is now disrupted in much of the midwest. Inhabits bogs and marshes in the northeast, prairie in the west and southwest.

These are secretive snakes that usually remain quiet or seek to escape when encountered but they will bite readily when provoked.

There are three subspecies recognized, the largest is the Eastern Massassauga of the Great Lakes region. The eastern race lives in marshes and woodland edges bordering meadows, and is usually quite dark in color. The Desert Massassauga is slimmer and much smaller and found in desert grasslands. In between is the Western Massassauga which inhabits grassland and marshland.

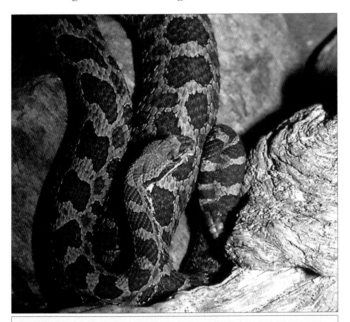

Photo 50. Eastern Massassauga, *Sistrurus catenatus catenatus*

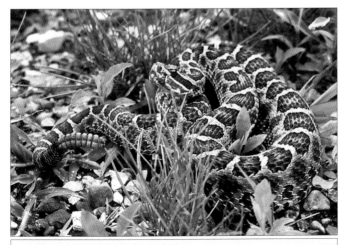

Photo 51. Western Massassauga, *Sistrurus catenatus tergiminus*

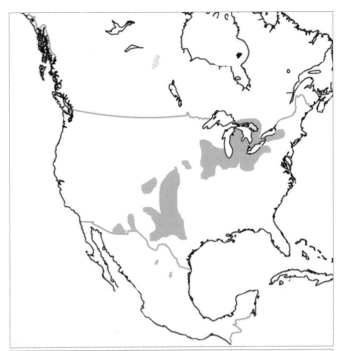

Map 49. Range of the Massassauga Rattlesnake, *Sistrurus catenatus.*

Venom and Bite: Although this is a small rattlesnake with limited amounts of venom, the venom is highly toxic for experimental animals, and there have been cases of fatal bites in man. Antivenom is not typically used in treating bites by this species, however, in the case of a serious envenomation or bites to children, antivenin may be warranted. "Antivipmyn" antivenom by Institudo Bioclone in Mexico is listed by the World Health Organization as effective in treating bites by this species. Known toxins include procoagulants and haemorragins.

Pygmy Rattlesnake,
Sistrurus miliarius

Description and Identification: This species and the Massassauga (S. catenatus) are the only United States rattlesnakes with the crown covered by large shields. In this species the tail is relatively long and slender, terminating in a tiny rattle that may be difficult to see under field conditions.

Ground color light gray, tan, reddish-orange, or dark gray often with an orange or rusty midline stripe; 5 rows of sooty spots or short dark crossbars; belly white heavily clouded and spotted with black; tail barred.

Average length 15-22 inches, maximum 32.5 inches.

Distribution, Habitat, and Biology: The southern lowlands and piedmont of the southeastern United

States from North Carolina to east Texas and north to southern Missouri and western Kentucky. Frequents pine woods and grassy marshes in the southern part of the range; rocky, wooded hills in the northwestern portions of its range. Strangely absent from most of the Mississippi Alluvial Plain.

The rattle of these snakes is audible only at very close range. They are rather alert and bad tempered.

Venom and Bite: The bite can be followed by severe pain and extensive swelling even when the snake is a small one only 6 to 9 inches long. Their venom is more toxic than that of many of the larger rattlesnake species, but their small size precludes injecting a fatal dose. No fatalities have been documented but small children or debilitated persons could present life threatening issues from a bite.

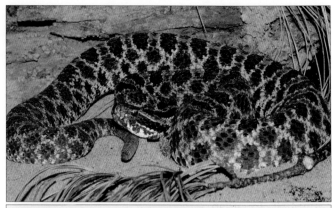

PHOTOS 52. Dusky Pygmy Rattlesnake, *Sistrurus miliarius miliarius*

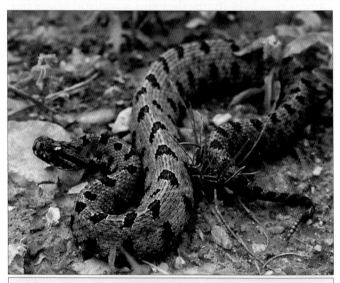

PHOTOS 53. Western Pygmy Rattlesnake, *Sistrurus miliarius streckeri*

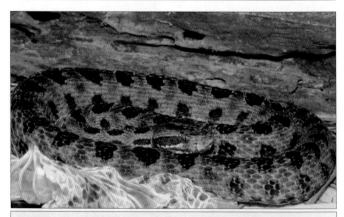

PHOTOS 54. Carolina Pygmy Rattlesnake, *Sistrurus miliarius miliarius*

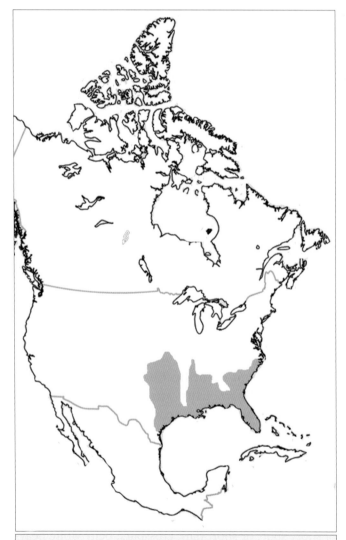

MAP 50. Range of the Pygmy Rattlesnake, *Sistrurus miliarius.*

Current References

Books

Bartlett, Richard D. and Allen Tenant. 2000. *Snakes of North America,* 2 Vols. Gulf Publishing Co. Houston, TX.

Brown, Phillip R. 1997. *A Field Guide to the Snakes of California.* Gulf Publishing Co. Houston, TX.

Campbell, Jonathan A. and William W. Lamar. 2004. *Venomous Reptiles of the Western Hemisphere* 2 Vols. Cornell University Press. Ithaca, NY.

Conant, Roger & Joseph T. Collins. 1998. *Reptiles and Amphibians of Eastern/Central North America.* Houghton Mifflin Co. New York, NY.

Dowling, Herndon G., Sherman A. Minton, and Findlay E. Russell. 1965. *Poisonous Snakes of the World.* Department of the Navy Bureau of Medicine and Surgery. Washington, DC.

Lee, Julien C. 1996. *The Amphibians and Reptiles of the Yucatan Peninsula.* Cornell University Press. Ithaca, NY.

Lowe, Charles H., Cecil R Schwalbe and Terry B Johnson. 1989. *The Venomous Reptiles of Arizona.* Arizona Game and Fish Department. Phoenix, AZ.

Palmer, William M. & Alvin L. Braswell. 1995. *Reptiles of North Carolina.* University of North Carolina Press. Chapel Hill, NC.

Roze, Janis A. 1996. *Coral Snakes of the Americas. Biology, Identification, and Venoms.* Krieger Publishing. Malabar, FL.

Rubio, Manny. 1998. *Rattlesnake, Portrait of a Predator.* Smithsonian Instituion Press. Washington, D.C.

Stebbins, Robert C. 2003. *Western Reptiles and Amphibians.* Houghton Mifflin Co. New York, NY.

Journals

Gold, Barry S., Robert A. Barish, & Richard C. Dart. 2004. "North American snake envenomation: diagnosis, treatment, and management." *Emergency Medical Clinics of North America*, Vol. 22, page 423-443.

Gomez H.F., and Dart, R.C. (1995). Clinical Toxicology of Snakebites in North America. In: Handbook of Clinical Toxicology of Animal Venoms and Poisons. Meier J and White J (Eds). CRC Press, Boca Raton, FL, pp 1-8.

Internet References

Clinical Toxinology Resources website - www.toxinology.com -The University of Adelaide

The Reptile Database - http//www.reptile-database.org-

Living Hazards Database - AFPMB - www.afpmb.org/content/living-hazards-database

Crofab website - www.crofab.com

Instituto Bioclone - www.bioclone.com

Original References

CONANT, Roger 1958. A Field Guide to Reptiles and Amphibians of the United States and Canada East of the 100th Meridian. Houghton Mifflin: Boston, xiii + 336 pp., pls. 1–40 (some color), figs. 1–62, Maps 1–248.

FITCH, Henry S. 1960. Autecology of the Copperhead. Univ. Kansas Publ. Mus. Nat. Hist., vol. 13, pp. 85–288, pls. 13–20. figs. 1–26, tables 1–26.

KLAUBER, LAURENCE M. 1956. Rattlesnakes: Their Habits, Life Histories, and Influence on Mankind. Univ. of California Press: Berkeley and Los Angeles. Vol. I, xxix + 1–708 pp., figs., tables, maps, frontis. (color). Vol. II, xvii + 709–1476 pp., figs., tables, frontis., (color).

STEBBINS, Robert C. 1954. Amphibians and Reptiles of Western North America. McGraw-Hill: New York, xxii + 1–528 pp., pls. 1–104.

WRIGHT, Albert H. and Anna A. WRIGHT 1957. Handbook of Snakes of the United States and Canada. Comstock: Ithaca, N.Y., 2 vols., 1105 pp., 305 figs., 70 maps.

PICADO, C. 1931. Serpientes venenosas de Costa Rica. Imprenta Alsina, San Jose, Costa Rica: 219 p., 58 figs.

SCHMIDT, Karl P. 1933. Preliminary Account of the Coral Snakes of Central America and Mexico. Zool. Ser. Field Mus. Nat. Hist., 20: 29–40.

SCHMIDT, Karl P. 1936. Notes on Central American and Mexican Coral Snakes. Zool. Ser. Field Mus. Nat. Hist., 20 (20): 205–216, figs. 24–27.

SCHMIDT, Karl P. 1941. The Amphibians and Reptiles of British Honduras. Zool. Ser. Field Mus. Nat. Hist., vol. 22, no. 8, pp. 475–510.

ALVAREZ del TORO, Miguel 1960. Los reptiles de Chiapas. Inst. Zool. Estado, Tuxtla Gutierrez, Chiapas, Mexico. 7–204 p., illustrated.

BURGER, W. Leslie 1950 A Preliminary Study of the Jumping Viper, *Bothrops nummifer*. Bull. Chicago Acad. Sci., 9 (3): 59–67, 1 pl.

CLARK, Herbert C. 1942 Venomous Snakes. Some Central American Records. Incidence of Snake-bite Accidents. Amer. Jour. Tropical Med., 22 (1): 37–49.

MERTENS, Robert. 1952. Die Amphibien und Reptilien von El Salvador, auf Grund der Reisen von R. Mertens und A. Zilch. Abh. Senckenbergischen Ges., 487: 1–120, 16 pls.

SCHMIDT, Karl P. 1955. Coral Snakes of the Genus *Micrurus* in Colombia. Fieldiana-Zool., 34 (34): 337–359, figs. 65–69.

SMITH, Hobart M., and E. H. TAYLOR. 1945. An Annotated Checklist and Key to the Snakes of Mexico. Bull. U. S. Natl. Mus. (187): 1–239 p.

STUART, L. C. 1963. A Checklist of the Herpetofauna of Guatemala. Misc. Pub. Mus. Zool. Univ. Michigan (122): 1–150, 1 pl., 1 map.

TAYLOR, Edward H. 1951. A Brief Review of the Snakes of Costa Rica. Univ. Kansas Sci. Bull., 34 (part 1, no. 1): 3–88, figs. 1–7, pls. 1–23.

CHAPTER **9**

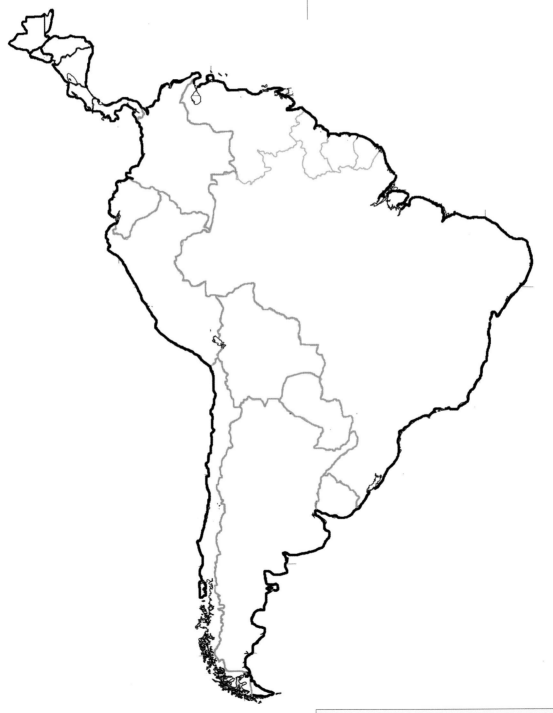

MAP 51. Definition of Region 2: United States Southern Command, Central America and the South American Continent.

Introduction

Most of the venomous snakes of the USSOUTHCOM region are tropical animals, and the tropics boasts a wide variety of species. In fact, the tropical regions of the Americas contains one of the richest snake faunas on earth. A total of 130 venomous snake species are found in this region, and many are quite dangerous. The popular view of the tropical jungles teeming with deadly serpents, however, is erroneous. In fact, finding these secretive animals in this habitat is often surprisingly difficult, and more snakes are likely to be encountered in parts of temperate North America than in much of this region.

The family Elapidae is represented here by two genus of coral snakes (*Micrurus* and *Leptomicrurus*). The unusual genus *Leptomicrurus* contains only 4 species, while *Micrurus* is well represented by at least 58 species. Generally coral snakes do not pose a significant threat because they are secretive and inoffensive animals. Most people bitten by coral snakes are handling the snake when bitten. These are pretty snakes that lack the broad head and vertically elliptical pupils characteristic of pit vipers. These features sometimes causes people to mistake a coral snake for a nonvenomous species.

The other venomous snakes are all pit vipers (family Viperidae, subfamily Crotalinae) and are easily recognized by the loreal pit, the broad head, eyes with vertical pupils, and the rough-scaled body.

There are but two species of rattlesnake in this region, the Middle American Rattlesnake (*Crotalus simus*) and the South American Rattlesnake or Cascabel (*Crotalus durrissus*). The latter is highly variable and widespread throughout much of South America. As with many species that have extensive ranges and numerous subspecies, the Cascabel varies not only in color and pattern but in venom toxicity as well, and some are among the most dangerous of all the rattlesnakes.

The most common, diverse, and wide-ranging venomous snakes in this region are the Lance-headed Vipers of the genus *Bothrops*. There are a total of 23 species listed by the Reptile Database. Some experts argue convincingly that the number should actually be a total of 42 species; arriving at that number by including in *Bothrops* the genera *Bothriopsis*, *Bothropoides* and *Rhinocerophis*. Several of the larger varieties of the Lancehead Vipers, such as the Terciopelo (*Bothrops asper)* and the Fer-de-lance (*Bothrops atrox*) are quite deadly.

In addition to the Lance-headed Vipers there are several other similar but less diverse genera of pit vipers found in the USSOUTHCOM region. When the original edition of *Poisonous Snakes of the World* was published back in 1965, nearly all were once considered to be members of the *Bothrops* group.

Ironically, more recently it has been suggested that several of these genera should be returned to their original designation within the *Bothrops* genus. Here the author has elected to follow the taxonomy of The Reptile Database (www.reptile-database-viewed 2012).

The Forest Pit Vipers, genus *Bothriopsis*, with 6 species; the *Rhinocerophis* genus with 6 species; and the *Bothropoides* genus (10 species) all were originally included in the *Bothrops* genus back in 1965, along with the Toad-headed Pit Vipers, genus *Bothrocophias*; 6 species,; the Hognosed Pit Vipers, genus *Porthidium,* 6 species; and *Atripoides,* the Jumping Vipers with 5 total species (of which 4 occur in the USSOUTHCOM region).

In addition to these pitvipers there are also the Palm Pit Vipers, genus *Bothriechis,* numbering 9 species (8 in this region). These are a group of small to medium sized, arboreal, *prehensile* tailed snakes that although less dangerous than most of the regions pit vipers, have been known to kill.

Perhaps the most legendary serpents in this region are the Bushmasters (genus *Lachesis*). Represented by four species, the Bushmasters are the largest venomous snakes in the western hemisphere (up to 11 feet). Despite the fact that their venom is less toxic than many other snakes in the region, their huge size makes them a highly dangerous snake. *Cerrophidian,* the Mountain Pit Vipers and *Agkistrodon*, the Moccasins, both with a single species in the region, round out the remainder of the pit vipers found in this region.

Maps 51 and 52 show the area covered by this chapter.

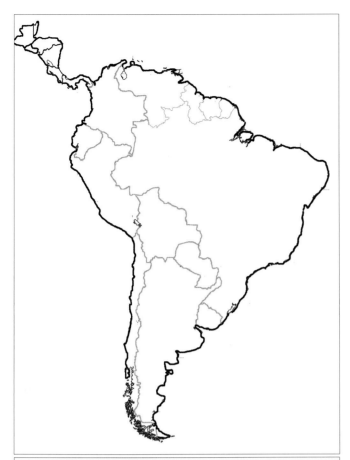

MAP 52. Region 2. United States Southern Command. Central and South America.

Generic And Species Descriptions

Family - Elapidae: Genus - Leptomicrurus.

Slender Coral Snakes

As with the more common and widespread American Coral Snakes (*Micrurus*), the Slender Coral Snakes are found only in the western hemisphere. There are only four species in this genus and all are found in tropical South America.

Unlike most members of the *Micrurus* genus which typically exhibit a classic coral snake pattern of tri-colored rings, the Slender Coral Snakes are mostly uniformly dark above. However, one species does exhibit the classic ringed pattern of the American Coral Snakes. All *Leptomicrurus* do have a *light colored ring encircling the head or neck*. There seems to be little information about the venom of these coral snakes, but any uniformly dark serpent with a yellow, whitish, or reddish ring around the head or neck may be a member of this genus and should thus be avoided.

Definition: Head small, not distinct from neck and about the same width as body, snout rounded no distinct canthus.

Eyes small; pupils round.

Head scales: The usual 9 on the crown, laterally nasal in contact with single preocular; mental scale in contact with chinshields.

Body scales: Dorsals smooth, in 15 nonoblique rows throughout body. Ventrals 212-382; anal plate divided; subcaudals paired 12-35. Body elongate and slender, tail short. Dorsal pattern uniformly dark with light ring around head or neck.

Maxillary teeth: Two relatively large tubular fangs; no other teeth on bone.

These snakes differ from Micrurus and Micruroides in that the yellow crossbands are incomplete dorsally; they are best defined on the ventral surface and appear as triangles on the sides. The contact of mental and anterior chin shields is also distinctive.

Some experts regard the Slender Coral Snake genus *Leptomicrurus* as being synonymous with the typical Coral Snakes (*Micrurus*). Here the author has maintained the status accorded these snakes by Campbell and Lamar in their epic work *The Venomous Snakes of the Western Hemisphere* published in 2004.

Andean Slender Coral Snake,

Leptomicrurus narduccii

Description and Identification: Formerly known as the Amazon Slender Coral Snake. A very elongate black coral snake with a broad yellow band on the back of the head. Adults average 24 to 30 inches. Occasional individuals exceed 3.5 feet. Belly pattern of red (or yellow/orange) and black crossbands, some of the red bands extending onto the sides as triangular blotches. Dorsal part of body solid black.

Ventrals 240-410. Subcaudals 17-35.

Distribution, Habitat, and Biology: The upper Amazon region, including northwestern Brazil, eastern Ecuador, Peru, and Bolivia. Inhabits lower slopes of the Andes Mountains within the Amazon drainage, as well as lowland rainforest.

Venom and Bite: Apparently, no bites by this species have been recorded. However, they attain a large enough size that they should be considered a dangerous animal.

Similar species: There are three other species of Slender Coral Snakes found in tropical South America. The Guyanan, Ringed, and Pygmy Slender Coral Snake. Map 54 shows the ranges of these other three species.

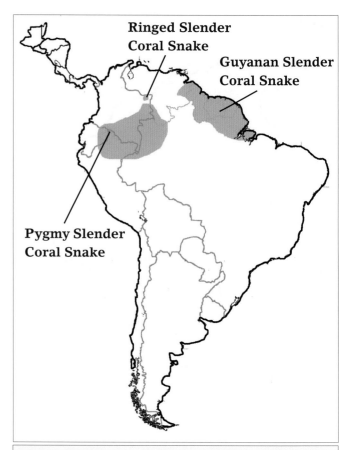

MAP 54. Range of various Slender Coral Snakes, *L. collaris* (Guyanan), *L. scutiventris* (Pygmy), and *L. renjifoi* (Ringed).

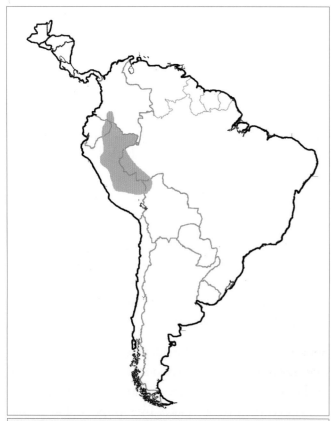

MAP 53. Range of the Andean Slender Coral Snake, *Leptomicrurus narduccii*.

Family - Elapidae: Genus - Micrurus

American Coral Snakes

When the book *Poisonous Snakes of the World* was published in 1965 there were about 40 species of *Micrurus* known to science. Today, that number has nearly doubled (some sources list up to 78 species) and new species are still being discovered. Some species boast several subspecies and many exhibit significant variation both geographically and within specific populations. To further complicate identification, there are numerous nonvenomous snake species that mimic the coral snakes in color and pattern. To say that this genus presents an identification problem for the lay individual is an understatement, but from a practical standpoint of snakebite treatment, the main concern is identifying an offending snake as a member of the *Micrurus* genus. This task is best accomplished by noting the *absence of a loreal scale and the 15 rows of smooth scales at midbody.*

This genus is contained entirely in the Western Hemisphere and most species occur in Central and South America. *Micrurus* is found from the Coastal Plain of the southeastern United States through much of Mexico, southward all the way to central Argentina in South America.

Definition: Head small, not distinct from neck; snout rounded, no distinct canthus. Body elongate , slender, not tapered; tail short.

Eyes small; pupils round.

Head scales: The usual 9 on the crown. Laterally, nasal scale in contact with single preocular (no loreal scale). Ventrally, mental scale separated from anterior chin shields by first infralabials.

Body scales: Dorsals smooth in 15 rows throughout body. Ventral scales 177-412, anal plate divided or entire; subcaudals 16-62, usually paired but more than 50 percent single in some species.

Maxillary teeth: Two relatively large tubular fangs with indistinct grooves; no other teeth on bone.

Remarks: Most coral snakes have color patterns made up of complete rings of yellow (or white), black, and red. In some species however, the typical triad pattern is replaced by black and red rings, black and white rings, black and orange, or black and yellow. Still others can have the red or black rings greatly expanded with only a few rings at either the head, the tail, or both; producing a nearly all red or all black snake. When threatened many species elevate the curled tip of the tail, presumably to fool a predator into thinking the snake's tail is the head. Coral snakes are inoffensive animals that do not coil and strike in the manner of the vipers or cobras. Bites from coral snakes invariably occur from the victim handling the snake, stepping on it barefoot, or carelessly placing a bare hand onto the snake's body. However, their venom is highly toxic and all species should be considered potentially deadly. There are a number of antivenoms produced for coral snakes in this region, including Coralmyn (by Institudo Bioclone in Mexico), Soro Antielapidico (by Instituto Butantan in Brazil), and Suero Antiofidico Anti-coral (made in Costa Rica).

Although many coral snake bites will not result in envenomation, some experts have recommended that any patient known to have been bitten by an American coral snake (*Micrurus*) be treated with antivenom without waiting for the development of symptoms (Gold et al. 2004). A lethal envenomation may not produce significant symptoms for up to 12 hours. A particulary complicated issue in the management of bites by *Micrurus*

species is the fact that once symptoms have appeared it may very difficult to reverse those symptoms, even with antivenom. Thus, persons bitten by coral snakes must always seek immediate medical attention and administration of antivenin is advised even in asymptomatic patients. With one exception (*M. corallinus*), the venom of all *Micrurus* species contains post-snyaptic neurotoxins. Systemic myotoxins are also usually present.

Pygmy Coral Snake,
Micrurus dissoleucus

Description and Identification: Averaging only 12 to 16 inches (record 26 inches), this is the smallest member of the *Micrurus* genus. The snout is black and with a white band just behind the eyes followed by another black band. The color sequence beginning just behind the head is red-black-white-black-white-black-red. This sequence of bands continues down the body. Ventrals 171-208; subcaudals 17-28.

Distribution, Habitat, and Biology: Found in dry habitats from southern Panama across northern Colombia and Venezuela.

Venom and Bite: The danger posed by this species to man is unknown, but they are a common animal within their range and thus a potential threat for snakebite. Due to their small size they may be less dangerous than most *Micrurus*.

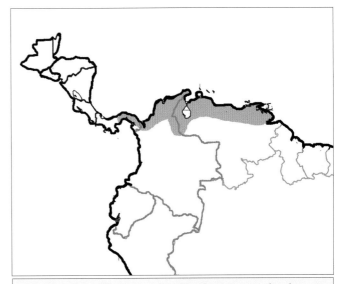

MAP 55. Range of the Pygmy Coral Snake, *Micrurus dissoleucus.*

Central American Coral Snake,
Micrurus nigrocinctus

Description and Identification: Pattern consists of broad red bands bordered by narrower yellow or white bands, followed by a black band that is narrower than the red but broader than the yellow or whitish bands. Pattern sequence beginning of the head is as follows; black, yellow, black. Body sequence is; yellow, red, yellow, black, yellow, red, yellow, black, yellow, etc. Adults average 2 to 3 feet in length; occasional individuals may attain lengths of over 4 feet.

Can be highly variable (6 subspecies) and some specimens may lack the light yellow or whitish rings completely, producing a black and red banded snake. The snout is always black extending back over frontal area in a point. A broad yellow band over posterior part of head and a black ring on neck. Scales of a red area often tipped with black.

Ventrals 180-230; subcaudals 31-58.

Distribution, Habitat, and Biology: Lowland rain forest areas and lower mountain slopes from southern Mexico (Chiapas and Oaxaca) southward to northwestern Colombia. This is one of the most common coral snake species within its range.

In the 1965 edition of *Poisonous Snakes of the World,* this species was known as the Black-banded Coral Snake.

Venom and Bite: Two fatal bites referable to this species are known from Costa Rica (S.A. Minton). Suero Antiofidico Anti-Coral antivenom made in Costa Rica is reported to be effective in treating bites by this species.

Similar Species: *Micrurus hippocrepis,* the Mayan Coral Snake is a similar species found in the southern half of Belize and a small part of northeastern Guatemala.

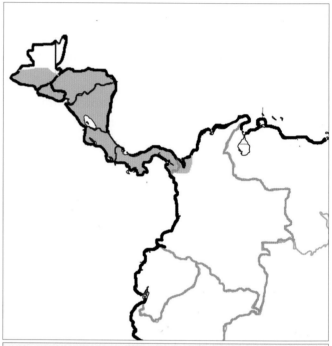

MAP 56. Range of Central American Coral Snake, *M. nigrocinctus*, in the USSOUTHCOM region.

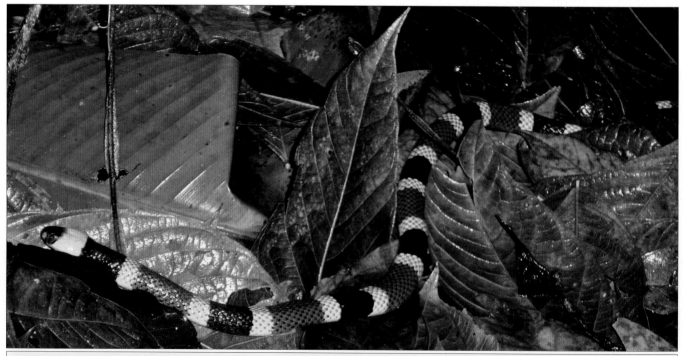

PHOTO 55. Central American Coral Snake, *Micrurus nigrocinctus*

Allen's Coral Snake,
Micrurus alleni

Description and Identification: This is a large coral snake, with a record length of 53 inches. With its classic triad pattern of broad red bands encircled by narrower yellow then slightly wider black bands, this species is readily recognized as a coral snake.

Distribution, Habitat, and Biology: A tropical rainforest species that ranges from eastern Honduras and eastern Nicaragua to central Panama.

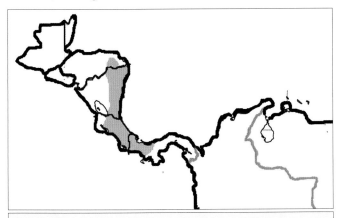

MAP 57. Range of the Allen's Coral Snake, *Micrurus alleni*.

Venom and Bite: Given the size attained by this species it is undoubtably a potentially deadly snake.

No specific antivenom, but Coralmyn by Instituto Bioclon, Antimicrurus, and Soro-Anti-Elapidico are listed under this species by Clinical Toxinology Resources website (www.toxinology.com-2012).

Similar Species: The Clark's Coral Snake, *Micrurus clarki* is a similar species that occurs sympatrically with *M. alleni* in northern Panama and southern Nicaragua. Its range also include southern Panama.

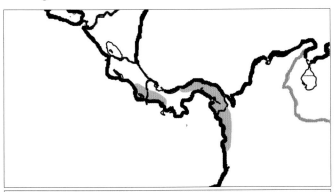

MAP 58. Range of the Clark's Coral Snake, *Micrurus clarki*.

Many Banded Coral Snake,
Micrurus multifasciatus

Description and Identification: This coral snake exhibits only black and red bands. The snout is black and there is a broad red band that encompasses most of the rest of the head. The rest of the body consists of alternating black and red bands. Several other coral snakes may show only black and red bands, but they are not sympatric with *multifasciatus*. Ventrals 233-311; subcaudals 22-38.

These are slender snakes that reach a maximum length of about 4 feet. Average size is about 3 feet.

Distribution, Habitat, and Biology: A rainforest species that inhabits both lowlands and mountain slopes. Found in Central America from Nicaragua to Panama.

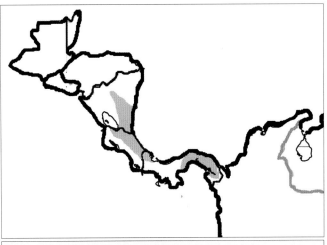

MAP 59. Range of the Many Banded Coral Snake, *Micrurus multifasciatus*.

Venom and Bite: Unknown but likely deadly. Antivenoms listed are the same as for the previous species.

Similar Species: *Micrurus multiscutatus,* the Cauca Coral Snake exhibits a pattern similar to the red and black forms of the Many Banded Coral Snake. It has a very limited range in southwestern Colombia.

Red-tailed Coral Snake,
Micrurus mipartitus

Description and Identification: A coral snake with broad black rings and numerous narrow white, or yellow rings between. Adults average about 24 inches in length; occasional individuals may exceed 3 feet.

Snout black, a broad red band passing just behind eye and covering posterior part of head. Body with 34-81 black rings separated by narrow, (usually) yellow rings; tail with 3-5 black rings and 2-5 red rings.

Ventrals 197-326; subcaudals 23-35.

In a deviation from the typical red, yellow/whitish, and black tri-color pattern, this snake is mostly a black and white (or black and yellow) animal with a reddish or orange ring on the head and several red/orange rings on the tail. On the body in between are rings of black and white.

Distribution, Habitat, and Biology: Rain forest areas from Nicaragua to northern Venezuela and Peru. In the original edition of this book published in 1965 this species was known as the Black-ringed Coral Snake.

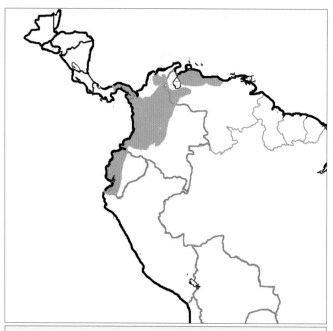

MAP 60. Range of the Red-tailed Coral Snake, *Micrurus mipartitus*.

Venom and Bite: This species is known to have been responsible for human fatalities. Suero Antifidico Anti-Coral Antivenom made in Costa Rica is listed as effective against the venom of this snake.

Annellated Coral Snake,
Micrurus annellatus

Description and Identification: This coral snake may exhibit the typical tri-colored pattern associated with most coral snakes, or it may show a pattern of only two color rings. If bi-colored it may be black and yellow, black and orange, or black and white. This is a small species, the largest specimen is a little less than 30 inches.

The total number of dark rings ranges from 17-83 on the body, 3 to 9 on the tail. Red is often visible on the belly.

Ventrals 186-225; anal plate divided; subcaudals 26-48.

Distribution, Habitat, and Biology: River valleys of the mountain regions of Peru, Bolivia, and Ecuador. This is a mountain species that lives at altitudes of 1,500 to 6,000 feet.

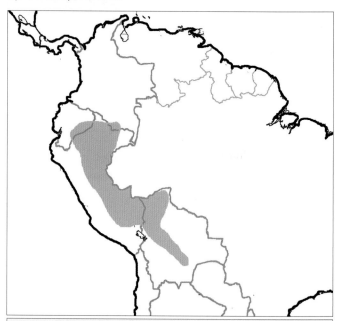

MAP 61. Range of the Annellated Coral Snake, *Micrurus annellatus*.

Venom and Bite: Although there are no known deaths from this snake's bite, the largest specimens are probably capable of killing a human.

Similar Species: The White-ringed Coral Snake, (*Micrurus albicinctus*) of the middle Amazon basin in northwest Brazil, and the Speckled Coral Snake (*Micrurus margaritiferus*) from northern Peru both exhibit a black and white bi-colored pattern similar to that seen on the above species.

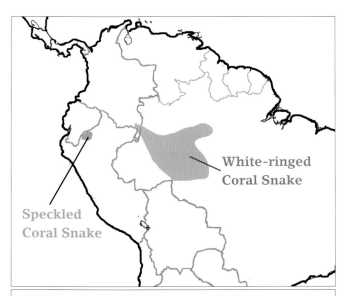

MAP 62. Range of the White-ringed Coral Snake, M. *albicinctus* and Speckled Coral Snake, M. *margaritiferus.*

Southern Coral Snake,
Micrurus frontalis

Description and Identification: A coral snake with triads of black rings and broad red interspaces; head black with edges of plates red. Adults average 3 to 4 feet; exceptional individuals exceed 50 inches.

Crown black to the posterior end of the parietals, labials and temporals spotted with yellow, crown scutes edged with red or yellow. Bod with 6-15 sets of black triads, separated with broad bands of red.

Ventrals 97-230; anal plate divided; subcaudals 15-26.

Distribution, Habitat, and Biology: Since the publication of *Poisonous Snakes of the World* back in 1965 this species has been divided into a total of six distinct species. However, all exhibit a relatively similar tri-color pattern and are difficult to distinguish by lay individuals. Thus, all six species are treated together in this account. For the professional reader of this account, the six new species are, in addition to the nominate species, *M. altirostris, M. baliocoryphus, M. brasilensis, M. diana,* and *M. pyrrhocryptus.*

The collective ranges of all six species include southwestern Brazil, northern Argentina, Uruguay, Paraguay, and Bolivia.

Venom and Bite: These are large snakes and they have been responsible for a number of deaths. Instituto Butantan in Brazil produces a specific antivenom for

M. frontalis (Soro Antielapidico). Instibudo National de Microbiologica in Argentina also produces an antivenom for *M. frontalis.* Campbell and Lamar (2004) report several cases of bites by this species that were successfully treated with neostigmine (an anticholinesterase drug).

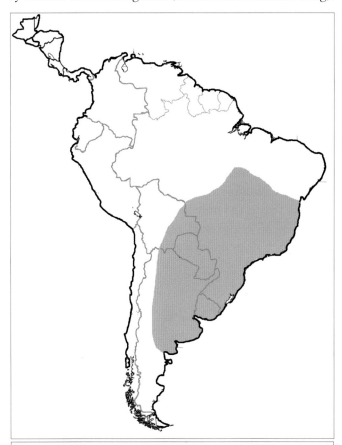

MAP 63. Collective range of the Southern Coral Snake group.

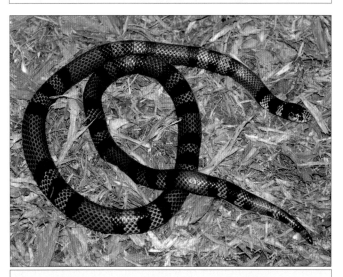

PHOTO 56. Southern Coral Snake, *Micrurus frontalis*

Hemprich's Coral Snake,
Micrurus hemprichii

Description and Identification: A coral snake with narrow yellow and red rings, and very broad black rings. Adults average 24 to 30 inches in length.

Snout and tip of chin black, with this color extending back over crown as a "cap." A red collar, narrowed above. Body with 5-10 triads of broad black rings separated by narrow red rings.

Ventrals 159-191; anal plate entire; subcaudals 23-30.

Distribution, Habitat, and Biology: Rim of the Amazon basin; northern Brazil, French Guiana, Surinam, Guyana, Colombia, Ecuador and Peru, and northern Bolivia. This is the only species of coral snake that normally has an entire anal plate. This and the triads of broad black rings make it a distinctive snake.

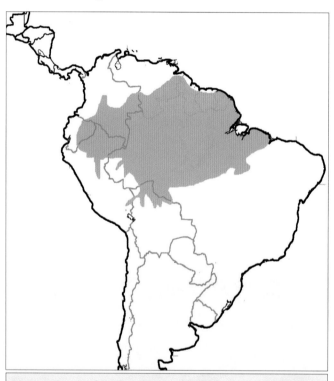

MAP 64. Range of Hemprich's Coral Snake, *Micrurus hemprichii.*

Venom and Bite: Little information is available on the effects of this snake's bite or the potency of its venom. Campbell and Lamar (2004) list two instances of bites by this species, neither of which were serious. However, Janis Roze in his definitive book *Coral Snakes of the Americas,* cautions that all *Micrurus* coral snakes should be regarded as potentially deadly.

Venezuelan Coral Snake,
Micrurus isozonus

Description and Identification: A large coral snake (maximum length up to 5 feet). This species exhibits the typical tri-color pattern of many coral snakes. In *isozonus* the orange/red rings are bordered by black and the color sequence of the rings is orange/black/white/black/white/black/orange.

Ventrals 199-231; subcaudals 24-33.

Distribution, Habitat, and Biology: Occupies both forested and open habitats in Venezuela and east central Colombia.

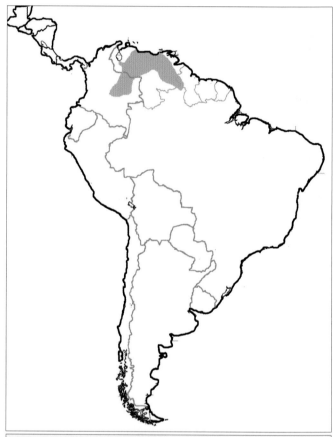

MAP 65. Range of the Venezuelan Coral Snake, *Micrurus isozonus.*

Venom and Bite: Although *isozonus* has a smaller range than some other coral snakes in South America, it is common within that range and its large size makes it a dangerous snake. Antivenoms listed by Clinical Toxinology Resources website- www.toxinolgy.com (2012). Anti-Micrurus by A.N.L.I.S. (Argentina), Soro Anti-elapidico by FUNED (Brazil), Coralmyn by Bioclon (Mexico), and Anti-Micrurus-Corales by PRO-BIOL (Columbia).

Amazonian Coral Snake,

Micrurus spixii

Description and Identification: A coral snake in which the black rings are all about equal in width and narrower than the yellow and red rings. Adults average 3 to 4 feet; occasional individuals attain a length of 5 feet.

Crown of head mainly black, often with shields edged and spotted with yellow; sides of head mostly light. Often a black collar followed by a yellow ring. Body with 4-9 complete triads of narrow and equal black rings separated by somewhat wider bands of yellow and red.

Ventrals 200-229; anal plate divided; subcaudals 15-25.

Distribution, Habitat, and Biology: The Amazon region; Brazil, Colombia, Equador, Peru, and Bolivia, southern Venezuela and northern Paraguay. An animal of the forest floor in tropical rainforest.

Venom and Bite: This is one of the largest of the coral snakes, and it has been responsible for several deaths. Soro Antielapidico antivenom by Instituto Butantan in Brazil is listed by as effective against South American *Micrurus*.

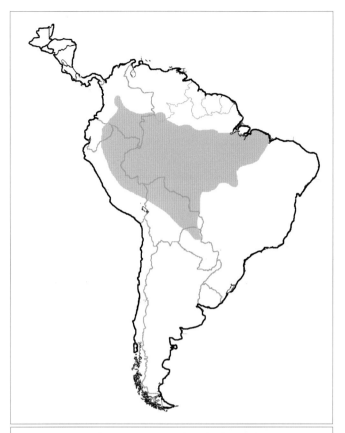

MAP 66. Range of Amazonian Coral Snake, *Micrurus spixii*.

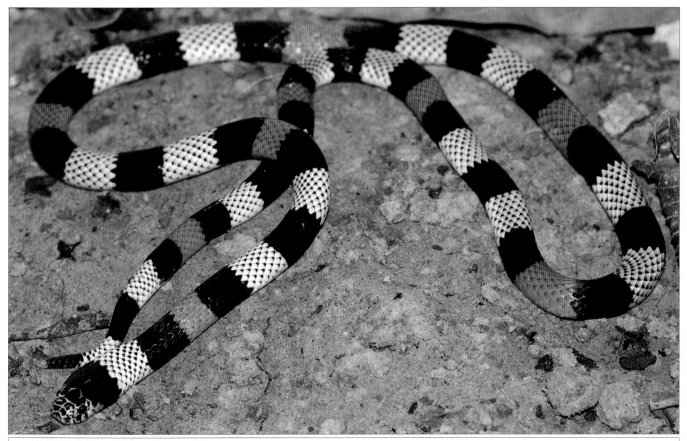

PHOTO 57. Amazonian Coral Snake, *Micrurus spixii*

Aquatic Coral Snake,
Micrurus surinamensis

Description and Identification: A coral snake with a red head and triads of black rings, of which the middle one is distinctly broader than the lateral ones.

Crown of head red, with each of the plates outlined in black. Body with 5-8 complete triads, each made up of a broad middle black band, with narrow bands laterally. Yellow rings narrowed dorsally. Dorsals 17-19 anteriorly, 15 at midbody and posteriorly.

In this coral snake the entire head is red, including the snout, and each scale is heavily edged in black. This is a unique feature seen only on this species of coral snake and thus is a significant diagnostic character that can be used to readily identify the Aquatic Coral Snake. Adults average about 3 feet in length; occasional individuals attain a length in excess of 4 feet. These are very stout bodied snakes by coral snake standards.

Distribution, Habitat, and Biology: Found throughout much of Brazil, northern Bolivia, eastern Peru, eastern Ecuador, southern Colombia and Venezuela, and all of Guyana, Suriname, and French Guiana. The name Aquatic Coral Snake is a reference to its preferred habitat in close proximity to streams and rivers. In fact, this species is known to be quite aquatic and feeds primarily on fish, an unusual lifestyle for a coral snake.

This species was formerly known as the Suriname Coral Snake.

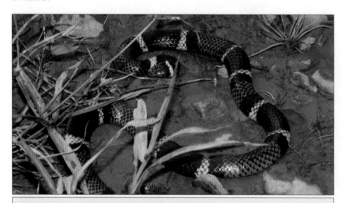

Photo 58. Aquatic Coral Snake, *Micrurus surinamensis*

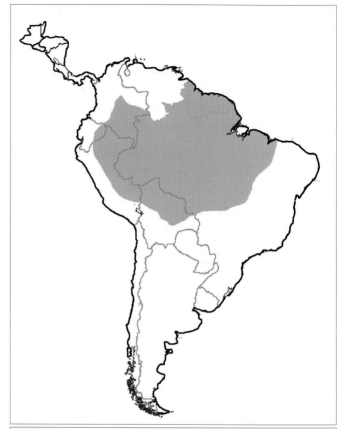

Map 67. Range of the Aquatic Coral Snake, *Micrurus surinamensis*.

Venom and Bite: These are large coral snakes with a rather large head. This combination means larger fangs and venom glands. Some lab studies using mice suggest the venom of this snake is highly potent. The estimated lethal dose for humans is 18-20 mg (dry weight). The maximum yield is 160 mg (Roze 1996) the highest yield of any coral snake. Fatalities have been recorded.

www.toxinology.com by Clinical Toxinology Resources (2012), lists the following antivenoms:

Product: Antimicrurus

Manufacturer: Instituto Nacional de Produccion de Biologicos

Country of Origin: Argentina

Product: Soro-Antielapidico

Manufacturer: Fundacao Ezequiel Dias-FUNED
Country of Origin: Brazil

Product: Coralmyn

Manufacturer: Instituto Bioclon

Country of Origin: Mexico

Product: Antimicruricos-Corales

Manufacturer: Laboratorios Biologicos PROBIOL

Country of Origin: Colombia

Painted Coral Snake,
Micrurus corallinus

Description and Identification: Medium large, averaging about 2-3 feet with a maximum of 40 inches. A classically tri-colored coral snake with broad red rings bordered by narrow white rings with a medium width black ring in between. The black of the snout extends posteriorly well beyond the eyes and often forms a point on the top of the head.

Ventrals 179-224; subcaudals 27-47.

Distribution, Habitat, and Biology: Found in rainforest areas from southeastern Brazil (outside the Amazon basin) southward into northern Uruguay.

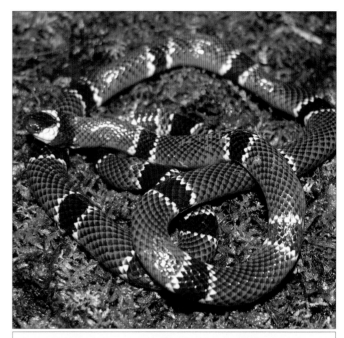

Photo 59. Painted Coral Snake, *Micrurus corallinus*

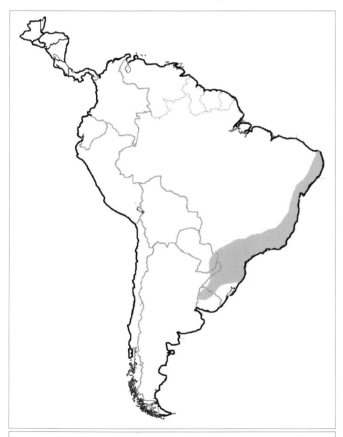

Map 68. Range of the Painted Coral Snake, *Micrurus corrallinus.*

Similar Species: A peruvian species of Coral Snake known as Bocourt's Coral Snake (*Micrurus bocourti*) is similar in appearance to the Painted Coral Snake.

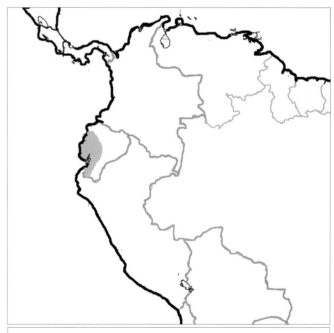

Map 69. Range of Bocourt's Coral Snake, *Micrurus bocourti.*

Venom and Bite: This snake accounts for a large number of coral snake bites within its range and has been responsible for numerous deaths. World Health Organization's antivenoms database lists antivenoms for the Painted Coral Snake as; Antielapidico Butantan (Brazil), Anti-elipidico FUNED (Brazil), and Antivenom *Micrurus* (Argentina). *M. corallinus* is the only coral snake known to have venom containing *pre-synaptic* neurotoxins (Roze 1996).

South American Coral Snake,
Micrurus lemniscatus

Description and Identification: Another tri-colored coral snake with a pattern of red, black, and yellow or whitish rings. As with many South American coral snakes the color sequence of the rings is red, black, light, black, light, black, red. The head pattern of this species is fairly distinctive, featuring a light ring around the snout (or light spots) followed by a black ring around the eyes and a red ring on the back of the head and the neck. Large individuals of this species can reach 4.5 feet.

Eyes notably small.

Ventrals 210-268; subcaudals 23-43.

Distribution, Habitat, and Biology: This is one of the most widespread species of coral snake in South America. It may be found in both lowland rainforest or on the lower slopes of forested mountains. It can also be found in more open areas such as areas cleared by man and it is often found around human habitations (Lamar and Campbell, 2004).

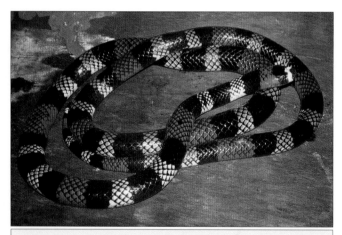

Photo 60. South American Coral Snake, *Micrurus lemniscatus*

Venom and Bite: A number of deaths have been recorded from the bite of the South American Coral Snake.

Antivenoms listed by Clinical Toxinology Resources website-www.toxinolgy.com (2012).

Product: Antimicrurus
Manufacturer: Instituto Nacional de Produccion de Biologics (A.N.L.I.S.)
Country of Origin: Argentina
Product: Soro Anti-Elapidico
Manufacturer: Fundaco Ezequiel Dias (FUNED)
Country of Origin: Brazil

Product: Coralmyn
Manufacturer: Instituto Bioclone
Country of Origin: Mexico
Product: Anti-*Micrurus* Corales
Manufacturer: Laboratories Biologicos
Country of Origin: Colombia

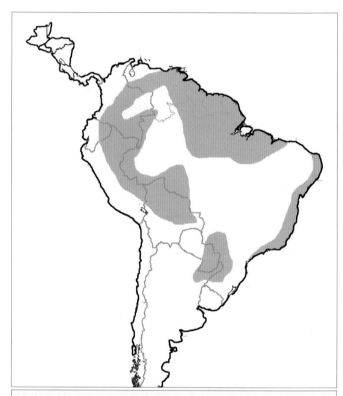

Map 70. Range of the South American Coral Snake, *Micrurus lemniscatus.*

Similar Species: The Caatinga Coral Snake, *Micrurus ibiboboca,* resembles the South American Coral Snake and is found sympatrically with that species in a few areas of Brazil.

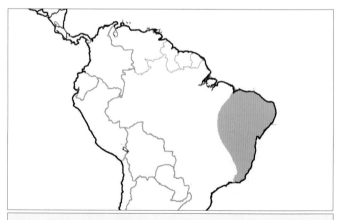

Map 71. Range of the Caatinga Coral Snake, *Micrurus iboboca.*

Argentinian Coral Snake,
Micrurus pyrrhocryptus

Description and Identification: Another coral snake with the typical South American tri-color pattern in which the color sequence of the rings is red, black, light, black, light, black, red. The black rings that are in contact with the red rings are significantly narrower than those in contact with the light rings. Average length 36 inches, maximum about 4 feet.

Ventrals 214-251; subcaudals 19-31.

Distribution, Habitat, and Biology: Inhabits the dry tropical forests and grassland habitats of north central Argentina. Also found in parts of Bolivia, Paraguay, and southern Brazil.

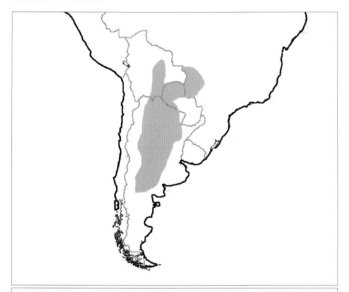

MAP 72. Range of the Argentinian Coral Snake, *Micrurus pyrrhocryptus.*

Venom and Bite: This is a dangerous species that has caused human deaths.

Antivenoms listed by Clinical Toxinology Resources website-www.toxinolgy.com (2012).

  Product: Antimicrurus
  Manufacturer: Instituto Nacional de Produccion de Biologics (A.N.L.I.S.)
  Country of Origin: Argentina
  Product: Soro Anti-Elapidico
  Manufacturer: Fundaco Ezequiel Dias (FUNED)
  Country of Origin: Brazil
  Product: Coralmyn
  Manufacturer: Instituto Bioclon
  Country of Origin: Mexico

Brazilian Coral Snake,
Micrurus decoratus

Description and Identification: The "fire engine red" bands on this species are bordered by narrow black, followed by yellow (cream), then a broad black band, then yellow (cream) again, then another narrow black band. There are commonly black specks within the red bands. The snout is black, followed by yellow, then black on the front edge of the parietals. These handsome little coral snakes grow to about 2 feet.

Distribution, Habitat, and Biology: In spite of its name this snake inhabits only a small portion of southern Brazil. Habitat is undisturbed and human altered woodlands from sea level about 3,000 feet

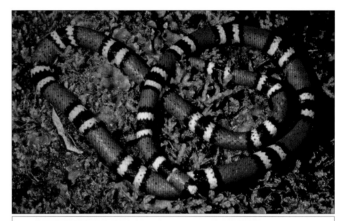

PHOTO 61. Brazilian Coral Snake, *Micrurus decoratus*

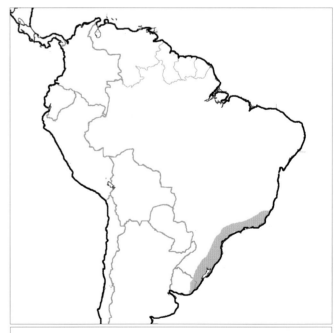

MAP 73. Range of the Brazilain Coral Snake, *Micrurus decoratus.*

The coral snake species described thus far are a representative example of the dangerously venomous Elapidae snakes that occur within the USSOUTHCOM region. However, this is by no means a complete picture of the Elapidae serpents of this region. For an account of all the region's coral snakes, the reader is referred to *The Venomous Reptiles of the Western Hemisphere* (2 vol.) by Jonathan Campbell and William Lamar; and to *Coral Snakes of the Americas: Biology, Identification, and Venoms* by Janis A. Roze.

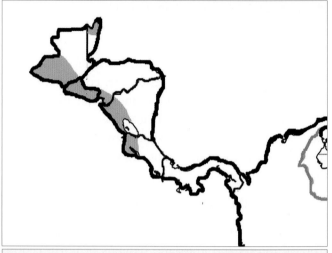

MAP 74. Range of the Common Cantil, *Agkistrodon bilineatus*, in the USSOUTHCOM region.

Family - Viperidae

Subfamily - Crotalinae: Pit Vipers

Genus - Agkistrodon: Moccasins

Four species are recognized. One is found in the US-SOUTHCOM region. The Copperhead, Cottonmouth, and Taylor's Cantil are all found in the USNORTHCOM region. The fourth species (Common Cantil) is primarily a Mexican species that also ranges into the USSOUTH-COM region in Central America. All have been responsible for human fatalities. The Copperhead is the least dangerous and most survive its bite. The Cottonmouth, Taylor's Cantil and Common Cantil, however, are all dangerous species.

Definition: Head broad, flattened, very distinct from narrow neck; a sharply distinguished canthus. Body cylindrical or depressed, tapered, moderately stout to stout; tail short to moderately long.

Eyes moderate in size, pupils vertically elliptical.

Head scales: The usual 9 on the crown.

Laterally, loreal pit separated from labials or its anterior border formed by second supralabial. Loreal scale present or absent.

Body scales: Dorsals keeled, with apical pits, in 23 to 27 rows. Ventrals 127-157, subcaudals single anteriorly, 19-71.

Common Cantil,
Agkistrodon bilineatus

Much of this species range is in the USNORTHCOM region. For information and photo of this species see Chapter 8, page 41. Map 74 shows the range of the Common Cantil in the USSOUTHCOM region.

Family - Viperidae

Subfamily - Crotalinae: Pit Vipers

Genus - Atropoides: Jumping Vipers

There are five species in this genus, four of which occur in USSOUTHCOM region.

Definition: Jumping Vipers are readily identified by their exceedingly stocky body shape. These are short, very thick bodied snakes with a series of dark, saddle shaped blotches down the back. The head is quite large with a broad snout and a prominent dark postocular stripe. These are short snakes, reaching a maximum length of only about 2 feet, but a large specimen may have a girth as big as a man's wrist. They have the ability to strike for an abnormally long distance, hence the name "Jumping Viper."

Dorsal scales heavily keeled in 21-29 rows; rostral scale concave and broader than high; ventrals 114-155; subcaudals undivided, 22-40.

Eyes comparatively small and separated from labials by several rows of small scales. Pupils ellipitical.

Jumping Vipers,
Atropoides mexicanus, Atropoides olmec, Atropoides occidus and *Atropoides picadoi*

Description and Identification: All four Jumping Viper species found within the USSOUTHCOM region are for the most part indistinguishable to the lay observer. In fact, until recently they were all considered to be a single species. Thus, the author has elected to treat all four of these similar snakes together in this account.

All are short, thick-bodied pit vipers with dark saddle-shaped blotches on a tan or gray background.

Adults average 18 to 24 inches in length.

Ground color tan, light brown or gray with about 20 dark brown or black rhomboid blotches down the back, these are often connected with lateral spots to form narrow cross bands. Top of head dark with oblique post orbital band forming upper limit of light color on sides of head. Ventral color whitish, sometimes blotched with dark brown. Snout rounded, canthus sharp. Body exceedingly stout; tail short.

Dorsal scales strongly keeled, tubercular in large individuals, in 23-27 rows at midbody; fewer (19) posteriorly. Ventrals 125-135; subcaudals 26-36; all or mostly single. Eye separated from labials by 3-4 rows of small scales.

Distribution, Habitat, and Biology: The name Jumping Viper is appropriate for this species, as its stout body can strike for a distance greater than its length. Ranging from southern Mexico to Panama, Jumping Vipers are rainforest animals and occur in a wide variety of elevations throughout their range. As with many other pit viper species, the young have bright yellow tail tips. Immature snakes are reported to feed heavily on grasshoppers, while mice appear to constitute the mainstay of the diet for adults.

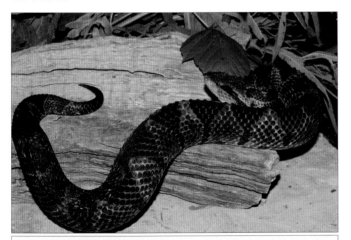

Photo 62. Central American Jumping Viper, *Atropoides mexicanus*

Venom and Bite: Haemorragins and myotoxins possibly present. The venom of jumping vipers is apparently not highly toxic, and they appear not to be deadly to humans. However, the venom is known to vary widely among snakes from different regions, and some may be more dangerous than others. These snakes also have a tendency to hang on after striking, a habit that can increase the amount of venom injected and thus increase the severity of the bite. Antivenom of choice for this species is Tri-Antivipmyn by Bioclon of Mexico..

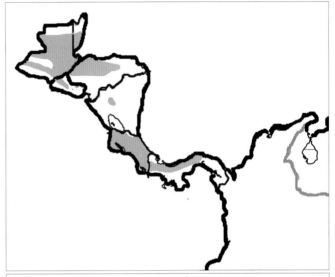

Map 75. Range of the Jumping Vipers, in the USSOUTHCOM region.

Family - Viperidae

Subfamily - Crotalinae: Pit Vipers

Genus - Bothriechis: Palm Vipers

There are a total of nine species and all are decidedly arboreal in habits. Eight of these species are found in the USSOUTHCOM region.

Definition: Average length about 2 feet but may reach 3 feet. Body moderate to slender. Tail moderate in length and *prehensile*. Head very distinct from neck with a sharply defined canthus.

Eyes moderate size with elliptical pupil.

Head Scales: Highly variable, some species have numerous small scales on top of the head while others have large, platelike scales. Two species have raised, spine-like scales above the eye.

Body Scales: Scale rows at midbody 17-25. Ventrals 134-175. Subcaudals 42-75, undivided.

Although less dangerous than the larger lance head pit vipers and the coral snakes, some species are known to have killed.

Coffee Palm Pit Viper,
Bothriechis lateralis

Description and Identification: A uniformly green tree viper with a *prehensile* tail. There is a light yellow lateral line along the tops of the ventrals and occasionally light yellow spots along the back.

Distribution, Habitat, and Biology: A tree dwelling snake of low forested mountain slopes in central Costa Rica and northwestern Panama.

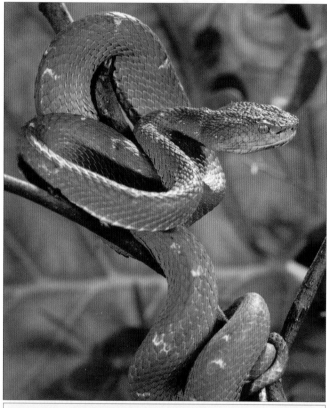

Photo 63. Coffee Palm Viper, *Bothriechis lateralis*

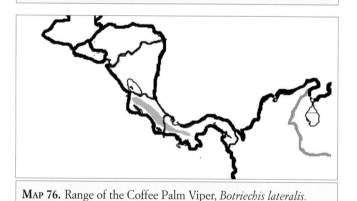

Map 76. Range of the Coffee Palm Viper, *Botriechis lateralis.*

Venom and Bite: Probably a potentially deadly species. Polyvalent Antivenom ICP manufactured in Costa Rica is listed for treating bites.

Black-speckled Palm Pit Viper,
Bothriechis nigroviridis

Description and Identification: Typical palm viper. Color green heavily speckled with black.

Distribution, Habitat, and Biology: Very similar to the preceding species, but ranging to higher elevations.

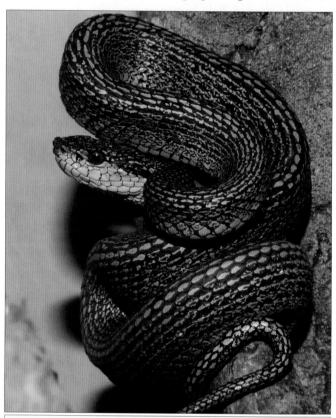

Photo 64. Black-speckled Palm Viper, *Bothriechis nigroviridis*

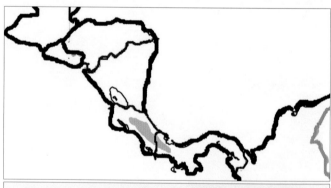

Map 77. Range of the Black-speckled Palm Viper, *Botriechis nigrovirids.*

Venom and Bite: "Implicated in human fatalities" (Campbell and Lamar, 2004). Polyvalent Antivenom ICP manufactured in Costa Rica is listed for treating bites.

Yellow-blotched Palm Viper,
Bothriechis aurifer

Description and Identification: Average length about 2.5 feet. May rarely reach 3 feet. Ground color is green with a series of black bordered pale blotches down the center of the back and extending onto the tail. A broad, dark postocular stripe is usually present. Immature specimens are greenish yellow. Scales on top of the head anterior of the eyes are large and plate-like. Keeled scales in 18 to 21 scale rows at midbody. Ventrals 148-167, 48-64 subcaudals, mostly undivided. The iris of the eye in this species is greenish yellow and heavily diffused with darks specks.

Distribution, Habitat, and Biology: Another primarily arboreal snake that hunts by day in trees and bushes in mountain cloud forests. Campbell and Lamar (2004) report treefrogs and rodents as prey, but small birds and lizards are probably also consumed. The range includes the southern tip of the USNORTHCOM region (see map 15 on page 47) as well as the northern tip of the USSOUTHCOM region (Guatemala only).

Venom and Bite: Deaths from the bite of this species have been recorded. Institudo Bioclon's "Tri-Antivip-myn" antivenom (manufactured in Mexico by Bioclon) is listed as having protective substances capable of neutralizing the toxic effects of the venom of *Bothriechis* species.

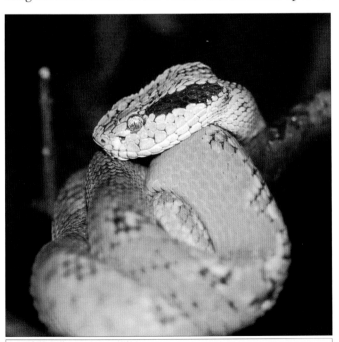

PHOTO 65. Yellow-blotched Palm Viper, *Bothriechis aurifer*

Similar species: Three additional members of this genus are restricted to northern Central America. All are relatively rare snakes with small ranges. The map below shows the ranges of *B. bicolor* (Guatemalan Palm Viper), *B. thalassinus* (Meredon Palm Viper) and *B. marchi* (Honduran Palm Viper).

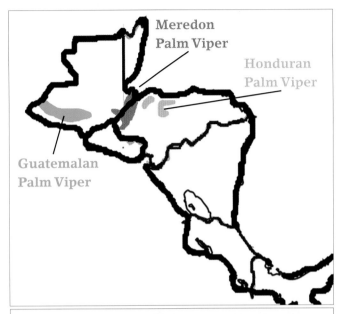

MAP 78. Range of the Honduran, Guatemalan and Meredon Palm Vipers.

Eyelash Viper,
Bothriechis schlegelii

Description and Identification: A green, tan, or yellow tree viper with raised and pointed scales above the eye. Body moderately stout, with a *prehensile* tail; head broad and distinct. Adults average 16 to 24 inches in length, with a maximum of 38 inches.

Ground color green, olive green, tan, salmon, or yellow with scattered black dots which may form irregular crossbands. Green and tan individuals commonly have narrow reddish and brown crossbands or a reticulated pattern of red. Belly green or yellow, spotted with black.

Canthus sharp; a row of small scales above eye, 2-3 of them raised and pointed. Dorsals 10-25, moderately keeled. Ventrals 138-169; subcaudals 42-64, all single.

Distribution, Habitat, and Biology: Ranges from southernmost Mexico to Colombia and Ecuador in northern South America. Found in tropical rainforest, mountain cloud forests, and wet mountain forests. Ranges from lowlands to over 6,000 feet in elevation. Common in cacao plantations. This is an arboreal snake that is usually found in trees and bushes.

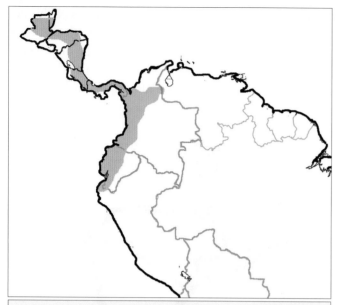

Map 79. Range of the Eyelash Viper, *Botriechis schlegelii* in the USSOUTHCOM region.

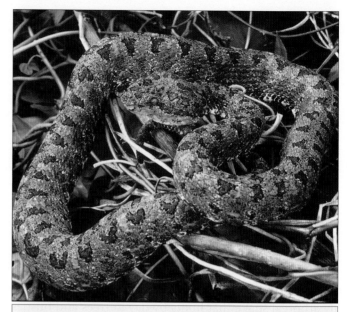

Photo 67. Eyelash Viper, *Bothriechis schlegelii*, green phase

Venom and Bite: Although back in 1965 this snake was not regarded as being particularly dangerous to man, there have since been a number of fatalities recorded from its bite.

Similar species: The Blotched Palm Viper, *Bothriechis supracilarius* is another arboreal, *prehensile* tailed snake that also possesses the raised scales above the eye and may be difficult to distinguish from the Eyelash Viper. This species is quite rare and is found only in a small region of Costa Rica. Clinical Toxinology Resources website lists haemorragins and procoagulants as possibly present in the venom of this species.

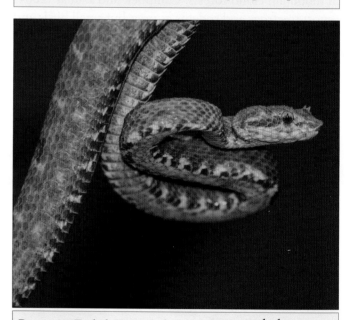

Photo 68. Eyelash Viper, *Bothriechis schlegeli*, red phase

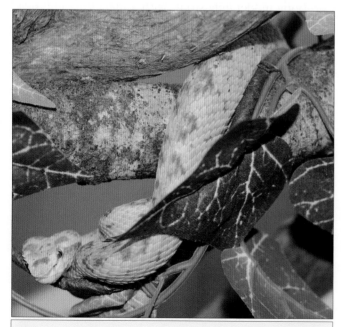

Photo 66. Eyelash Viper, *Bothriechis schlegelii,* yellow phase

Family - Viperidae

Subfamily - Crotalinae: Pit Vipers

Genus - Bothriopsis - Forest Pit Vipers

There are six species of these pit vipers and all are endemic to South America. They range in size from 32 inches to over 5 feet in length. All are forest animals and they are mostly arboreal in habits. They are found in both lowland and montane habitats. In the first edition of this volume back in 1965 this genus had not yet been described.

Definition: Body moderately slender to slender; head broad and distinct from neck; canthus well defined; rostral scale as tall or taller than wide; *tail prehensile*.

Eyes moderately large in size; pupil ellipitical.

Head scales: crown of head with 5-9 scales; supralabials 6-9.

Body scales: 19-29 rows of keeled scales at midbody, 153-254 ventrals, 41-91 mostly divided subcaudals.

Two-striped Forest Pit Viper

Bothriopsis bilineata

Description and Identification: A green tree viper that usually exhibits a yellow ventro-lateral stripe. Ground color green, blueish gray, or greenish blue with numerous small dorsal spots that are tan or reddish brown. Tip of tail usually red or reddish brown. Belly yellow, without markings. Adults average 24 to 30 inches, maximum about 4 feet. The labial scales are normally yellow and a yellow or cream colored line defines the border of the ventral scales on each side.

Snout rounded; canthus rostralis sharp and slightly raised. Dorsals strongly keeled in 23-35 nonoblique rows, fewer posteriorly. Ventrals 190-218, subcaudals 55-73 all or nearly all divided. *Tail prehensile*.

Distribution, Habitat, and Biology: Found in the Amazon regions of Brazil, Colombia, Bolivia, Peru, Ecuador, Venezuela as well as Guyana, French Guiana and Suriname. Habitat is lowland forests from sea level to about 3,000 feet. Reportedly fond of tree-lined forest watercourses where it lives an arboreal lifestyle.

Venom and Bite: Although most victims receiving proper treatment will survive a bite by this species, it is a dangerous snake that is capable of killing.

There is no specific antivenom available for this species. Venom contains procoagulants in the form of fibrinogenases as well as possible haemorragins.

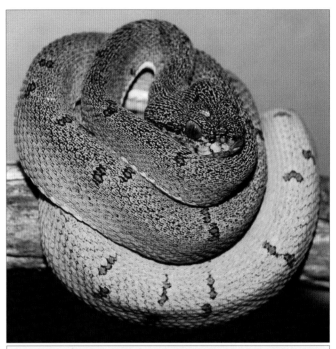

PHOTO 69. Two-striped Forest Pit Viper, *Bothriopsis bilineata*

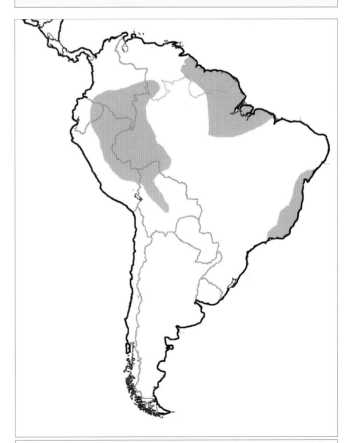

MAP 80. Range of the Two-striped Forest Viper, *Bothriopsis bilineata*.

Speckled Forest Pit Viper,
Bothriopsis taeniata

Description and Identification: This is the largest of the Forest Pit Vipers, and occasional specimens exceed 5 feet in length. Ground color brownish, yellowish, or grayish with numerous small dark spots on the dorsum, often alternating with areas of lighter pigment. There is a row of white spots on the lateral edge of the ventrals. The entire dorsal surface is heavily diffused with dark speckling.

Body fairly slender; 25-29 rows of scales at midbody; head elongate, larger than and distinct from the neck.

Ventrals 203-254; subcaudals 66-91, mostly single.

Distribution, Habitat, and Biology: As with other Forest Pit Vipers, this is an arboreal species that lives mostly in trees and bushes. Its habitat is tropical lowland and foothill rainforests from sea level to just over 4,000 feet.

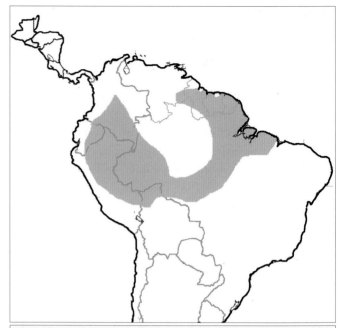

MAP 81. Range of the Speckled Forest Pit Viper, *Bothriopsis taeniata.*

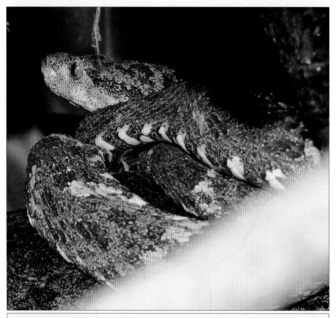

PHOTO 70. Speckled Forest Pit Viper, *Bothriopsis taeniata*

Venom and Bite: Campbell and Lamar (2004) detail several instances of snakebite by this species.

Although those authors mention no fatalities, the symptoms described were quite severe and this is undoubtably a dangerous snake. Venom toxins are like the previous species.

Similar Species: There are four other species of Forest Pit Vipers in equatorial South America. All have rather small ranges. *B. pulchra,* the Andean Forest Pit Viper, lives on the eastern slope of the Andes Mountains in Ecuador and northern Peru. *B. chloromelas*, the Inca Forest Pit Viper is found the Andes of central Peru, and *B. oligolpis,* the Peruvian Forest Pit Viper inhabits a small region in southern Peru and northwestern Bolivia. Finally, *B. medusa*, the Venezuelan Forest Pit Viper is found in a tiny area on the coast of Venezuela.

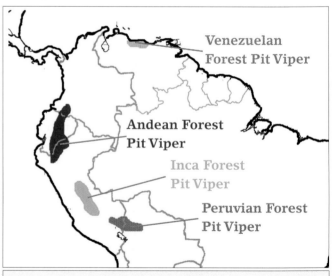

MAP 82. Range of other Forest Vipers, *Bothriopsis* species

Family - Viperidae

Subfamily - Crotalinae: Pit Vipers

Genus - Bothrocophias

Toadheaded Pit Vipers

Five species found in northwestern South America. All are terrestrial animals of equatorial rainforests both in lowland and mountain habitats. In the original edition of this book published in 1965 this genus was as yet undescribed

Definition: Body moderately slender to stout; posterior portion of head exceptionally broad and very distinct from neck. Top of head covered with small scales, canthus sharp. Tail not *prehensile*. Snout often upturned.

Eyes small; pupils elliptical.

Dorsal scales 21-25 at midbody (keeled); ventrals

118-177, subcaudals 38-54.

Toadheaded Pit Vipers,

Bothrocophias myersi
Bothrocophias micropthalmus
Bothrocophias hyoprora
Bothrocophias campbelli
Bothrocophias colombianus
Bothrocophias rhombeatus

Description and Identification: The five species of this genus are similar enough in appearance and habits as to warrant treating all five together in this account. The five species of Toadheaded Pit Vipers are the Colombian (*B. colombianus*), the Small-eyed (*B. micropthalmus*), the Ecuadorian (*B. campbelli*), the Amazonian (*B. hyopora*), the Chocoan (*B. myersi*), and *B. rhombeatus,* which has no common name. These snakes average about 2.5 feet in length as adults. Two species can exceed 4 feet (*B. colombianus, B. campbelli*). Coloration is dark brown, tan, reddish brown, or gray with a series of darker hourglass shaped crossbands (often with lighter centers) which extend the entire length of the body and tail. The top of the head is uniformly colored and matches the ground color. The side of the head is usually lighter in color with a dark postocular stripe.

Body stout to moderately slender, head distinctly wide, eyes moderately small to small in one species (*micropthalmus*), snout slightly upturned. Dorsal scales at midbody 21-25. Ventrals 118-177; subcaudals 38-54 (divided except in *hyoprora*).

Distribution, Habitat, and Biology: These are all terrestrial species. Three are found on the western slopes of the Andes and two occur on the eastern side of the continental divide. They range from Colombia through Ecuador and Peru into Bolivia and a large portion of western Brazil (see range map 83 below). Cloud forest, lower wet montane forest, and lowland rainforest is given as habitat by Lamar and Campbell (2004).

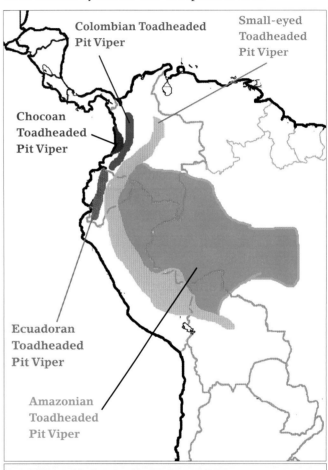

Map 83. Range of the Toadheaded Pit Vipers, *Bothocophias* species.

Venom and Bite: Some species reportedly have a highly toxic venom and all should be considered as a potentially lethal. The website www.toxinology.com (viewed 2012) lists as venom toxins procoagulants and possibly haemorragins.

Family - Viperidae

Subfamily - Crotalinae: Pit Vipers

Genus - Bothrops, Bothropoides,

and Rhinocerophis

Lancehead Pit Vipers

This group of 39 species of South American pit vipers were formerly all grouped into the genus *Bothrops*. Recent changes to the taxonomy of the *Bothrops* genus has resulted in that one genus being split into three. The three new genera are: the neuwiedi group (genus *Bothropoides*) containing 10 species; the alternatus group (genus *Rhinocerophis*) containing 6 species, and the original Lancehead Viper genus *Bothrops* retaining the remaining 23 species plus two newly described species. Collectively these three genera kill more people than any other types of venomous snakes in the Western Hemisphere.

It should be noted here that some experts have argued convincingly that all three of these genera (along with the genus *Bothriopsis*) should all be lumped together in the *Bothrops* genus. In this volume the author has elected to follow the current taxonomy of the Reptile Database (viewed 2012).

Genus - Bothrops

True Lancehead Vipers

There are 23 species of True Lancehead Pit Vipers (some experts recognize more). All are dangerous snakes and several species rank among the most deadly snakes in the Western Hemisphere. They range from tropical regions of southern Mexico throughout Central America to southern South America. Most are snakes of lowland regions and they are primarily nocturnal in habits. A few species range high into mountains where they may be more diurnal in movements.

Most average 3 to 4 feet in length but some species can exceed 6 feet. The largest can approach 9 feet in length.

Definition: Head broad, flattened, very distinct from narrow neck. Postocular stripe usually present. Body slender to moderately stout. Tail moderately long, non-*prehensile*. Scales on top of head small and keeled.

Eyes moderate in size, elliptical pupil.

Loreal pit present. Dorsal scales keeled, 21-33 rows at midbody. Ventrals 141-240. Subcaudals (divided) 33-95.

Terciopelo,
Bothrops asper

Description and Identification: Head triangular and distinct from the neck. Body moderately slender. Eyes moderately large, pupils elliptical. Scale rows at midbody 25-29, heavily keeled. Subcaudals 56-70, mostly undivided. Ventrals 185-220.

Adults average about 4 feet but can reach a length in excess of 8 feet. The color of these snakes is confusingly variable, and they may be brown, gray, yellowish, reddish, olive, or very dark charcoal. The dorsal pattern varies somewhat in discernability, however it is consistently a pattern of dark triangles on each side of the body which meet at the top of the back. These dark markings are edged in a lighter pigment that also highlights the center of each triangle. This pattern runs the entire length of the body and onto the tail. A narrow, dark postocular stripe is nearly always present from the eye to the angle of the jaw.

Young snakes may have a yellow tail tip.

Distribution, Habitat, and Biology: The Terciopelo is mostly a lowland animal, found in rainforests from sea level to moderate elevations of up to 3,600 feet. It is most often found in the vicinity of rivers and streams. These are ground dwelling snakes and the color and pattern of the Terciopelo is highly cryptic. They are nearly invisible when coiled atop the leaf litter on the forest floor. They are ambush predators that as adults feed mostly on small mammals and birds. Young snakes will eat invertebrates, frogs, and lizards. These snakes are often referred to as "Fer-de-lance," but that name should be reserved for the very similar species *Bothrops atrox.*

This is a wide-ranging species, being found from southern Mexico through Central America and well into northern South America.

Venom and Bite: Venom contains procoagulants, haemorragins, and systemic myotoxins. Its large size, long fangs, and extended reach when striking along with its propensity to defend itself at the slightest provocation make this one of the most dangerous snakes in the Western Hemisphere. In addition, it possesses a highly toxic venom and can deliver large doses deep into tissues. The venom can cause severe necrosis and inhibits the clotting factor of the blood (hemorrhage is often a cause of death).

Severe envenomations that do not receive prompt and proper medical attention often result in death. The Terciopelo is a fairly common snake throughout its range and it sometimes occurs around human habitations. It is thus responsible for a significant number of snakebite deaths. Antivenoms for treating bites from this snake are: "Tri-Antivipmyn" produced by Institudo Bioclon (Mexico) and "Antiofidico Bothropico Polivalente" made by Instituto Nacional de Higiene y Medicina Tropical (Ecuador).

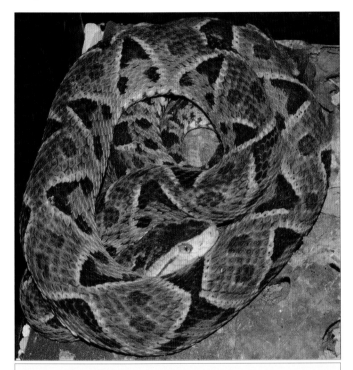

Photo 71. Terciopelo, *Bothrops asper*

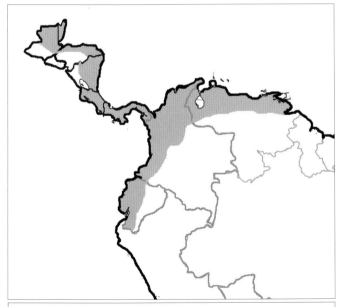

Map 84. Range of the Terciopelo, *Bothrops asper*, in the USSOUTHCOM region.

Common Lancehead,

Bothrops atrox

Description and Identification: An olive green, gray, or brownish (rarely reddish) snake with a pattern of lateral darker black edged triangles whose apices meet, or nearly meet, at the vertebral line.

Adult snakes average about 4 feet and the largest specimens can exceed 6 feet. Face is lighter with a moderately narrow postocular stripe.

The dorsum has a series of paired lateral triangles. Each triangle is lighter in the center and usually has a light edging to the dark triangle. The ventral surface is light cream to yellow with dark blotches becoming more numerous posteriorly.

In many respects this snake is very similar to the preceding species (*B. asper*). One distinguishing character is the lighter color of the side of the head and narrower postocular stripe on asper. *B. asper* also usually shows a stronger contrast between the dark triangles and the ground color.

Ventrals 169-214; subcaudals 52-72, all divided.

These snakes are also commonly known as the Fer-de-Lance, but most experts agree that name should be reserved for *Bothrops lanceolatus* from the Caribbean island of Martinique.

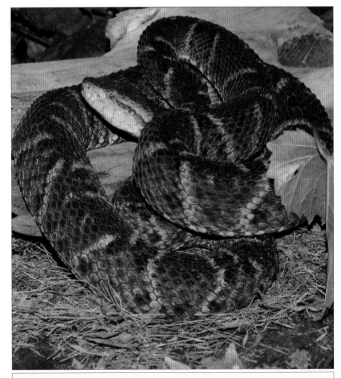

Photo 72. Common Lancehead, *Bothrops atrox*

Distribution, Habitat, and Biology: A terrestrial, lowland species of equatorial rainforests from southern Colombia and Venezuela to northern Bolivia; including all of Guyana, Suriname, French Guiana, and the northern half of Brazil. Habitat includes overgrown areas in urban environments as well as true wilderness.

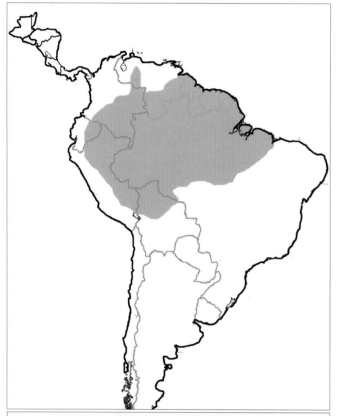

MAP 85. Range of the Common Lancehead, *Bothrops atrox.*

Venom and Bite: This is a deadly species. Like the preceding species (the Terciopelo), the Common Lancehead possess a highly toxic venom, long fangs, large size, and an athletic striking ability. Together the two snakes share the distinction of killing more humans than any other snake in the Western Hemisphere. A number of antivenoms are produced for the bite of this species including "Antibotropico-laquetico" and "Antibotropico-crotalico" (Brazil), "Antibotropico polivalente" (Peru), "Antifidico Bothropico Polivalente" (Ecuador), and "Antifidico Polivalente Botropico Laquetico" (Bolivia). Venom toxins are the same as those listed for the Terciopelo.

Similar species: *Bothrops marajoensis*, the Marajo Lancehead is very similar to the Common Lancehead. It occuppies a very limited range within the Amazon Delta of northern Brazil.

Brazilian Lancehead,
Bothrops moojeni

Description and Identification: This is one of the larger lanceheads with a record length of over 7 1/2 feet. The color and pattern is typical of most lanceheads with the ground color usually brown, grayish brown, tan, or reddish brown. There are a series of dark, hourglass shaped bands that are narrowest vertebrally and have lighter centers and lighter borders. The top of the head matches the ground color and the face is light and usually has a dark postocular stripe.

Ventrals 179-210 subcaudals 44-70, divided; midbody scale rows 23-29.

Distribution, Habitat, and Biology: Most of the range of this species is contained in Brazil where it inhabits savannas and grasslands.

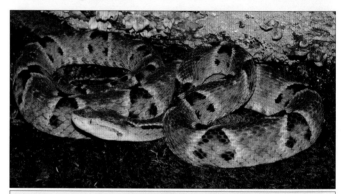

PHOTO 73. Brazilian Lancehead, *Bothrops moojeni*

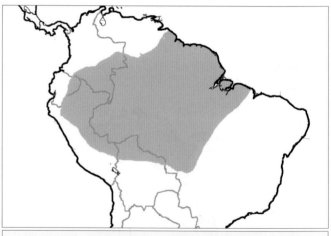

MAP 86. Range of the Brazilian Lancehead, *Bothrops moojeni.*

Venom and Bite: Another large and dangerous lancehead that is responsible for numerous deaths and amputations. "Antibotropico-laquetico" antivenom is manufactured in Brazil.

St. Lucia Lancehead,

Bothrops caribbaeus

Description and Identification: A pale gray, yellowish gray, or reddish pit viper; the only venomous snake on the West Indian island of St. Lucia. Adults average 3 to 4 feet in length, occasional individuals are recorded at about 7 feet.

Head dark gray with a black postocular stripe. Body blotches obscure, little darker than the ground color which is light gray, often with rust red suffusion. Chin white or cream, belly yellowish.

Dorsals strongly keeled, in 25-29 rows at midbody, fewer (19) posteriorly. Ventrals 197-212; subcaudals divided, 64-72.

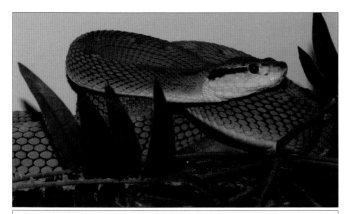

PHOTO 74. St. Lucia Lancehead, *Bothrops caribbaeus*

Distribution, Habitat, and Biology: Found in lowland rainforest, cacao, and coconut plantations. Range restricted to the Caribbean island of St. Lucia.

Venom and Bite: Another large and highly dangerous lancehead that has caused human deaths. "Bothrofav" antivenon produced in France by Sanofi-Pasteur is recommended for treating bites by this species. Myotoxins and haemorragins listed as possibly present.

Jararacussu,

Bothrops jararacussu

Description and Identification: A dull-colored black and yellowish pit viper with a broad, lance-shaped head. Adults average 3 to 4 feet; maximum length about 5.5 feet.

Crown of head *unicolor* black and dark brown with dark yellowish lines over the temporal regions which separate the black postorbital stripe from the dark color of the crown; side of head mostly yellowish.

About 15 pairs of lateral upside-down U-shaped black body blotches may alternate with one another or oppose and connect across the back. Often much of back covered with irregular patches of dark pigment, leaving lateral blotches irregularly outlined with dark yellow. Belly yellow, irregularly blotched with dark brown or black.

Prefrontals (canthals) broader than long, separated from one another by 1-2 rows of small scales. Dorsals strongly keeled, keels tending to be tuberculate along back, in 23-27 rows at midbody, fewer posteriorly.

Ventrals 170-186; subcaudals 44-66 all or nearly all divided.

Distribution, Habitat, and Biology: Found near rivers and streams in southern Brazil, Paraguay, and northern Argentina. This is an amphibious species and may be found in the water. Primarily a lowland species, it is not a very common snake.

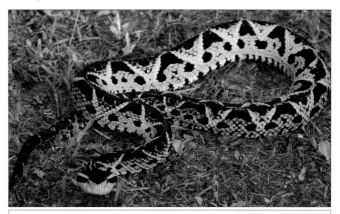

PHOTO 75. Jararacussu, *Bothrops jararacussu*

Venom and Bite: Produces a very toxic venom (perhaps the most toxic of any *Bothrops*), in large amounts (averaging nearly 250 mg. in a milking); it is one of four species of snakes which cause the most fatalities from snakebite in Brazil.

Many polyspecific antivenoms appear to be less than satisfactory in neutralizing this snakes highly toxic venom.

The World Health Organization lists several Antivenoms for treating bites of *B. jararacussa.* All but one are made in Brazil. Instituto Nacional de Produccion de Biologicos in Buenos Aires, Argentina makes "Antiveneno Bothropico." In Brazil Instiudo Butantan in Sao Paulo, Brazil produces "Antibotropico-laquetico," and "Antibotropico Butantan." In addition, the following Brazilian facilities make an antivenom that is listed as useful against the bite of the Jararacussa. Centro de producao e Pesquisas de Immunobiol makes "Antibotropico CPPI," and Fundaco Ezequiel Dias makes "Antibotropico FUNED"

Antibbotropico-laquetico FUNED" and "Antibotropico-Crotalico FUNED."

Venom is principally procoagulants and systemic myotoxins responsible for myonecrosis.

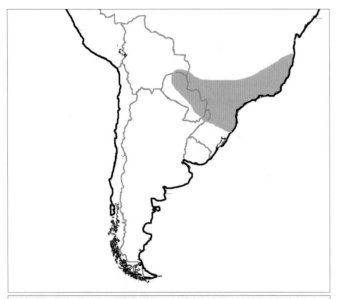

Map 87. Range of the Jararacussu, *Bothrops jararacussu.*

Fer-de-Lance,
Bothrops lanceolatus

Description and Identification: A lancehead recognized by its dark truncated lateral blotches and high numbers of dorsals and ventrals; the only venomous snake on the island of Martinique. Adults average 4 to 5 feet; occasional individuals attain lengths of about 7 feet.

Head brown with a sharply defined darker postorbital band that extends down to the corner of the mouth. Body gray, olive, or brown with an obscure series of 22-27 hourglass shaped blotches down the back. Ventral surface white or cream with a few grayish or brown stipple marks anteriorly, more posteriorly.

Dorsals strongly keeled, in 31-33 rows at midbody, fewer (29) anteriorly and posteriorly (21-23).

Ventrals 215-230; subcaudals divided, 56-67.

Distribution, Habitat and Biology: Although the name "Fer-de-Lance is widely used by lay persons in referring to nearly any tropical lancehead pit viper. The name was originally used for this species, *lanceolatus,* which is found only on the West Indies Island of Martinique. It was formerly found throughout the island but now is restricted to the less inhabited forested regions.

Venom and Bite: This highly dangerous snake has caused many deaths. The specific antivenom "Bothrofav" is produced by Sanofi-Pasteur in France specifically for treating bites by this species.

Known toxins are a mixture of potent procoagulants.

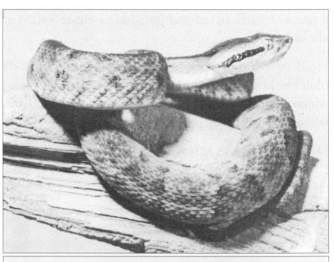

Photo 76. Fer-de-Lance, *Bothrops lanceolatus*

Whitetail Lancehead,
Bothrops leucurus

Description and Identification: This is a large lancehead that may reach 6.5 feet. Four feet is average. Apparently the "white tail" of the Whitetail Lancehead is only evident in young snakes. In color and pattern this species is a typical lancehead with a series of trapezoidal dark blotches on a brown, grayish, or reddish body. Very old specimens are said to sometimes be quite dark (Lamar & Campbell-2004).

Distribution, Habitat, and Biology: A terrestrial species of the eastern coastal forests of Brazil.

Venom and Bite: Little information available. Given its size this is surely a very dangerous snake.

The World Health Organization lists no specific antivenom for this species but Clinical Toxinology Resources webstite lists several of the widely used pit viper antivenoms manufactured in the Americas, including those listed here:

Product: Soro-antibotropico laquetico
Manufacturer: Instituto Butantan
Country of Origin: Brazil
Product: Soro-antibotropico
Manufacturer: Fundaco Ezequiel Dias (FUNED)
Country of Origin: Brazil

Product: Soro Antibiotropico
Manufacturer: Instituto Butantan
Country of Origin: Brazil
Product: Soro-antibotropico-crotalico
Manufacturer: Instituto Butantan
Country of Origin: Brazil
Product: Antivipmyn
Manufacturer: Instituto Bioclon
Country of Origin: Mexico

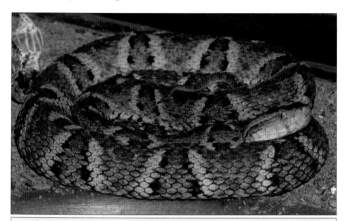

Photo 77. Whitetail Lancehead, *Bothrops leucurus*

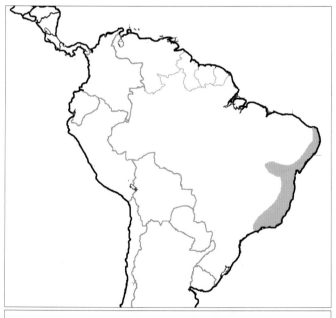

Map 88. Range of the Whitetail Lancehead, *Bothrops leucurus*

Barnett's Lancehead,
Bothrops barnetti

Description and Identification: While these snakes are smaller than some other *Bothrops*, only about 4 to 4 1/2 feet as adults, they are heavy-bodied serpents. The dorsal pattern is typical of most *Bothrops* snakes, with a series of triangular dark blotches on the side (which in this species are dramatically edged in white) with the top of the triangle approaching the top of the back. Ground color is some shade of brown or grayish.

Distribution, Habitat, and Biology: A desert-arid scrub species that occurs in a relatively small region along the coast of northwestern Peru.

Venom and Bite: Little information available. Probably quite dangerous. Antivenoms are the same as for the preceding species.

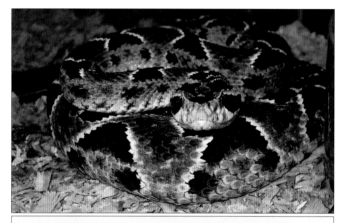

Photo 78. Barnett's Lancehead, *Bothrops barnetti*

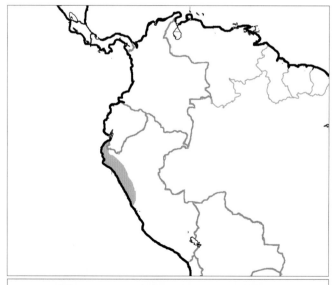

Map 89. Range of the Barnett's Lancehead, *Bothrops barnetti.*

Brazil's Lancehead,
Bothrops brazili

Description and Identification: Ground color brown to reddish brown with a series of darker, hourglass shaped bands across the back. The color and pattern of some specimens is remniscent of the North American Copperhead (*Agkistrodon controtrix*). Unlike most members of the *Bothrops* genus, this species usually lacks a postocular stripe, or if present it is narrow and poorly defined. Average length 2 to 3 feet, maximum nearly 5 feet.

Body stout; 25-27 scale rows at midbody is typical, but may have as few as 23 or as many as 29. Ventrals 151-202; subcaudals 42-68 usually divided.

Distribution, Habitat, and Biology: A rainforest species native to the Amazon basin. This is a terrestrial snake that lives among the damp leaf litter on the floor of the rainforest.

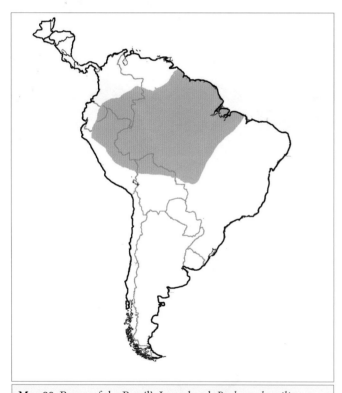

MAP 90. Range of the Brazil's Lancehead, *Bothrops brazili.*

Venom and Bite: The World Health Organization website (viewed 2012) lists a single antivenom for treating bites by this species. Antibiotropico Polyvalente is manufactured by Instituto Nacional de Salud in Peru.

Venom is known to contain procoagulants in the form of fibrogenases.

Venezuelan Lancehead,
Bothrops venezuelensis

Description and Identification: Ground color is brown or brownish gray. Dorsal pattern variable but always with a series of darker transverse, more or less hourglass shaped bands (narrowest vertebrally, widest ventro-laterally). On some specimens the bands are quite distinct while on others the pattern may be obscured by dark stippling. These are fairly large snakes that average about 4 feet as adults and can reach a maximum of 5.5 feet.

Distribution, Habitat and Biology: This species has a relatively small range in northern and central Venezuela. Habitat is lower montane wet forest and cloud forest (Lamar and Campbell 2004).

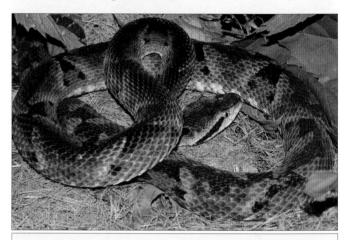

PHOTO 79. Venezuelan Lancehead, *Bothrops venezuelensis*

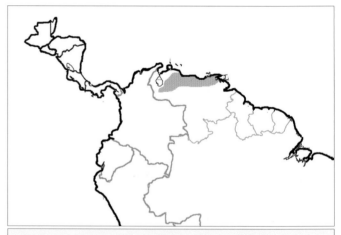

MAP 91. Range of the Venezuelan Lancehead, *Bothrops venezuelensis.*

Venom and Bite: There appears to be little information available on the effects of this species' bite, but it is undoubtably a very dangerous snake.

Additional species: In addition to those species that are described heretofore, there are an additional 14 snakes belonging to the *Bothrops* genus that are found in the USSOUTHCOM region (some experts may recognize more). Most of these omitted species have limited ranges and therefore do not pose a significant snakebite threat. All members of the *Bothrops* genus, however, are dangerous snakes with the potential to kill, and some are quite deadly.

The additional *Bothrops* species not included in the preceding text are:

Bothrops andianus - Andean Lancehead

Bothrops columbiensis - Colombian Lancehead

Botrhops isabelae - Common Lancehead

Bothrops lojanus - Lojan Lancehead

Bothrops osbornei - Osborne's Lancehead

Bothrops muriciensis - Murici Lancehead

Bothrops pictus - Desert Lancehead

Bothrops pirajai - Piraja's Lancehead

Bothrops punctatus - Chocoan Lancehead

Bothrops roedingeri - Roedinger's Lancehead

Bothrops sanctaecrucis - Bolivian Lancehead

Bothrops marmoratus - Marbled Lancehead

Family - Viperidae

Subfamily - Crotalinae: Pit Vipers

Genus - Bothropoides

Neuwiedi Lancehead Vipers

Included by some experts in the *Bothrops* genus, 10 species are recognized in this genus. They are a confusing group from a taxonomic standpoint and further changes may occur in this genus in the future.

Definition: Head broad, flattened, very distinct from narrow neck. Body slender to moderately stout. Tail moderately long, non-*prehensile.*

Scales on top of head small and keeled. Eyes moderate to large in size, elliptical pupil.

Loreal pit present.

Dorsal scales keeled, 19-29 rows at midbody.

Ventrals 139-216. Subcaudals 32-71.

Jararaca,

Bothropoides jararaca

Description and Identification: An olive-green, brown-blotched pit viper with a rather long, but short-snouted head. Adults average 3 to 4 feet; occasional individuals approach 6 feet in length.

Crown of head dark olive, usually with some dark brown irregular markings which may be light-edged. A well defined dark brown post orbital stripe present; remainder of side of head light. About 25 pairs of lateral brown blotches on the body; they are well defined midbody and quite irregular in shape posteriorly. Ground color olive, grayish, or brownish. Belly yellowish, blotched with gray, often entirely gray posteriorly.

Prefrontals small, longer than broad, separated from one another by 4-5 rows of small scales. Dorsals weakly keeled, keels extending entire length of scales, in 20-27 rows at midbody. Ventrals 170-216; subcaudals 51-74, all or nearly all divided.

Distribution, Habitat, and Biology: Grasslands and open country through southern Brazil, northeastern Paraguay, and northern Argentina.

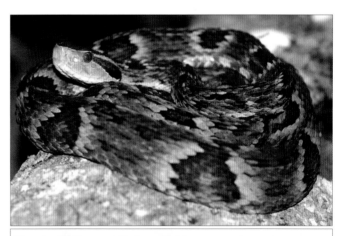

Photo. 80. Jararaca, *Bothropoides jararaca*

Venom and Bite: Venom contains procoagulants (fibrinogenases) and haemorragins. *B. jajaraca* is one of the most common venomous snakes throughout its range. Probably for that reason, rather than because of its venom quantity and toxicity, it is second only to the Cascabel (*Crotalus durissus*) as a source of deaths from snakebite within its range. Several South American antivenoms are listed as effective in treating its bite. Two of those antivenoms are Antibiotropic laquetico and Antibiotropico by Fundacao Ezequiel manufactured in Brazil. Also listed are Polyspecfic Antibiotropic by Institute Butantan (Brazil); Antibothrops Tetravalenta by Instituto Nacional de Microbiologia (Argentina); Soro Antitropico and Soro Antifidico Polyvalente by Instituto Vital Brazil (Brazil).

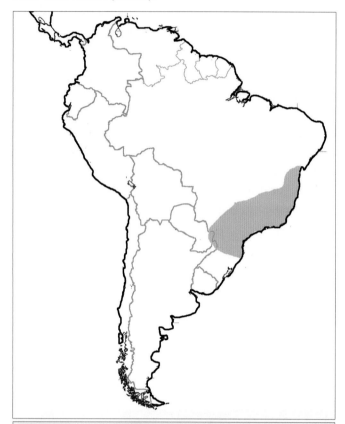

MAP 92. Range of the Jararaca, *Bothropoides jararaca.*

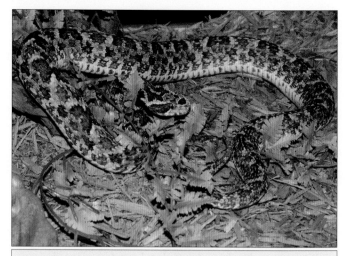

PHOTO 81. Caatinga Lancehead, *Bothropoides erythromelas*

Caatinga Lancehead,
Bothropoides erythromelas

Description and Identification: A medium sized pit viper with a maximum length of about 3 feet.

Body moderately stout; eyes large; broad dark postocular stripe bordered on top by a distinct white or pale line. Ground color is brown to reddish and the typical cryptic pattern of the lancehead vipers is present with a good deal of alternating dark/light mottling in between the dorso-lateral blotches.

Scale rows at midbody 19-21; ventrals 139-158; subcaudals divided, 32-42.

Distribution, Habitat, and Biology: Frequents drier habitats within its range, including thorn forests and dry deciduous woodlands. Reportedly fond of upland, rocky areas. The name Caatinga is derived from a particular eco-region that is endemic to northeastern Brazil.

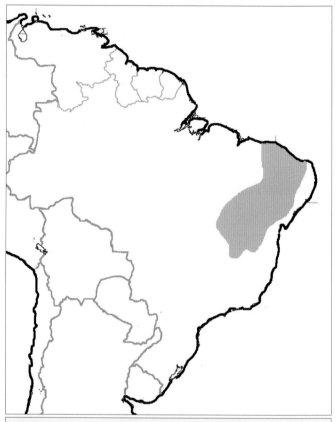

MAP 93. Range of the Caatinga Lancehead, *Bothropoides erythromelas.*

Venom and Bite: Despite its small size relative to most South American lanceheads, this snake is probably capable of killing a human. Lamar and Campbell (2004) report that these snakes are a significant source of snakebites within their range. Venom toxins similar to other *Bothropoides.*

Mato Grosso Lancehead,
Bothropoides mattogrossensis

Description and Identification: A medium-large pit viper reaching a maximum length of just over 4 feet. The ground color is typically some shade of brown and there is a series of darker brown blotches down the center of the back which are narrowest at the top of the back. There are also a series of smaller lateral blotches that match the dorsal blotches in color.

22-27 scale rows at midbody; ventrals 162-187; 37-61 divided subcaudals.

Distribution, Habitat, and Biology: This snake's range coincides with the Brazilian states of Mato Grosso and Mato Grosso del Sur, hence the name. It is also found in Paraguay and Bolivia.

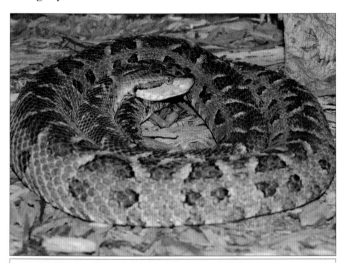

Photo 82. Mato Grosso Lancehead, *Bothropoides mattogrossensis*

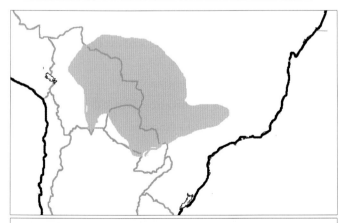

Map 94. Range of the Mato Grosso Lancehead, *Bothropoides mattogrossensis.*

Venom and Bite: There is little information available on the effects of this snake's bite in humans. It is probably a dangerously venomous species.

Jararaca Pintada,
Bothropoides neuwiedi

Description and Identification: A distinctly-patterned tan or grayish pit viper with a distinctive pattern on the crown. Adults average 2 to 3 feet in length.

Crown of head light tan or brown with a series of distinct spots; often a U-shaped mark on the rear part of the head, the two arms of the "U" sometimes connected with the body pattern. Pattern geographically variable but basically a paired series of small triangular or rhomboidal black or dark brown dorsal blotches that alternate or fuse across the back to form small X-shaped markings. Rounded dark spots may fall between mains series on the midline and a lateral series of small spots alternates with the dorsal blotches. All of the markings may be outlined with bright yellow. Ground color tan or light gray. Belly yellowish, some ventrals edged with gray.

Dorsals strongly keeled, in 22-27 rows at midbody. Ventrals 158-185, subcaudals divided, 34-56.

Distribution, Habitat, and Biology: Drier forest habitats are preferred by this species and it is found throughout much of southern Brazil.

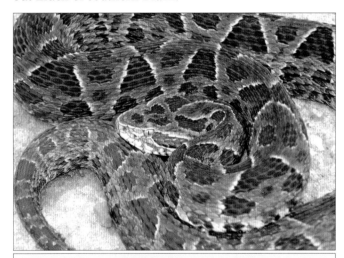

Photo 83. Jararaca Pintada, *Bothropoides neuwiedi*

Venom and Bite: This is a rather small snake but it ranges over a large area of southern Brazil where it is a significant threat to the local populace. Fortunately properly treated bites are not likely to be fatal.

Antivenoms listed for this species are the polyvalent "Antibiotropico" antivenoms made by Instiudo Butantan and Fundaco Ezequiel Diaz (both in Brazil), bivalent "Suero antiofidico bivalente anti-bothropico" by Instituto de Higiene (Uruguay), and "Tropical trivalente" made by Instituto Nacional de Microbiologia in Argentina.

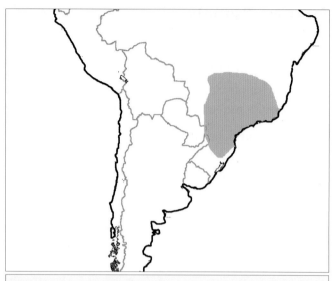

MAP 95. Range of the Jararaca Pintada, *Bothropoides neuwiedi.*

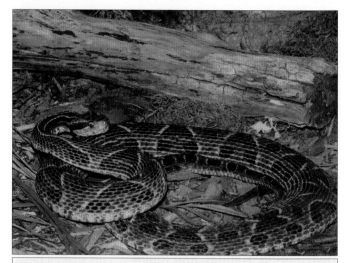

PHOTO 84. Chaco Lancehead, *Bothropoides diporus*

Chaco Lancehead,

Bothropoides diporus

Description and Identification: A medium brown snake with chocolate brown trapezoid dorsal blotches. Easily confused with the Urutu (page 110). Average adult size just under 3 feet, with a maximum of 44 inches.

Distribution, Habitat, and Biology: Found in northern Argentina, eastern Paraguay, and southwestern Brazil. Habitat is humid temperate forests and savanna. Fairly common in suitable habitat.

Venom and Bite: Another highly dangerous species that has been responsible for a significant number of snakebite fatalities.

World Health Organization's list of antivenoms for treating bites by this species (www.int/bloodproducts/snakeantivenoms/database-2012):

Product: Antibiotropico bivalente
Manufacturer: Laboratorio Central de Salud Publica
Country of Origin: Argentina
Product: Antifidico polivalente BIOL
Manufacturer: Instituto Biologico Argentino
Country of Origin: Argentina
Product: Antiveno Bothropico Crotalico
Manufacturer: Instiudo Nacional de Produccion de Biologicos
Country of Origin: Argentina
Product: Antiveno Bothropico Bivalente
Manufacturer: Instiudo Nacional de Produccion de Biologicos
Country of Origin: Argentina
Product: Antiveno Bothropico Tetravalente
Manufacturer: Instiudo Nacional de Produccion de Biologicos
Country of Origin: Argentina

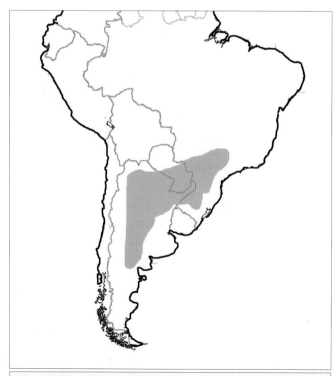

MAP 96. Range of the Chaco Lancehead, *Bothropoides diporus.*

Pampas Lancehead,
Bothropoides pubescens

Description and Identification: Can reach a length of 4 feet. The ground color is gray or brown with dark, light edged trapezoidal or triangular dorsal blotches that are offset on each side of the vertebral line.

Distribution, Habitat, and Biology: Ranges throughout Uruguay and the southernmost region of Brazil (Rio Grande do sul). A terrestrial species of open grasslands. The term "Pampas" refers to a particular habitat that is endemic to South America in northern Argentina, Uruguay, and southern Brazil. It is a largely treeless region where the vegetation is dominated by grasses.

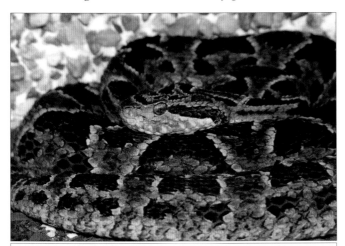

Photo 85. Pampas Lancehead, *Bothropoides pubescens*

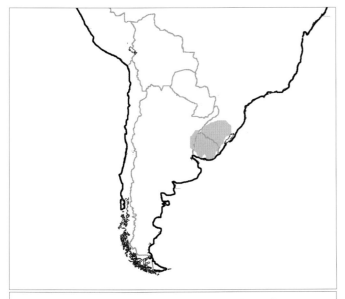

Map 97. Range of the Pampas Lancehead, *Bothropoides pubescens.*

Venom and Bite: Known deaths from the bite of this snake have been recorded in Uruguay.

The World Health Organization lists a single antivenom for treating envenomations by this species.

Product: Antifidico Bivalente Antibothropico
Manufacturer: Instituto de Higiene
Country of Origin: Uruguay

Additional species: Four other *Bothropoides* species are found in South America. Two of these, the Alcatraz Island Lancehead (*B. alcatraz*) and the Golden Lancehead (*B. insularis*) occur on islands off the coast of Brazil and pose little threat to man, though one (*B. insularis*, the Golden Lancehead) is known to have an extremely toxic venom.

In additon to the 2 insular species named above the other 2 species are:

Bothropoides pauloensis - Black-faced Lancehead (southern Brazil and n.w. Paraguay)

Bothropoides lutzi - Cerrado Lancehead (eastern Brazil)

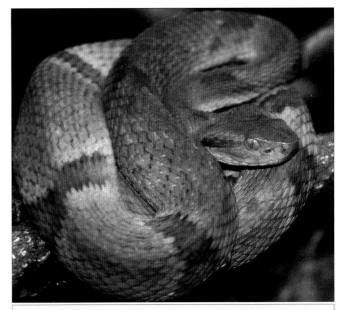

Photo 86. Golden Lancehead, *Bothropoides insularis*

This rare island species is known to exist on a single tiny island off the coast of Brazil (Ilha Quimada Grande). It has perhaps the most toxic venom of any lancehead species.

Family - Viperidae

Subfamily - Crotalinae: Pit Vipers

Genus - Rhinocerophis

Alternatus Lancehead Vipers

The 6 species of this genus are found only in the southern half of South America. One species, *Rhinocerophis ammodytoides* (Patagonian Lancehead) is the world's southernmost venomous snake ranging as far as 47 degrees south latitude.

Dorsal pattern consists of a series of dark blotches that are usually triangular and narrowest vertebrally (except in *R. alternatus* whose pattern is a distinctive sideways "C" shape that is more laterally placed (see Photo 87 on the right), and in *R. ammodytoides* whose pattern is more spotted than blotched. Ground color some shade of brown (grayish, tan, or chocolate).

Head usually has distinct marking and there is a distinct to faded postocular stripe, tail short.

Pupils elliptical, eyes moderate in size, loreal pit present.

Midbody scale rows 23-33 (keeled), ventrals 147-183 subcaudals 25-57

Urutu,

Rhinocerophis alternatus

Description and Identification: A brown lancehead with rounded blotches which are narrowly edged with yellow. Adults average 3-4 feet; occasional individuals exceed 5 feet.

Head brown with distinctive marking on the crown. About 20 pairs of rounded lateral markings shaped like an upside down U whose apices meet on the dorsal midline. Ground color brown, slightly lighter than blotches which have lighter centers.

Dorsals strongly keeled, in 25-35 rows at midbody, ventrals 155-183; subcaudals divided, 30-53.

Distribution, Habitat, and Biology: Along watercourses through southern Brazil, all of Uruguay, eastern Paraguay, and northeastern Argentina.

Venom and Bite: This is a dangerous snake and it causes a large number of bites each year. Ordinarily the bite is not lethal, but it causes severe local effects which if untreated can lead to septicemia and death. The World

Health Organization lists the following antivenoms (all manufactured in Argentina). "Antibiotropica bivalente" by Laboratorio Cnetral de Salud Publica, "Antifidico Polyvalente BIOL" by Instituto Biologico Argentina Argentina, "Antiveneno Bothropico Bivalente" by Instituto Nacional de produccion de Biologicos, and "Anitveneno Bothropico Tetravalente." Anitvenoms effective against this species are also produced in Brazil ("Antibotropico Butantan" by Instituto Butantan) and in Uruguay by Instituto de Higiene ("Antifidico Bivalente Antibothropico").

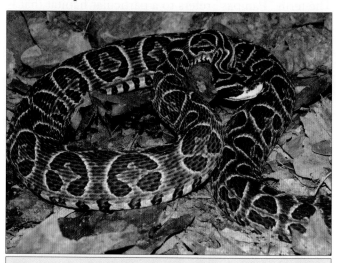

PHOTO 87. Urutu, *Rhinocerophis alternatus*

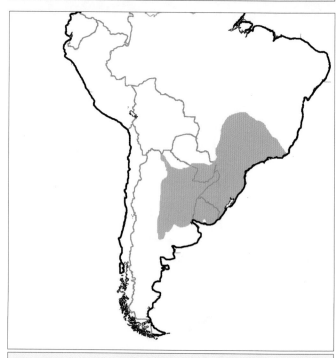

MAP 98. Range of the Urutu, *Rhinocerophis alternatus.*

Patagonian Lancehead,

Rhinocerophis ammodytoides

Description and Identification: Maximum length about 3 feet. Ground color tan or gray with a profusion of small, rounded dark brown spots all along the top of the back and smaller rounded spots on the sides. The appearance is usually of a spotted rather than blotched or banded snake, a condition unusual among the lancehead pit vipers. On some individuals the larger spots on the back may coalesce to form a zigzag vertebral stripe. The distinctly upturned snout may be its most diagnostic characteristic.

Tail short and darker in color, scales keeled in 23-25 rows at midbody. Ventrals 147-160; subcaudals 30-41 (divided).

Distribution, Habitat, and Biology: This is the world's most southerly ranging venomous snake, being found as far south as 43 degrees latitude. Its range is contained entirely within the country of Argentina, where it occurs from the eastern slope of the Andes Mountains to the Atlantic coast. The most temperately adapted of the lancehead pit vipers, its habitat includes the grasslands of the Argentine Pampas and open deciduous shrublands.

Venom and Bite: Despite is small size, this snake may be capable of killing a human. Suggested antivenoms for this species are manufactured in Argentina by Instituto Nacional de Produccion de Biologicos and include "Antiveneno Bothropico Bivalente and Antiveneno Bothropico Tetravalente".

Additional Species: In addition to the Urutu and the Patagonian Lancehead there are at least five more members of the Alternatus Lancehead group (*Rhinocerophis*). Three of these, the Cotiara (*R. cotiara*) and the Fonseca's Lancehead (*R. fonsecai*) resemble the Urutu in color and pattern. Meanwhile the Sao Paulo Lancehead (*R. itapetiningae*) is more similar in pattern to the Patagonian Lancehead. A fifth species, Jonathan's Lancehead, *R. jonathani* is a very rare, newly described species. The ranges of these additional *Rhinocerophis* species is shown below.

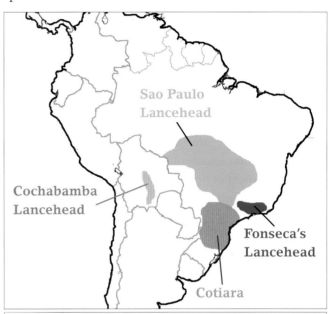

MAP 100. Range of *R. cotiara, R. fonsecai, R. jonathani,* and *R. itapetiningae.*

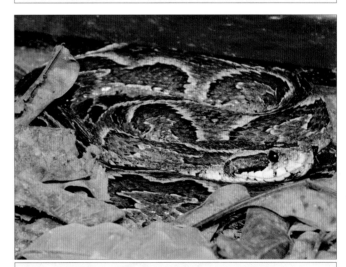

PHOTO 88. Fonseca's Lancehead, *Rhinocerophis fonsecai*

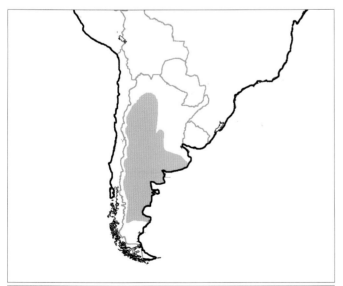

MAP 99. Range of the Patagonian Lancehead, *Rhinocerophis ammodytoides.*

Family - Viperidae

Subfamily - Crotalinae: Pit Vipers

Genus - Cerrophidian

Mountain Pit Vipers

There are five species, three of which are quite rare and have very restricted ranges in southern Mexico (see US-NORTHCOM). One species, *C. godmani* (Godman's Mountain Pit Viper) is fairly common and ranges from southern Mexico into the USSOUTHCOM region in Guatemala. Another species, *C. wilsoni* (Wilson's Mountain Pit Viper) is endemic to Honduras. A third species *C. sasai* (Costa Rican Mountain Pit Viper) is fairly widespread in Central America from El Salvador to western Panama. They are all mountain species that are primarily diurnal in habits.

Definition: These are small to medium sized snakes with a maximum length of about 30 inches. The head is large with a distinct neck. Body is only moderately stout and the tail is short.

Eyes moderate in size, pupils elliptical.

Head Scales: Variable. Some exhibit a few large plates similar to *Agkistrodon* (moccasins) while others have many small head scales remniscent of *Crotalus* (rattlesnakes).

Body scales: There are 17-21 scale rows at midbody. Dorsal scales are moderately keeled. Ventrals 120-150, subcaudals 22-36 (undivided).

A map showing the combined ranges of the *Cerrophidian* species found in the USSOUTHCOM region appears below. For a photograph and information regarding these snakes see Chapter 8, page 49, USNORTHCOM.

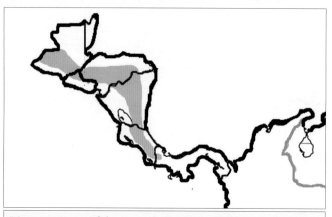

MAP 101. Range of the *Cerrophidian* Mountain Pit Vipers in the USSOUTHCOM region.

Family - Viperidae

Subfamily - Crotalinae: Pit Vipers

Genus - Porthidium

Hognosed Pit Vipers

Most of the nine species of these small to medium sized pit vipers have a distinctive upturned snout. This character is more apparent in some species than others, but all have some degree of "hognosed" appearance. These snakes range from southern Mexico to northern South America. There are five species found within the US-SOUTHCOM region.

Definition: Triangular head very distinct from neck. Body slender to moderately stout. Canthus sharply defined. Rostral scale always higher than wide.

Eyes moderately large, pupil elliptical.

Dorsal scales heavily keeled in 21- 27 rows at midbody. Ventrals 136-176, subcaudals 25-44.

Adult range from about 20 inches to 2.5 feet in length.

The venom of this genus is probably mostly procoagulants and some haemorragins.

Rainforest Hognosed Pit Viper,
Porthidium nasutum

Description and Identification: A small brownish pit viper with a pronounced upturned snout. Average adult size about 18 inches, maximum 2 feet. Ground color is usually some shade of brown (tan, reddish, yellowish), occasionally gray. Dorsal pattern a series of angular dark brown or black blotches on each side of the mid-dorsum.

Body moderately stout, head very distinct from neck, rostral twice as tall as wide.

Dorsal scale rows at midbody 21-25; ventral scales 123-145; subcaudal scales 23-41 (undivided).

Distribution, Habitat, and Biology: This is a terrestrial species that inhabits lowland, tropical rainforests. It is both diurnal and nocturnal in habits. This species ranges from southernmost Mexico (Chiapas and Tabasco) through Central America to northern South America (Colombia and Ecuador).

Venom and Bite: Although the *Porthidium* genus is generally regarded as less dangerous than most Central and South American pit vipers, this species has caused human deaths.

Antivenoms for this species are as follows:

Product: Antivipmyn
Manufacturer: Institudo Bioclon
Country of Origin: Mexico
Product: Polyvalent Antivenom ICP
Manufacturer: Institudo Clodomiro Picado
Coountry of Origin: Costa Rica

From the World Health Organization Venomous Snake Antivenom website (www.who/bloodproducts/snakeantivenoms/database - 2012).

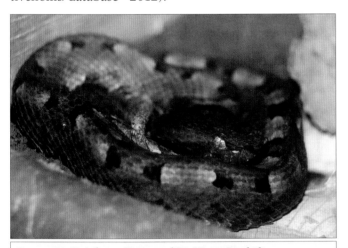

PHOTO 89. Rainforest Hognosed Pit Viper, *Porthidium nasutum*

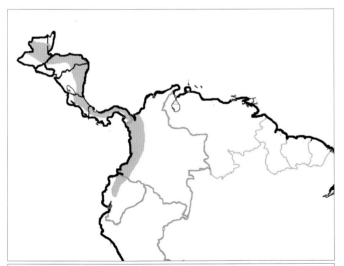

MAP 102. Range of the Rainforest Hognosed Viper, *Porthidium nasutum*, in the USSOUTHCOM region.

Similar species: The Manabi Hognosed Viper *P. arcosae* of the southern coast of Colombia, Lansberg's Hognosed Viper, *P. lansbergii,* of southern Panama, northern Colombia, and northern Venezuela; the Ujaran Hognosed Viper, *P. volcanicum* and the White-tailed Hognosed Viper, *P. porrasi*, of Costa Rico are all very similar to the species described above. Of these, only *P. lansbergii* (below) occupies a large enough range to pose a significant threat of snakebite.

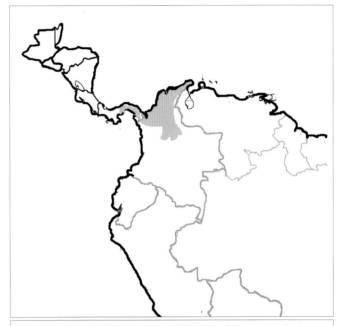

MAP 103. Range of the Lansberg's Hognosed Viper, *Porthidium lansbergii.*

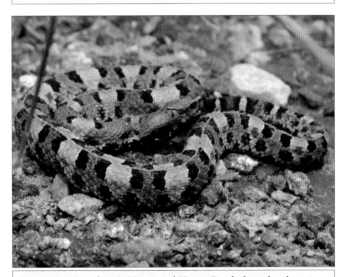

PHOTO 90. Lansberg's Hognosed Viper, *Porthidium lansbergii*

Slender Hognosed Viper,
Porthidium ophryomegas

Description and Identification: An abundant terrestrial pit viper which unlike most other members of its genus has a typical rostral that is not significantly upturned in "hognosed" fashion. This is one of the larger *Porthidium,* reaching a maximum of about 30 inches.

Body moderately slender; ground color brown, tan, or grayish brown. Dorsal pattern a series of dark brown to black dorsal blotches with a light, middorsal stripe.

Midbody scale rows 23-28, ventrals 155-176; subcaudals 32-45 (undivided).

Distribution, Habitat, and Biology: Prefers drier habitats within its range. Rodents, lizards, frogs, and invertebrates are listed as food items by Lamar and Campbell (2004).

Venom and Bite: It is likely not deadly, but bites should be treated cautiously.

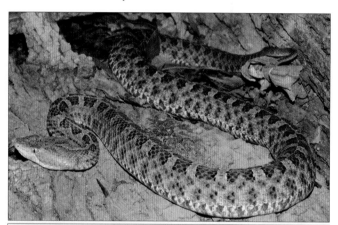

PHOTO 91. Slender Hognosed Viper, *Porthidium ophryomegas*

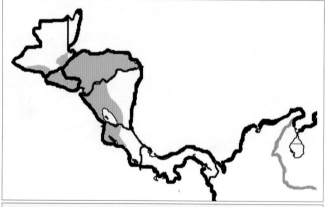

MAP 104. Range of the Slender Hognosed Viper, *Porthidium ophryomegas.*

Family - Viperidae

Subfamily - Crotalinae: Pit Vipers

Genus - Lachesis

Bushmasters

There are 4 species of Bushmasters and all are found in tropical America. They were once all considered to comprise a single species. All 4 species are very similar in appearance and all are treated as one in this account. These are large snakes that attain lengths of 9 to 10 feet, making them the longest of the pit vipers (older reports of 12-14 foot snakes are difficult to verify). Needless to say, they are quite dangerous to man.

Definition: Head broad, very distinct from narrow neck; snout broadly rounded, no canthus. Body cylindrical, tapered, moderately stout; tail short.

Eyes small; pupils vertically elliptical.

Head scales: A pair of small internasals separated from one another by small scales; a pair of narrow supraoculars; other parts of crown covered with very small scales. Laterally, the second supralabial forms the anterior border of the loreal pit, third supraocular very large; eye separated from supralabials by 4-5 rows of small scales.

Body scales: Dorsals heavily keeled with bulbous tubercles, feebly imbricate, in 31-39 nonoblique rows at midbody, fewer posteriorly. Ventrals 191-236; subcaudals mainly paired, 31-56, followed by 13-17 rows of small spines and a terminal spine.

These snakes are unique among the pit vipers of the western hemisphere in that they are egg layers rather than live bearers.

Bushmasters,
Lachesis muta, Lachesis melanocephala,
Lachesis stenophrys, and Lachesis acrochorda

In the original edition of *Poisonous Snakes of the World* (1965) a single species of Bushmaster was recognized.

Description and Identification: These large tan or brown snakes with black or dark brown rhombs are easily recognized. The peculiar burr of pointed spines near the end of the tail is distinctive. Adults average 5 to 7 feet in length; occasional individuals attain a length of 9 feet; a maximum length of 12 feet has been reported (unverified).

Ground color tan, reddish, grayish yellow, creamy, or pinkish with 23-35 black or brown rhombs on body. Markings with light centers; tail dark with light cross-bands. A dark postorbital stripe which continues onto the neck. White or light yellowish below.

Scientists now recognize 4 species of Bushmasters and they are: the South American Bushmaster, *L. muta* (the most widespread), the Chocoan Bushmaster *L. acrochorda* (Panama and northeastern South America), the Black-headed Bushmaster, *L. melanocephala* (western Costa Rica), and *L. stenophrys,* the Central American Bushmaster (Nicaragua through Panama).

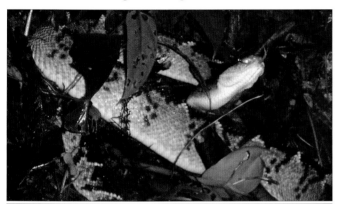

PHOTO 92. Central American Bushmaster, *Lachesis stenophrys*

Distribution, Habitat and Biology: Rainforest and tropical deciduous forest from southern Nicaragua to the coastal lowlands of Ecuador and the Amazon basin of Peru, Bolivia, and Paraguay. Primarily nocturnal in habits adult snakes feed on small and medium sized mammals including rats and marsupials. These are ambush predators that may spend several days (even weeks) quietly coiled amid leaf litter waiting for passing prey. Small mammal burrows and hollow logs may be used as refuge.

Venom and Bite: With the largest fangs of any pit viper and enormous venom glands, the Bushmasters are deadly snakes that kill a high percentage of their victims. The following are Antivenoms listed by the World Health Organization for treating bites by this snake. "Soro Antiboropico-Laquetico" from Instituto Butantan (Sao Paulo, Brazil), "Antifidico Polyvalente" by Labortatorios PROBIOL S.A., in Bogota, Colombia, and "Antilachesico Monovalente," a monospecific antivenom produced by Instituto Nacional de Salud in Lima, Peru.

Bushmaster venom contains a mixture of procoagulants, haemorragins, and possibly myotoxins.

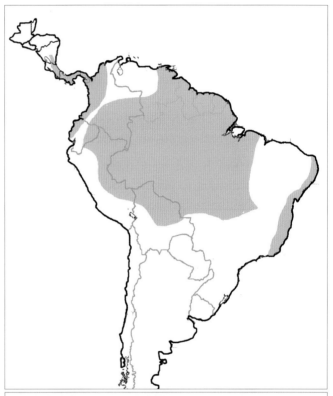

MAP 105. Range of the Bushmasters, *Lachesis species.*

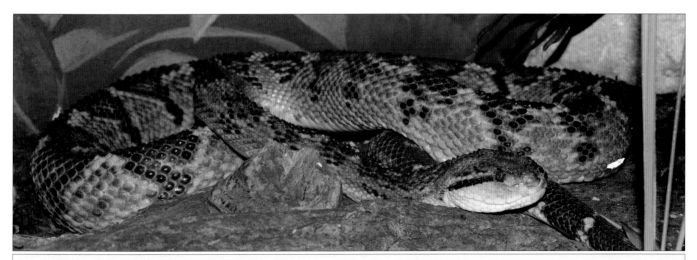

PHOTO 93. South American Bushmaster, *Lachesis muta*

Family - Viperidae

Subfamily - Crotalinae: Pit Vipers

Genus - Crotalus

Rattlesnakes

About 38 species of rattlesnakes are currently recognized. Rattlesnakes are found mostly in North America and Mexico, and only two species (*C. durissus* and *C. simus*) can be found in the USSOUTHCOM region. The South American Rattlesnake (*C. durissus*) is widespread throughout South America from Colombia to Argentina. *C. simus*, the Central American Rattlesnake, occupies northern Central America. Both these rattlesnakes are dangerous animals. Antivipmyn and Tri-Antivipmyn antivenoms by Bioclone of Mexico are effective antivenoms for treating most bites by the Central American Rattlesnake *C. simus*, but the South American Rattlesnake *C. durissus* is a highly dangerous species for which several additional antivenoms are produced.

Definition: Head broad, very distinct from narrow neck, canthus distinct to absent. Body cylindrical, depressed, or slightly compressed, moderately slender to stout; tail short with a horny segmented rattle.

Eyes small, pupils vertically elliptical.

Head scales: Supraoculars present, a pair of internasals often distinct, occasionally a pair of prefrontals; enlarged canthal scales often present; other parts of crown covered with small scales. Laterally , eye separated from supralabials by 1-5 rows of small scales.

Body scales: Dorsals keeled, with apical pits, in 19-33 non-oblique rows at midbody. Ventrals 132-206, subcaudals 13-45, all single or with some terminal ones paired.

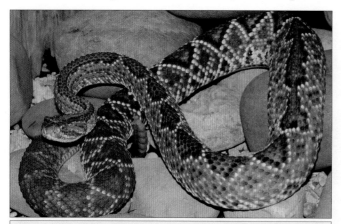

Photo 94. South American Rattlesnake, *Crotalus durissus- subspecies terrificus*

South American Rattlesnake,

Crotalus durissus

Description and Identification: This is the only rattlesnake species found in South America, but it is highly variable and there are a total of 11 subspecies recognized. Several of these subspecies, including *C. vegrandis*, the "Uracoan Rattlesnake," and *C. unicolor,* the "Aruba Island Rattlesnake" are regarded by some experts as distinct species. Throughout much of its range this species is often known by its Spanish name, "Cascabel."

The series of large rhombic blotches (diamonds) down the back, stripes on the neck, and the large rattle are distinctive. Body stout and slightly compressed, especially anteriorly. Adults average 4 to 5 feet; maximum length about 6 feet.

Body brown or olive with 18-32 darker, light edged rhomb-shaped markings down the back. Those on neck sometimes elongate into stripes. Tail usually *unicolor* dark brown or black. White or cream colored below.

Scale rows at midbody usually 27. Dorsal scales along the top of the back are exceptionally heavily keeled, with the keels forming a tubercular shape, especially anteriorly. There are 155-190 ventral scales and 25-32 mostly undivided subcaudals.

Distribution, Habitat, and Biology: These widespread snakes are found in every South American country except Ecuador and Chile. Dry areas, grasslands, and thorny scrub are the preferred habitats. Some subspecies inhabit dry forested regions where their overall color becomes darker.

Venom and Bite: The South American Rattlesnakes are one of the few pit vipers to possess a neurotoxic venom in the form of *pre-synaptic* neurotoxins. Other pathologies of the venom are secondary nephrotoxicity and secondary myotoxicity. This is one of the most dangerous of the rattlesnakes and is one of the most dangerous snakes in the Americas. The toxicity of the venom varies throughout its large range. In Brazil, where it is the main cause of death from snakebite, it is extremely toxic. The venom of this rattlesnake has minor local effect but very grave systemic symptoms. These include blindness, paralysis of the neck muscles, cessation of breathing and heartbeat, and finally, death.

Specific antivenoms are "Anticrotalico Butantan" (Institudo Butantan, Brazil), "Anticrotalico FUNED (Fundacao Ezequiel Dias, Brazil), "Antiveno Crotalico" (Instituto Nacional de produccion de Biologicos, Argentina), and "Anticrotalico IVB" by Instituto Vital Brazil S.A. (Brazil).

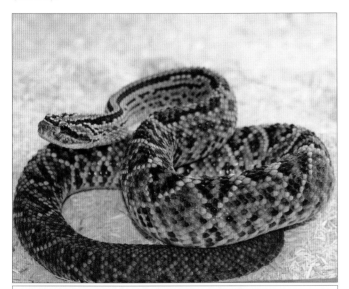

PHOTO 95. South American Rattlesnake, *Crotalus durissus-subspecies durissus*, "Neotropical Rattlesnake"

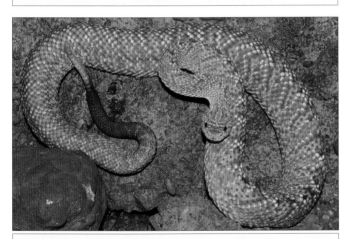

PHOTO 96. South American Rattlesnake, *Crotalus durissus subspecies vegrandis*, "Uracoan Rattlesnake"

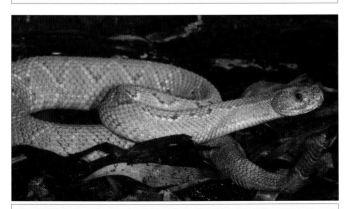

PHOTO 97. South American Rattlesnake, *Crotalus durissus*, subspecies unicolor, "Aruba Island Rattlesnake"

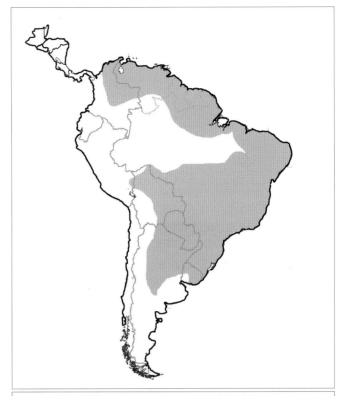

MAP 106. Range of the South American Rattlesnake, *Crotalus durissus.*

Middle American Rattlesnake,
Crotalus simus

Description and Identification: A large, stout bodied rattlesnake that can reach a length of up to 6 feet (average 4-5). One of the most characteristic features of this rattlesnake are the tubercle-like keels of the vertebral scales, which produce a pronounced ridge along the spine (especially anteriorly). In this respect it is similar to the South American Rattlesnake and was in fact once considered to be a subspecies of that snake. The dorsal markings consist of a "diamondback" pattern. The ground color is brownish or grayish with hues of red, yellow, greenish, blue-gray, or orange.

Scale rows at midbody 25-33; ventrals 170-191; subcaudals 18-26, mostly undivided.

Distribution, Habitat, and Biology: Ranges through most of Central America from southern Mexico southward to Costa Rica. Prefers drier habitats in mountain pine forests, savannas, and scrub.

Venom and Bite: Like the preceding species, *C. simus* venom contains *pre-synaptic* neurotoxins and like the preceding species, this is a large and highly dangerous snake.

World Health Organizations Venomous Snake Antivenoms Database list of antivenoms for treating bites by this species: (www.int/bloodproducts/snakeantivenoms/database-2012).

Product: Antivipmyn
Manufacturer: Instituto Bioclon
Country of Origin: Mexico
Product: Polyvalent Antivenom ICP
Manufacturer: Instituto Clodomiro Picado
Country of Origin: Costa Rica

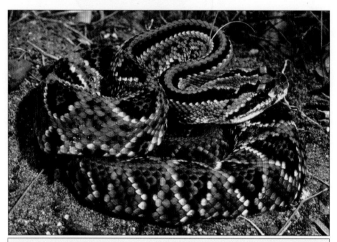

Photo 98. Middle American Rattlesnake, Crotalus simus

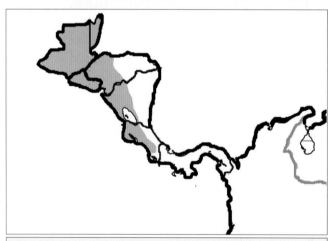

Map 107. Range of the Middle American Rattlesnake, Crotalus simus in the USSOUTHCOM region.

Current References

Books

Campbell, Jonathan A. and William W. Lamar. 2004. *Venomous Reptiles of the Western Hemisphere* 2 Vols. Cornell University Press. Ithaca, NY.

Dowling, Herndon G., Sherman A. Minton, and Findlay E. Russell. 1965. *Poisonous Snakes of the World.* Department of the Navy Bureau of Medicine and Surgery. Washington, DC.

Lee, Julien C. 1996. *The Amphibians and Reptiles of the Yucatan Peninsula.* Cornell University Press.

Ithaca, NY.

Roze, Janis A. 1996. *Coral Snakes of the Americas. Biology, Identification, and Venoms.* Krieger Publishing. Malabar, FL.

Rubio, Manny. 1998. *Rattlesnake, Portrait of a Predator.* Smithsonian Instituion Press. Washington, D.C.

Journals

Carrasco, Paola A., Camilo I. Mattoni, Gerardo C. Leynaud & Gustav J. Scrocchi. 2012. "Morphology, phylogeny, and taxonomy of South Amereican bothropoid pitvipers (Serpentes, Viperidae)." Zoologica Scripta 41, 2, 109-124.

Websites

The University of Adelaide - Clinical Toxinology Resouces Website (2012) - www.toxinology.com

The Reptile Database - http//www.reptile-database.org

Armed Forces Pest Management Board - www.afpmb.org/content/living-hazards-database

World Health Organization - www.who.int/bloodproducts/snakeantivenoms/database

www.faunaparaguay.com

The MAVIN Antivenom Index - www.toxininfo.org/antivenoms/index

Original References

PICADO, C. 1931. Serpientes venenosas de Costa Rica. Imprenta Alsina, San Jose, Costa Rica: 219 p., 58 figs.

SCHMIDT, Karl P. 1933. Preliminary Account of the Coral Snakes of Central America and Mexico. Zool. Ser. Field Mus. Nat. Hist., 20: 29–40.

SCHMIDT, Karl P. 1936. Notes on Central American and Mexican Coral Snakes. Zool. Ser. Field Mus. Nat. Hist., 20 (20) : 205–216, figs. 24–27.

SCHMIDT, Karl P. 1941. The Amphibians and Reptiles of British Honduras. Zool. Ser. Field Mus. Nat. Hist., vol. 22, no. 8, pp. 475–510.

ALVAREZ del TORO, Miguel 1960. Los reptiles de Chiapas. Inst. Zool. Estado, Tuxtla Gutierrez, Chiapas, Mexico. 7–204 p., illustrated.

BURGER, W. Leslie 1950 A Preliminary Study of the Jumping Viper, *Bothrops nummifer*. Bull. Chicago Acad. Sci., 9 (3) : 59–67, 1 pl.

CLARK, Herbert C. 1942 Venomous Snakes. Some Central American Records. Incidence of Snake-bite Accidents. Amer. Jour. Tropical Med., 22 (1) : 37–49.

MERTENS, Robert. 1952. Die Amphibien und Reptilien von El Salvador, auf Grund der Reisen von R. Mertens und A. Zilch. Abh. Senckenbergischen Ges., 487: 1–120, 16 pls.

SCHMIDT, Karl P. 1955. Coral Snakes of the Genus *Micrurus* in Colombia. Fieldiana-Zool., 34 (34) : 337–359, figs. 65–69.

SMITH, Hobart M., and E. H. TAYLOR. 1945. An Annotated Checklist and Key to the Snakes of Mexico. Bull. U. S. Natl. Mus. (187) : 1–239 p.

STUART, L. C. 1963. A Checklist of the Herpetofauna of Guatemala. Misc. Pub. Mus. Zool. Univ. Michigan (122) : 1–150, 1 pl., 1 map.

TAYLOR, Edward H. 1951. A Brief Review of the Snakes of Costa Rica. Univ. Kansas Sci. Bull., 34 (part 1, no. 1) : 3–88, figs. 1–7, pls. 1–23.

AMARAL, Afranio do. 1925. A General Consideration of Snake Poisoning and Observations on Neotropical Pit-Vipers. Contr. Harvard Inst. Tropical Biol. Med., 2: 64 p., 16 pls.

AMARAL, Afranio do. 1930. Lista remissiva dos ophidios da regiao neotropica. Mem. Inst. Butantan, 4: 127–271.

DUNN, Emmett R. 1944. Los genereos de anfibios y reptiles de Colombia, III. Tercera Parte: Reptiles; orden de las serpientes. Caldasia, 3 (12) : 155–224.

FONSECA, Flavio da. 1949. Animais peconhentos. Publ. Inst. Butantan, Sao Paulo. 376 p., 129 figs., 13 color pls.

HOGE, Alphonse R. 1965. Preliminary Account on Neotropical Crotalinae (Serpentes, Viperidae). Mem. Inst. Butantan 32:109–184, pls. 1–20, maps 1–10.

LAZELL, James D., Jr. 1964. The Lesser Antillean Representatives of *Bothrops* and *Constrictor*. Bull. Mus. Comp. Zool., 132 (3) : 245–273, figs. 1–5.

MOLE, R. R. 1924. The Trinidad Snakes. Proc. Zool. Soc. London: 235–278, pls. 1–10.

PETERS, James A. 1960. The Snakes of Ecuador: A Check List and Key. Bull. Mus. Comp. Zool., 122 (9) : 491–541.

ROZE, Janis A. 1955. Revision de las corales (Serpentes: Elapidae) de Venezuela. Acta Biol. Venezuelica, 1 (art. 17) : 453–500, 4 figs. (2 color).

ROZE, Janis A. 1966. La Taxonomia y Zoogeografia de los ofidios de Venezuela. Universidad Central de Venezuela, Caracas. 362 pp. 79 figs., 80 maps.

SANDNER MONTILLA, F. 1965. Manual de las serpientes ponzonosas de Venezuela. (Pub. by author) Caracas. 108 p. 69 figs., 9 col. pls.

SANTOS, Eurico. 1955. Anfibios e repteis do Brasil (vida e costumes). 2nd ed. F. Briguiet & Cia., Rio de Janeiro. 262 p., 65 figs., 10 color pls.

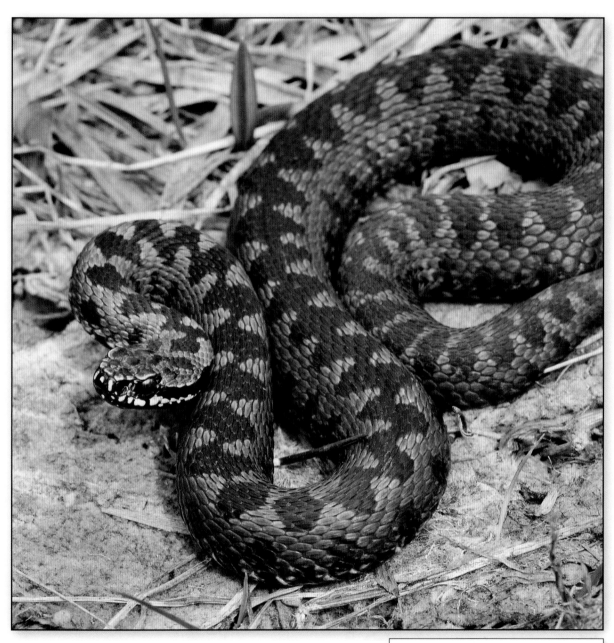

European Viper, *Vipera berus*

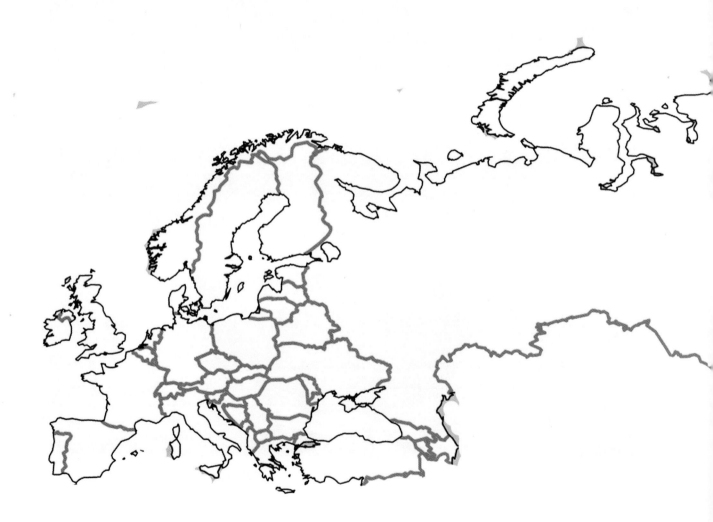

CHAPTER **10**

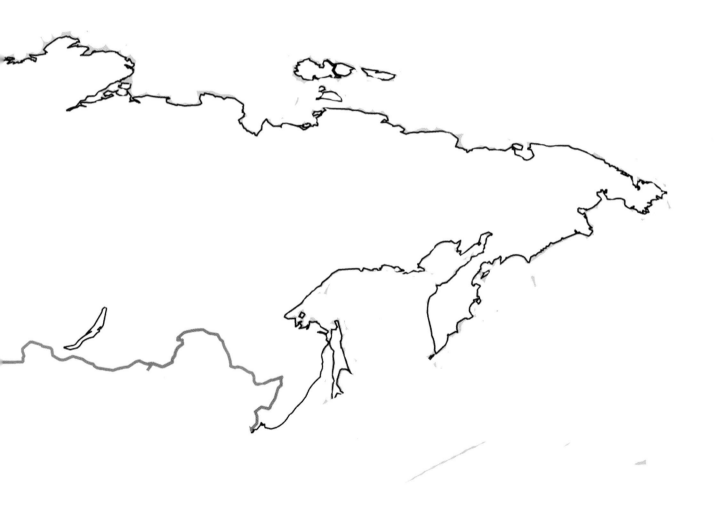

MAP 108. Region 3, The United States European Command.

Introduction

Despite the fact that this region contains a huge land mass (all of Europe and Russia, plus Turkey and the Caucasus), it has a relative paucity of venomous snake species. There are only 31 venomous snakes found here (not counting two species belonging to the mainly harmless families Colubridae and Lamprophiidae whose bites have caused pronounced symptoms of envenomation).

In Europe and Russia, the generally cool present day climate, the scarcity of habitat for snakes, and the geological history of glaciation that eliminated all reptiles from much of the region some 10,000 to 20,000 years ago, has created an area of the world that has comparatively few snake species. Many of the species found in the USEUCOM region have ranges that barely enter into the region in areas like the Caucasus or extreme southeastern Russia. Thus, in much of Europe and western Russia there are but a handful of venomous snakes, and only a few are widespread.

All the venomous snakes of Europe and western Russia present a strikingly similar appearance. They are small to medium sized snakes of moderately stout build and short tails. All are easily recognized by the presence of an elliptical pupil.

By far the largest group of venomous snakes in this region are the "vipers," family Viperidae, subfamily Viperinae, represented by 26 species, although only a few of these have extensive ranges. There are three genera of vipers in the region covered by this chapter, the largest being the genus *Vipera* with 21 species, 19 of which are found in the USEUCOM region. The second largest group (with 6 total species, 4 in the region) are the *Montivipera* vipers that are found mostly in Turkey and the Caucasus, and the *Macrovipera* vipers with only 2 total

species, both of which are in the USEUCOM region and one of those is restricted to a few small islands in the Mediterranean Sea.

The pit viper subfamily of vipers (Crotalinae) is represented by 5 species belonging to a single genus, *Gloydius.* Primarily an Asian genus with 12 total species, 4 of the *Gloydius* found in this region are in eastern Russia only. One species however is wide-ranging in the region. Usually known by the common name "Mamushi" these pit vipers are similar morphologically to the Moccasins (*Agkistrodon*) of North and South America.

There is but one member of the cobra family (Elapidae) found in the USEUCOM region (the Desert Cobra), and its range in this region is restricted to a small area in Turkey.

There are two other genera of snakes in this region whose bites range from mildly venomous to possibly life threatening. They are the Montpeliar Snake (*Malpolon-* family Lamprophiidae) and the Keelbacks (*Rhabdophis-* family Colubridae). Neither are regarded as a significant threat to man and are not included in this book.

The map below shows the area contained in the USEUCOM region covered in this chapter.

The venomous snakes of this region are well studied, particularly in Europe, and much has been written about their natural history and the effects of their venoms. Most European species are not highly dangerous to man, though some do rarely cause deaths.

More recently, the impact of centuries of human alteration of natural habitats has caused significant declines in the populations of many species, and most snake populations in Europe and the Caucasus are in decline. Many are now endangered.

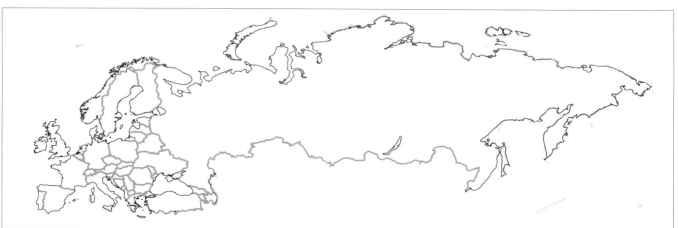

MAP 109. Region 3, United States European Command. All of Europe and Russia, plus Turkey, Armenia, Georgia, and Azerbaijan.

Family - Viperidae

Subfamily - Viperinae -True Vipers

Genus -Vipera

True Adders

The genus *Vipera* contains a minimum of 20 species and some experts recognize up to 23. At least 18 species are found in USEUCOM region. These "True Adders" are the only venomous snakes in most of Europe, western Russia, and the Mediterranean region. With the exception of a few species they are restricted to this region. Two species range into north Africa, another is endemic to Iran, and 2 more have ranges that reach into the US-CENTCOM region.

Definition: Head broad; distinct from narrow neck; canthus distinct. Body cylindrical, varying from moderately slender to stout; tail short.

Eyes moderate in size to small; pupils vertically elliptical.

Body scales: Dorsals keeled with apical pits in 19 to 23 nonoblique rows at midbody. Ventrals rounded 114 to 170; subcaudals paired , 18-49. Anal scute not divided.

Most Vipera are relatively small snakes and although several species are known to have caused human fatalities, deaths from their bites are not common.

Many members of this genus are remarkably similar in appearance, especially so to the untrained eye. Most species exhibit similar markings, patterns, and colors. To add to the confusion, several species have numerous subspecies and many may display more than one color scheme even among individuals within the same population. The easiest way to begin the task of identifying *Vipera* snakes is by consulting the range maps and eliminating all those species not found within the area where the snake in question has been seen. This tactic works well with many species which have small ranges, if not for those more widespread species such as the European Viper (*V. berus*).

European Viper,

Vipera berus

Description and Identification: Head distinct from neck but ovoid rather than distinctly triangular; snout blunt, flat, not upturned; top of head with 5 large smooth shields.

Ground color pale gray, olive, or yellow to russet or brown, the darker colors generally in males. Down the entire length of the back runs a black or dark brown zigzag line rarely broken into spots for all or part of its length and even more rarely straight edged. Top of head behind eyes with a dark "X" or chevron-mark. Belly pale gray with darker suffusion. Uniformly black or very dark brown individuals are often seen, especially in some mountainous regions. At least 3 subspecies (sometimes 4 or more) are recognized.

Average length 20 to 24 inches. Maximum 3 feet; females larger than males.

Distribution, Habitat, and Biology: This is the only venomous snake found in northern Europe but it is widely distributed there and is in fact the most northerly ranging venomous snake in the world, being found even within the Arctic Circle. It also has an extreme east west distribution, ranging from 5 to 145 degrees east longitude (Great Britain to southeastern Russia) making it the most widely distributed venomous snake in the USEU-COM region. It is also found in parts of the USCENT-COM and USPACOM regions. In central and southern Europe is largely confined to mountains where it occurs to at least 9,000 feet elevation. It is the only venomous snake in Great Britain. In northernmost areas of their range they may hibernate for 7 months of the year.

Nocturnal in habits during warm weather; diurnal in cool; has considerable tolerance for cold and has been seen basking near patches of snow. Disposition usually timid, but strikes quickly and repeatedly if provoked. Hisses audibly when threatened.

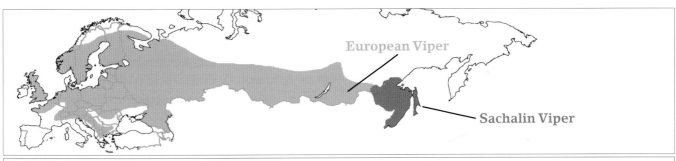

Map 110. Range of the European Viper, *V. berus*, and the Sachalin Viper, *V. sachalinensis* in USEUCOM region.

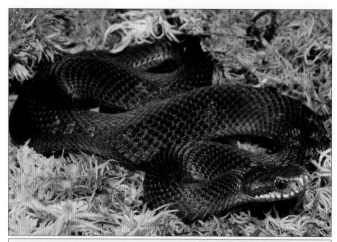

PHOTO 99. European Viper, *Vipera berus*, Melanistic phase

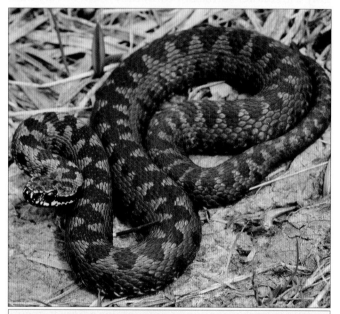

PHOTO 100. European Viper, *Vipera berus*, Typical zigzag phase

Venom and Bite: The European Viper is a fairly common snake in northern Europe where it is responsible for a large number of snakebites (a 1995 study in Sweden revealed 231 bites in that country alone). The venom is primarily haemotoxic, and recorded deaths from myocardial infarction following bites suggests the possibility of a cardiotoxin in some populations. Although deaths have been recorded, the European Viper is not generally regarded as being deadly to a healthy adult who receives medical treatment. They can pose a significant threat to small children however.

The venom is probably procoagulants and haemorragins. Small amounts of neurotoxins may also be present, but they are apparently not clinically significant.

World Health Organization list of antivenoms for treating bites by this species (www.int/bloodproducts/snakeantivenoms/database-2012):

Product: Viper Venom Antitoxin (polyvalent).

Manufacturer: Institute of Virology, Vaccine and Sera TORLAK

Country of Origin: Serbia

Product: Viper venom antitoxin European (polyvalent)

Manufacturer: Immunoloski Zavod

Country of Origin: Croatia

Product: Viperfav (polyvalent)

Manufacturer: Sanofi-Pastuer

Country of Origin: France

Product: Anti-viper (anti-adder) venom (monovalent)

Manufacturer: Federal State Company for Immunobiological Medicines

County of Origin: Russia

Product: Viper Venom Antitoxin (monovalent).

Manufacturer: Biomed

Country of Origin: Poland

Similar Species: The Sakhalin Island Viper, *V. Sakhalinensis* is a similar species regarded by some as a subspecies of *V. berus*. It inhabits extreme southeastern Russia and Sakhalin Island off the Pacific coast of Russia.

Portuguese Viper,

Vipera seoanei

Description and Identification: Very similar to the European Viper, but with a larger head. Ground color gray or brown. The dark middorsal stripe varies from wavy, zig-zag, or broad with irregular edges. Nearly solid black individuals are known.

Distribution, Habitat, and Biology: Found only in the northern part of the Iberian Peninsula and extreme southwest France. Lives in both woodlands and meadows from sea level to about 4,500 feet. Fond of rocky slopes. Micro-habitats include hedgerows and stone walls / fences. Feeds on rodents and lizards.

Venom and Bite: Although this species has the potential to cause human fatalities, there is no specific antivenom available and no antivenom recommended by the World

Health Organization. The venom is primarily haemotoxic and probably has both procoagulant and hemorrhagic properties. Polyvalent antivenoms produced for other European *Vipera* may have some efficacy in treating bites by this species.

List of polyvalent antivenoms that may be useful in treating bites by the Portuguese Viper:

Product: Viper Venom Antitoxin (polyvalent)

Manufacturer: Institute of Virology, Vaccine and Sera TORLAK

Country of Origin: Serbia

Product: Viper venom antitoxin European (polyvalent*)*

Manufacturer: Immunoloski Zavod

Country of Origin: Croatia

Product: Viperfav (polyvalent*)*

Manufacturer: Sanofi-Pastuer. Country of Origin: France

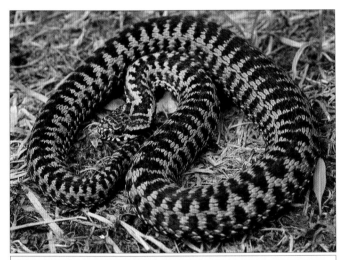

PHOTO 101. Portuguese Viper, *Vipera seoanei*

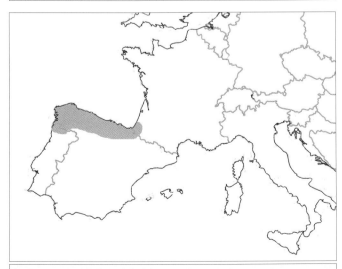

MAP 111. Range of the Portuguese Viper, *Vipera seoanei.*

Asp Viper,
Vipera aspis

Description and Identification: Head more triangular than in European Viper, snout slightly but distinctly upturned at the tip. Shields on crown fragmented, usually only 2 or 3 enlarged.

Color similar to European Viper but generally more apt to be reddish or brown. Dorsal pattern of dark spots more or less fused into narrow bars across the back, sometimes forming zigzag band; dark head mark not well defined; belly dark gray with lighter flecks; underside of tail tip yellow or orange.

Size about the same as European Viper, averaging about 24 inches; females average larger than males and really large individuals may reach nearly 3 feet.

Distribution, Habitat, and Biology: Found in southeastern Europe from the Pyrenees Mountains of northern Spain across most of the southern two-thirds of France, western Switzerland, and most of Italy. Prefers dry hilly areas at lower elevations but also ranges up to 9,000 feet in the Pyrenees. Diurnal in cool weather and nocturnal in warm weather.

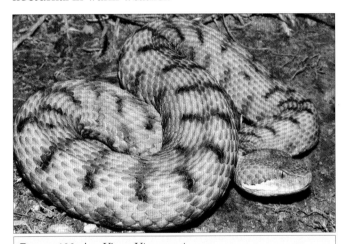

PHOTO 102. Asp Viper, *Vipera aspis.*

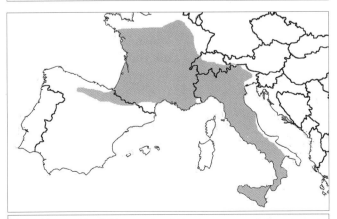

MAP 112. Range of the Asp Viper, *Vipera aspis.*

Venom and Bite: The venom of *V. aspis* is primarily hemotoxic with procoagulants and haemorragins probably present. One recent study suggests that there is a neurotoxic component in at least some populations (Ferquel et al 2007). Antivenom is frequently required in treating bites and the fatality rate is probably about 1 percent.

World Health Organization list of antivenoms for treating bites by this species (www.int/bloodproducts/snakeantivenoms/database-2012):

Product: Viper Venom Antitoxin (polyvalent)
Manufacturer: Institute of Virology, Vaccine and Sera TORLAK
Country of Origin: Serbia
Product: Viper venom antitoxin European (polyvalent)
Manufacturer: Immunoloski Zavod
Country of Origin: Croatia
Product: Viperfav (polyvalent)
Manufacturer: Sanofi-Pastuer
Country of Origin: France

Similar Species: The Anatolian Steppe Viper, *V. anatolica* is considered a member of the Asp Viper complex but now enjoys full species status. It is found only in a small area within the Anatolian region of Turkey.

Snub-nosed Viper,
Vipera latastei

Description and Identification: Similar to the European Viper but snout more upturned and pointed, shield of crown much fragmented and usually not symmetrical. Also similar to the Long-nosed Viper but on that species the upturned snout is more pronounced and its anterior surface is covered by numerous small scales rather than having its anterior surface formed only from the rostral. Neither of these two similar species are found on the Iberian Peninsula. Adults average 20 inches with a maximum of 30 inches.

Distribution, Habitat, and Biology: In the USEUCOM region this species is restricted to the Iberian Peninsula where it is widespread south of the Pyrenees Mountains. It is also found across the strait of Gibraltar in northern Africa. It prefers drier habitats on dry rocky hillsides or open forests. Ranges from near sea level to over 5,000 feet.

Venom and Bite: There seems to be little information available on the venom of this species, although its bite has caused death it is not generally regarded as highly dangerous to man. There is no specific antivenom available, but it is likely that some of the polyvalent *Vipera* antivenoms produced in Europe would be effective in treating severe bites.

List of polyvalent antivenoms likely to have some cross reactivity with Vipera latastei venom.

Product: Viper Venom Antitoxin (polyvalent)
Manufacturer: Institute of Virology, Vaccine and Sera TORLAK
Country of Origin: Serbia
Product: Viper venom antitoxin European (polyvalent)
Manufacturer: Immunoloski Zavod
Country of Origin: Croatia
Product: Viperfav (polyvalent)
Manufacturer: Sanofi-Pastuer
Country of Origin: France

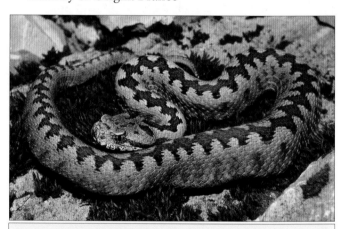

Photo 103. Snub-nosed Viper, *Vipera latastei*

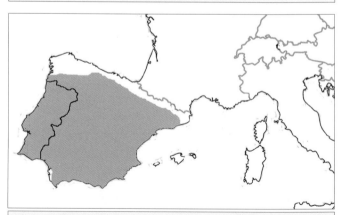

Map 113. Range of the Snub-nosed Viper, *Vipera latastei*, in the USUECOM region.

Long-nosed Viper,
Vipera ammodytes

Description and Identification: Most readily identified by the snout which terminates in a strongly upturned appendage, its anterior surface formed from several small scales (rather than by the single rostral scale). The crown is covered by small scales of irregular size and arrangement.

Color ash-gray, yellow, pale orange, coppery, or brownish; zig-zag dorsal line very prominent; pattern more vivid in male; head without distinct dorsal markings; belly yellow or brownish more or less heavily clouded with dark gray; tail tip orange or reddish. There are at least 4 subspecies of *V. ammodytes,* and some experts recognize more.

This is the largest viper in Europe; average length 25 to 30 inches; maximum about 40 inches.

Distribution, Habitat, and Biology: Ranges across much of southern Europe from northern Italy to Georgia. A primarily terrestrial species that may sometimes climb into small bushes. Mainly nocturnal. Fond of arid or semi-arid habitats and open slopes with rocky outcrops. Ranges from low plains up to over 7,000 feet in elevation.

Usually described as sedentary and retiring but quick to strike if molested or aroused.

Venom and Bite: Long-nosed Vipers possess a toxic venom and proportionately long fangs and they are regarded as the most dangerous of the European vipers.

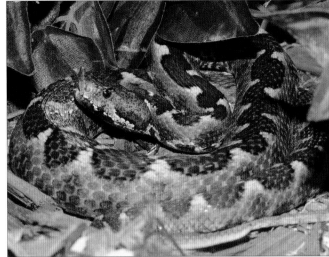

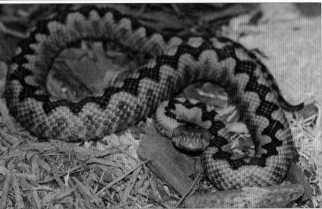

PHOTOS 104 & 105. Long-nosed Viper, *Vipera ammodytes*. Red phase (top) gray phase (bottom).

Uniquely for a European viper, the venom is known to include pre-synaptic neurotoxins. Numerous deaths from the bite of this snake have been recorded.

World Health Organization's Venomous Snake Antivenoms Database list of antivenoms for treating bites by this species (www.who.int/bloodproducts/snakeantivenoms/database-2012):

> Product: Viper Venom Antitoxin (polyvalent)
>
> Manufacturer: Institute of Virology, Vaccine and Sera TORLAK
>
> Country of Origin: Serbia
>
> Product: Viper venom antitoxin European (polyvalent)
>
> Manufacturer: Immunoloski Zavod
>
> Country of Origin: Croatia
>
> Product: Viperfav (polyvalent)
>
> Manufacturer: Sanofi-Pastuer
>
> Country of Origin: France

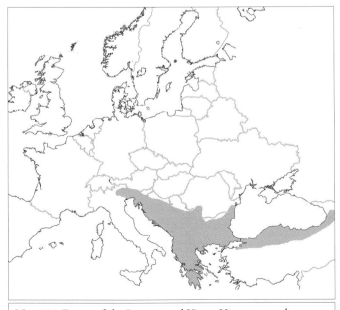

MAP 114. Range of the Long-nosed Viper, *Vipera ammodytes.*

Transcaucasian Viper,
Vipera transcaucasiana

Description and Identification: Rostral scale raised into pronounced nasal horn makes this snake very similar to the preceding species and some consider it to be a subspecies of *Vipera ammodytes*. Dorsal pattern consists of narrow dark bars that are slightly offset on each side of the vertebral line. Ground color grayish or reddish.

Distribution, Habitat, and Biology: A rare species found in parts of the Caucasus region.

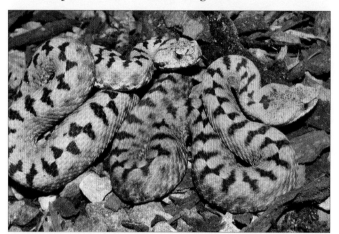

Photo 106. Transcaucasian Viper, *Vipera transcaucasiana*

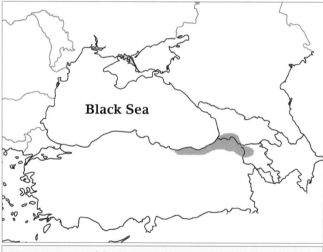

Map 115. Range of the Transcaucasian Viper, *Vipera transcaucasiana.*

Venom and Bite: Nothing much is known about the venom of this rare snake. The fact that it is a close relative of the Long-nosed Viper suggests that its venom may be quite toxic. No specific antivenom is produced for this snake but antivenoms listed under Long-nosed Viper probably have cross reactivity against the venom of this species.

Meadow Viper,
Vipera ursinii

Description and Identification: One of the smallest of the European Vipers averaging 18 to 20 inches and reaching a maximum of about 32 inches. Body rather slender with only 19 scale rows. Ground color variable from gray to brown with a dark zig-zag or wavy dorsal stripe.

Distribution, Habitat, and Biology: This species is spottily distributed in southern Europe in widely disjunct localities constituting 5 subspecies. It was once probably much more wide-ranging. Lives mainly in mountainous regions in open, grassy habitats. Several disjunct populations of this snake are regarded by some experts as distinct new species.

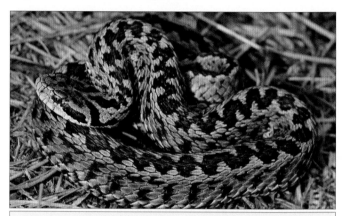

Photo 107. Meadow Viper, *Vipera ursinii*

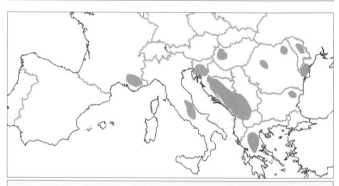

Map 116. Range of the Meadow Viper, *Vipera ursinii.*

Venom and Bite: The venom of the Meadow Viper is presumed to be the least toxic of any of the European Adders. In addition, this is a small species with small fangs, low venom yields, and a tolerant disposition. It is thus widely regarded as the least dangerous of the *Vipera* genus and there are no known fatalities from its bite. Viper Venom Antitoxin European manufactured by Immunoloski Zavod in Croatia is one of the suggested antivenoms for treating severe bites.

Caucasus Viper,
Vipera kaznakovi

Description and Identification: Ground color yellow, reddish, gray, or black. Often there are two narrow longitudinal dorso-lateral stripes on each side of a broad, dark vertebral stripe. The dorso-lateral stripes are light in color and may be yellow, reddish, tan, or gray. The head is short and broad.

Distribution, Habitat, and Biology: Ranges along the eastern end of the Black Sea in northeast Turkey, western Georgia, and the western end of the Russian Federation's Caucasus Mountains. Habitat is forested foothills to nearly 3,000 feet in elevation. This species occupies a very small geographic range in a part of the world where natural habitats are under assault. It is an IUCN endangered species and its future is uncertain.

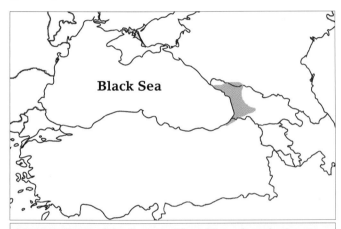

MAP 117. Range of the Caucasus Viper, *Vipera kaznakovi.*

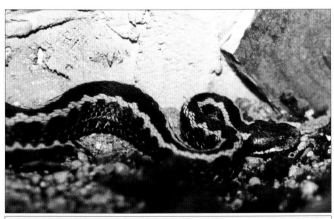

PHOTO 108. Caucasus Viper, *Vipera kaznakovi*

Venom and Bite: There is little information available on the venom of this species or the severity of its bite in humans. Several of the polyvalent antivenoms for *Vipera* (such as Viper Venom antitoxin European) are probably useful in treating serious bites.

Caucasus Subalpine Viper,
Vipera dinniki

Description and Identification: The ground color is olive, gray, or yellowish and in sharp contrast to the dark, irregular mid-dorsal stripe, producing a strikingly colored serpent. Reaches 20 inches.

Distribution, Habitat, and Biology: Found at elevations between 4,500 and 8,500 feet on both the northern and southern slopes. It ranges from the Black Sea in southern Russia to Azerbaijan near the eastern terminus of the Caucasus. Lives in mountain meadows, rocky slopes, and talus. Active from April through September.

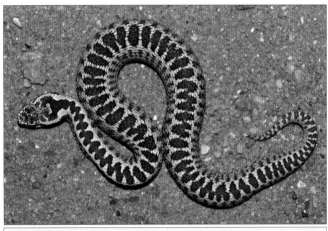

PHOTO 109. Caucasus Subalpine Viper, *Vipera dinniki*

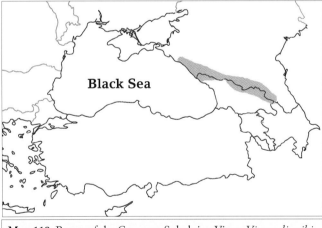

MAP 118. Range of the Caucasus Subalpine Viper, *Vipera dinniki.*

Venom and Bite: No known fatalities from its bite. Venom probably haemotoxic. Viper Venom antitoxin European is likely effective in treating serious bites.

Similar Species: The Caucasian Meadow Viper (*V. lotievi*) occupies much of the same area on the northern slope of the Caucasus Mountains.

Nikolsky's Viper,
Vipera nikolskii

Description and Identification: Similar to the European Viper *(V. berus)* and considered by some to be a subspecies. Generally this is a much darker snake, and nearly solid black specimens are common. Ground color may also be gray, charcoal, or brownish with a dark, irregular (often zig-zag) middorsal stripe. These are small snakes, averaging only about 14-16 inches in length.

Distribution, Habitat, and Biology: Found in forest-steppe in much of central Ukraine and parts of western Russia. Like most *Vipera* a terrestrial species. Mainly diurnal in habits.

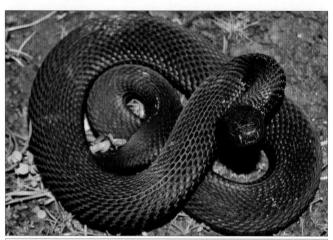

Photo 110. Nikolsky's Viper, *Vipera nikolskii*

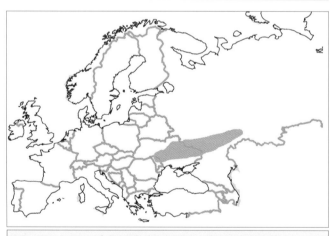

Map 119. Range of the Nikolsky's Viper, *Vipera nikolskii.*

Venom and Bite: This is probably a potentially deadly species. No antivenom is recommended by the World Health Organization's Venomous Snakes Antivenom Database. Viper Venom antitoxin European is a polyvalent antivenom effective against the bite of several European *Vipera,* and possibly a good choice for treating bites by this species.

Steppe Viper,
Vipera renardi

Description and Identification: Another small viper species that averages 14-18 inches with a maximum length of 2.5 feet. Body color gray, tan, or brown with the dark zig-zag middorsal stripe typical of *Vipera* snakes. Edges of the mid-dorsal stripe often rounded.

Distribution, Habitat, and Biology: Wide-ranging across eastern Europe and western Asia. In the USEU-COM region it is an uncommon snake that lives at lower to moderate elevations (up to 3,000 feet) in classical Steppe (grassland) habitats.

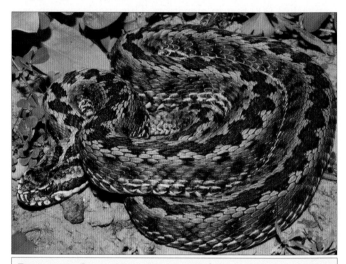

Photo 111. Steppe Viper, *Vipera renardi.*

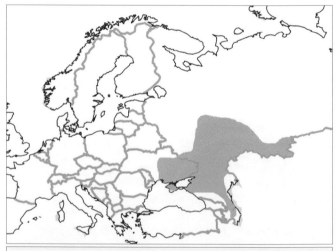

Map 120. Range of the Steppe Viper, *Vipera renardi,* in the USEUCOM region.

Venom and Bite: There are no known deaths from its bite, but otherwise little is known about the venom of this species or its effect on humans. Viper Venom antitoxin European is likely effective in treating serious bites.

Armenian Steppe Viper,

Vipera eriwanensis

Description and Identification: A grayish snake with a dark, zig-zag, middorsal stripe, the corners of its zig-zags are usually rounded. Maximum length is about 20 inches.

Distribution, Habitat, and Biology: Found only in Armenia, eastern Turkey, and western Azerbaijan. Even within this small region it occurs only in pockets of suitable habitat in widely disjunct localities.

It is classified as vulnerable by the IUCN. Inhabits rocky outcrops, talus and grassy slopes of mountains from 5,000 to 8,500 feet.

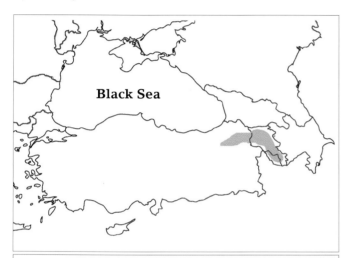

Black Sea

MAP 121. Range of the Armenian Steppe Viper, *Vipera eriwanensis.*

Venom and Bite: An uncommon species that is not a significant source of snakebite injuries. No known deaths are recorded. Viper Venom antitoxin European is likely effective in treating serious bites.

Additional Species: In additon to those species profiled previously, 5 other *Vipera* species occur in the USUEUCOM region. All these additional species have small, restrictive ranges in the Caucasus region.

These additonal species are:

   Turkish Viper - *V. barani*
   Magnificent Viper - *V. magnifica*
   Orlov's Viper - *V. orlovi*
   Darveski's Viper - *V. darveskii*
   Black Sea Viper - *V. pontica*

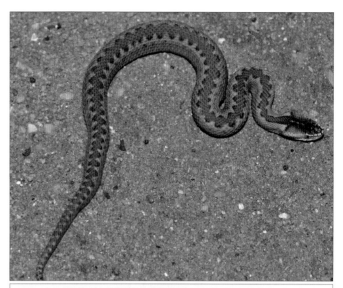

PHOTO 112. Orlov's Viper, *Vipera orlovi*

Family - Viperidae

Subfamily - Viperinae - True Vipers

Genus - Montivipera

Eurasian Mountain Vipers

This genus of medium sized snakes are intermediate in size between the two very similar genera *Vipera* (True Adders) and *Macrovipera* (large Near Eastern Vipers). The *Montivipera* today constitute 8 species, but the taxonomic status of several species is questioned by some experts. In fact, this group is so controversial among herpetologists at present that some do not even recognize the genus *Montivipera,* and instead lump all these snakes into the genus *Vipera*. Historically they were assigned to that genus, but the newer taxonomic designation of *Montivipera* is gaining popularity among experts. 5 species are found in USEUCOM region from Greece through Turkey and into Armenia. Two of these also range in the USCENTCOM region where there are an additional three other species.

Definition: Head broad; distinct from narrow neck; canthus distinct. Body cylindrical, varying from moderately slender to stout; tail short.

Eyes moderate in size to small; pupils vertically elliptical.

Head scales: Head covered in numerous small scales. Supraoculars are large and often raised to create a small ridge above the eye.

Body scales: Dorsals keeled with apical pits in 21 to 25 nonoblique rows at midbody. Ventrals rounded 142 to 181; subcaudals paired , 23-39. Anal scute entire.

Ottoman Viper,
Montivipera xanthina

Description and Identification: Body gray or brownish with darker dorsal markings consisting of a series of ovoid blotches anteriorly that combine into a broad, wavy dorsal stripe posteriorly. This is the largest of the Eurasian Mountain Vipers and it averages about three feet; maximum 4.5 feet.

Distribution, Habitat, and Biology: Most of this species' range is in western Turkey, but it is also found in northeast Greece and several islands in the Aegean Sea. It may be found from sea level to over 6,000 feet. Habitat is listed as grassy mountain slopes and scrub. A fairly common species in undisturbed habitats.

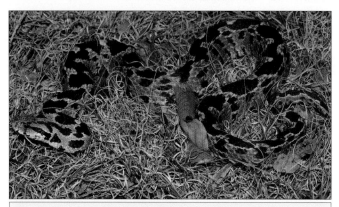

Photo 113. Ottoman Viper, *Montivipera xanthina*

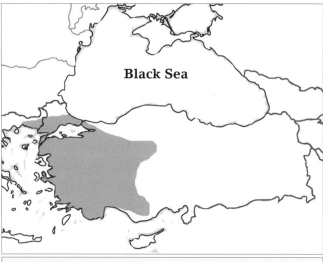

Map 122. Range of the Ottoman Viper, *Montivipera xanthina.*

Venom and Bite: No specific antivenom is recommended by the World Health Organization. Viper Venom Antitoxin European (Croatia) and Viper Venom Antitoxin (Yugoslavia) are listed by Clinical Toxinology Resources Website (2012) at *www.toxinology.com.* Deaths have been recorded.

Armenian Viper,
Montivipera raddei

Description and Identification: Can reach about 3 feet. The ground color is smoky gray with a series of reddish to orange vertebral blotches. Sides with series of dark vertical bars.

Distribution, Habitat, and Biology: Found in mountains areas of Armenia and adjacent Turkey, Iran, and Azerbaijan. Lives at altitudes of 3,000 to 7,000 feet in brushy or wooded areas. Rocky habitats are preferred but may also be found in areas of human alteration, (i.e., pastures and field edges).

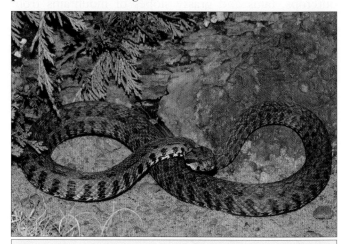

Photo 114. Armenian Viper, *Montivipera raddei*

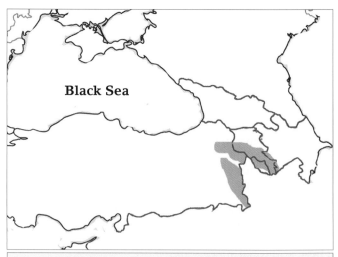

Map 123. Range of the Armenian Viper, *Montivipera raddei*, in the USEUCOM region.

Venom and Bite: The venom is reputed to be quite toxic and deaths have occurred within a few hours of its bite. WHO recommended antivenoms, Polyvalent Snake Antivenom manufactured by Razi Vaccine & Serum Institute, Iran. Venom toxins are probably procoagulants and haemorragins with some neurotoxins possibly present.

Central Turkish Mt. Viper,
Montivipera albizona

Description and Identification: Maximum length 30 inches, but averages smaller. Color and pattern similar to the Armenian Viper but with lighter body color and larger (brownish) vertebral blotches.

Distribution, Habitat, and Biology: Reportedly has extensive period of hibernation (Phelps, 2010).

Inhabits dry, rocky mountain slopes.

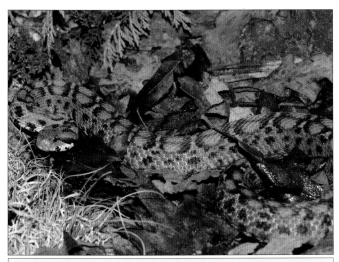

PHOTO 115. Central Turkish Moutain Viper, *Montivipera albizona*

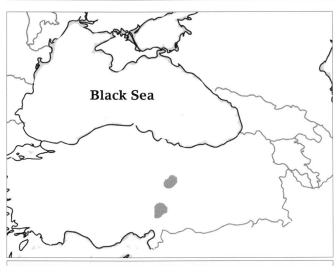

MAP 124. Range of the Central Turkish Mt. Viper, *Montivipera albizona.*

Venom and Bite: Neither the World Health Organization or Toxinology Resources websites list an antivenom for this species. Polyvalent Snake Antivenom manufactured by Razi Vaccine & Serum Institute, Iran may have some effectiveness against this species.

Wagner's Viper,
Montivipera wagneri

Description and Identification: These are one of the larger members of the genus, and they can reach a length of just over 3 feet. Ground color gray, dorsal blotches irregular in shape and usually reddish brown or yellowish brown to gold and edged in black.

Distribution, Habitat, and Biology: Found in both the USEUCOM and USCENTCOM regions, its known range is restricted to a small mountainous area of eastern Turkey and northwestern Iran.

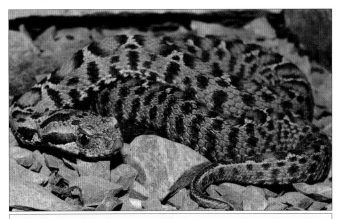

PHOTO 116. Wagner's Viper, *Montivipera wagneri*

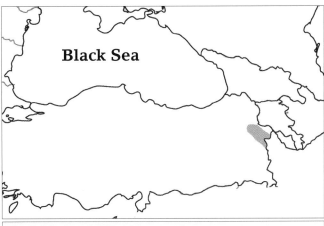

MAP 125. Range of the Wagner's. Viper, *Montivipera wagneri* in the USEUCOM region.

Venom and Bite: Little information is available on the venom of this species, but it should be considered a potentially deadly species. No specific antivenom is produced but Polyvalent Snake Antivenom by Razi Vaccine (Iran) is probably a good cover for all members of this genus.

Additional Species: *M. bulgardica,* the Bulgardagh Viper is another similar mountain viper that has a very small range in the USUECOM region within Turkey.

Family - Viperidae

Subfamily - Viperinae -True Vipers

Genus -Macrovipera

Blunt-headed Vipers

These vipers are found in deserts and mountains both in the Caucasus and the Middle East. They are similar in many respects to both the *Vipera* and *Montivipera*, but they are the largest of the three genera and are by far the most dangerous to man. Some specimens can reach 6 feet in length. This is a small genus, with only 2 species. They are found in both the USCENTCOM and the USEUCOM region which has both species. One of these is found in Turkey, the Caucasus, and the Mediterranean island of Cyprus. Another is restricted to a group of small islands in the Aegean Sea off the coast of Greece (Cyclades Islands).

Definition: Pupil elliptical. Head broad with numerous small scales, snout rounded.

Body scales: Dorsal scales 23-25, strongly keeled. Ventrals rounded 146 to 177; subcaudals paired , 35-51. Anal scute entire.

Levantine Viper,

Macrovipera lebatina

Although it is found in southern Turkey and in parts of all three Caucasus states, the bulk of this species' range is contained in the USCENTCOM region. For more information on this species see Chapter 11 (USCENTCOM), page 145.

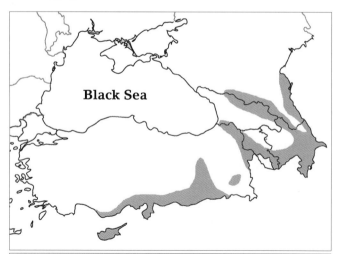

MAP 126. Range of the Levantine Viper, *Macrovipera lebatina*, in the USEUCOM region.

Similar Species: The Blunt-nosed Viper, *Macroviper schweizeri* (below) is a similar species found only in the USEUCOM region on the Cyclades Islands (Greece) in the Aegean Sea.

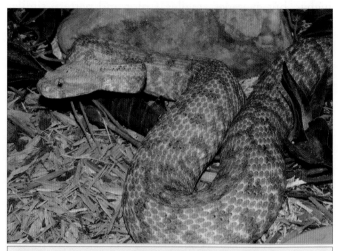

PHOTO 117. Levantine Viper, *Macrovipera lebatina*

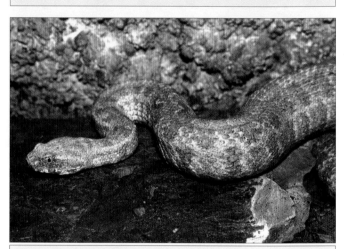

PHOTO 118. Blunt-nosed Viper, *Macrovipera schweizeri*

Family - Viperidae

Subfamily - Crotalinae - Pit Vipers

Genus - Gloydius

Asian Moccasins

At least 12 species are recognized. These pit vipers are primarily Asian in origin and they are found mostly in the USPACOM region. They are also found in the USCENTCOM region. Three are found in the USEUCOM region and 2 of those barely enter the region in extreme southeastern Russian. One species (*G. halys*) ranges westward as far as the Caspian Sea in southeastern Russian and southern Azerbaijan, and is also fairly widespread across southern Russia.

They are usually called "Asian Moccasins" because they were once included in the genus *Agkistrodon* with the North American Copperheads and Cottonmouths. They are also sometimes known by the name "Mamushi," which is the Japanese name for the *Gloydius* species that is native to Japan (*G. blomhoffi*). The members of this genus are the only pit vipers found in the USEUCOM region, and thus are readily identified by the presence of a loreal pit.

Definition: Head broad, flattened, very distinct from narrow neck; a sharply distinguished canthus.

Eyes moderate in size, pupils vertically elliptical.

Head scales: 9 large plates on the crown.

Body scales: Dorsal scales keeled in 20-15 rows at midbody.

Haly's Pit Viper,
Gloydius halys

Description and Identification: The presence of a loreal pit distinguishes this genus from all other snakes of the USEUCOM region.

Color yellowish, tan, reddish, or grayish with many dark brown or gray crossbands alternating with spots on the sides or with cross bands and spots fusing to produce an irregular network; belly cream to yellow with fine black punctuation especially toward the tail; top of head with dark spot above each eye and at nape. Tip of tail yellowish. Average length 22 to 28 inches; maximum about 35 inches.

Distribution, Habitat, and Biology: A snake of the vast Asian steppe where it occurs in grassland and desert; often abundant around rocky bluffs that probably are hibernating dens. Much of this snakes' range is just to the south of Russia in the USCENTCOM and USPACOM regions.

Venom and Bite: Bites by this species are apparently not usually life threatening, however the Clinical Toxinology Resources Website (www.toxinology.com) states that "lethal potential cannot be excluded" (viewed 2012).

The World Health Organization Snake Antivenoms Database lists a specific antivenom "Agkistrodon halys antivenin" produced by the Shanghai Institute Biological Technology Co., Ltd, Shanghai, China.

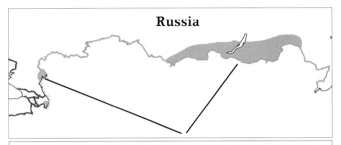

MAP 127. Range of the Haly's Pit Viper, *Gloydius halys*, in the USEUCOM region.

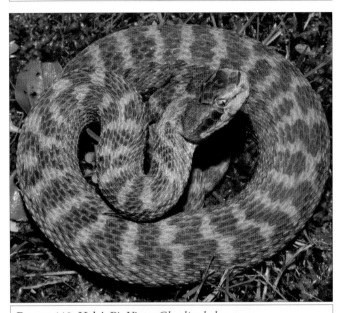

PHOTO 119. Haly's Pit Viper, *Gloydius halys*

Similar Species: Two other similar species have ranges that extend northward from the USPACOM region into a portion of the USEUCOM region. Both the Central Asian Pit Viper (*G. intermedius*) and the Ussurian Mamushi (*G. ussuriensis*) can be found in extreme southeastern Russia. For information on these two species see Chapter 13, (USPACOM-Part 1).

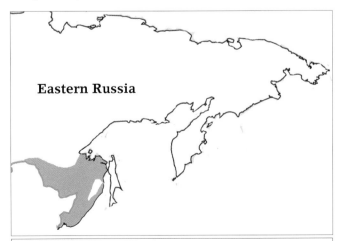

MAP 128. Combined ranges of the Central Asian Pit Viper, *Gloydius intermedius*, and Ussurian Mamushi, *Gloydius ussuriensis*.

Family - Viperidae

Subfamily - Viperinae - True Vipers

Genus - Pseudocerastes

False Horned Vipers

This genus is widespread in the USCENTCOM region but occurs in the USEUCOM region only in extreme southeastern Turkey. A single species can be found here. For information on these snakes see page 153, Chapter 11 (USCENTCOM).

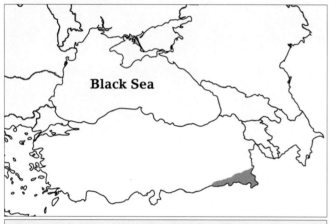

MAP 129. Range of the Eastern False Horned Viper, *Pseudocerastes persicus,* in the USEUCOM region.

Family - Elapidae Genus -Walterinnesia

Desert Cobras

The cobra family is represented in this region by a single species, and it barely occurs in the area. Morgan's Desert Cobra is found mostly in the USCENTCOM region but does barely range into a small area of southwestern Turkey. For information on this species see Chapter 11 (USCENTCOM) page 156.

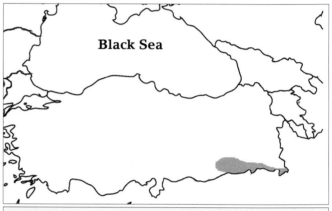

MAP 130. Range of the Morgan's Desert Cobra, *Walterinnesia morgani,* in the USEUCOM region.

NOTES

Current References

Books

David, Patrick & Gernot Vogel. 2010. *Venomous Snakes of Europe, Northern, Central, and Western Asia.* TERRALOG Vol 16. Edition Chimaira, Frankfort, Germany.

Dowling, Herndon G., Sherman A. Minton, and Findlay E. Russell. 1965. *Poisonous Snakes of the World.* Department of the Navy Bureau of Medicine and Surgery. Washington, DC.

Phelps, Tony. 2010. *Old World Vipers, A Natural History of the Azemoipinae and Viperinae.* Edition Chimaira. Frankfurt, Germany.

Jounals

Ferquel E., de Haro L., Jan V., Guillemin I., Jourdain S., et al. (2007) "Reappraisal of *Vipera aspis* venom neurotoxicity". Plos ONE 2(11): doi:10.1371/journal.pone.001194.

Karlson-Stiber, Christine M.D., Helene Salmonson, M.Sc., and Hans Persson, M.D. (2006) "A Nationwide Study of *Vipera berus* Bites During One Year--Epidemiology and Morbidity of 231 Cases". *Clinical Toxicology* 44: 25-30.

Stumpel N. and Joger U. (2009) "Recent advances in phylogeny and taxonomy of Near and Middle Eastern vipers an update". ZooKeys 31: 179-191.

Web References

World Health Organization - www.who.int/bloodproducts/snakeantivenoms/database

The Reptile Database, http//www.reptiledata-base.org

Armed Forces Pest Management Board, www.afpmb.org/content/living-hazards-database

www.herpfrance.com

www.reptarium.cz/en/taxonomy

University of Adelaide, Clinincal Toxinology Resources Wesbsite (2012), www.toxinology.com

International Union for Conservation of Nature, www.iucnredlist.org

Munich Antivenom Index, www.toxinof.org

Original References

HELLMICH, Walter. 1956. Die Lurche und Kriechtiere Europas. Carl Winter: Heidelberg, pp. 1–166, pls. 1–68 (color), figs. 1–9.

MERTENS, Robert and H. WERMUTH. 1960. Die Amphibien und Reptilien Europas. Dritte Liste nach dem Stand vom 1. Januar 1960. Waldemar Kramer: Frankfurt-am-Main, xi + 264 pp., figs. 1–45.

SCHWARZ, E. 1936. Untersuchungen uber Systematik und Verbreitung der europaischen und mediterranen Ottern. Behringwerk-Mitteilung: Marburg-Lahn, vol. 7, pp. 159–362, pl. 1.

TERENTJEV, P. V. and S. A. CERNOV. 1949. Apredelitelj Presmykajuschcichsja i Semnowodnych. [Distribution of Reptiles and Amphibians] Third Ed. [in Russian] Government Printing Office: Moscow, 339 pp., 123 figs., 37 maps.

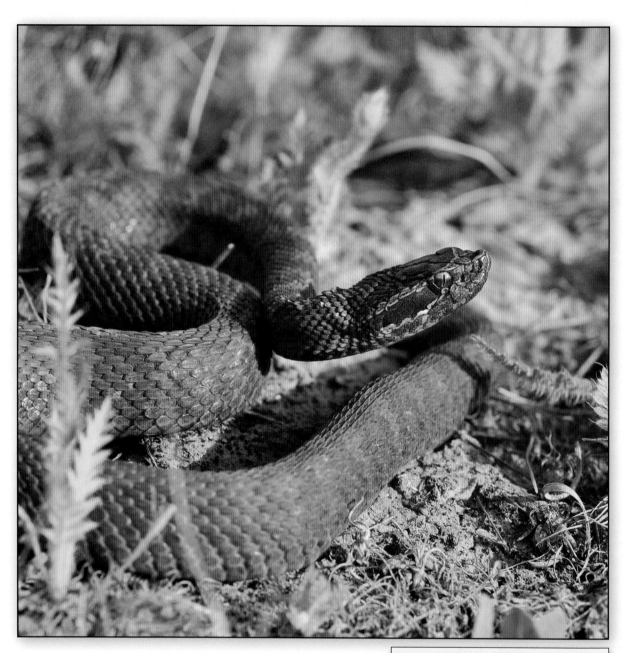

Haly's Pit Viper, *Gloydius halys*

CHAPTER **11**

REGION **4**
USCENTCOM
United States Central Command

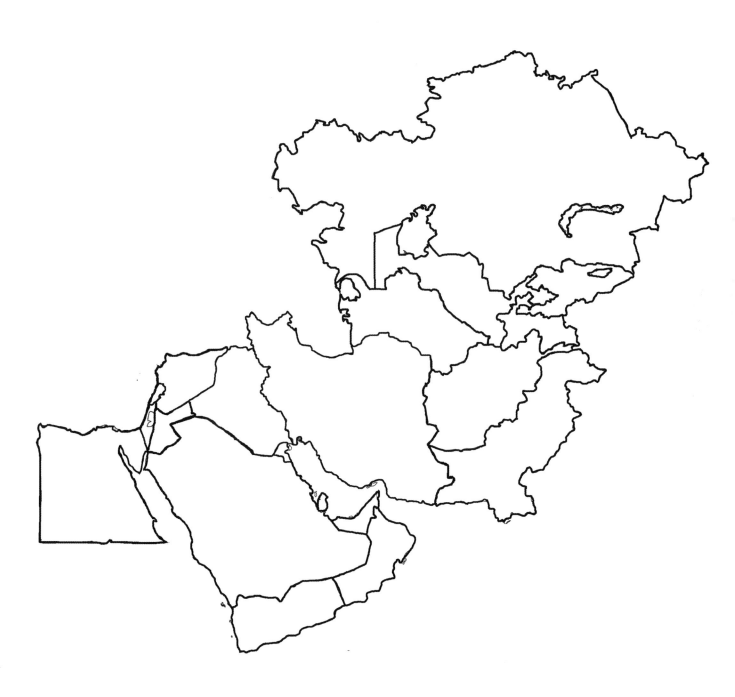

MAP 131. Region 4. The United States Central Command.

Introduction

In terms of its snake fauna this region is a bridge between three continents. Europe, Asia, and Africa converge in the region, and snakes from all three continents can be found here. Despite this fact, the numbers of venomous snake species here is relatively low compared to other regions in this book. This is due in large part to the fact that in this section the geographic area covered is significantly smaller than any other chapter in this book.

Although the actual number of venomous snake species found here is not as great as in some other regions (35 species), the diversity is fairly high. Four of the world's five snake families that have dangerously venomous genera can be found in this region. The true vipers family-Viperidae / subfamily Viperinae with 9 genera and 24 species are the most well represented. Next is the cobra family (family-Elapidae), with 2 genera totaling 8 species. By contrast, the pit vipers Family Viperidae / subfamily-Crotalinae has but a single genus each within this region, and the unusual family Lamprophiidae has two species.

By contrast, the USEUCOM region contains, for all practical purposes only two families (a third barely enters that region), and 26 of its 31 species are in a single family (Viperidae). Although this region shares three of its genera and several of its species with the generally less dangerous snakes of the USEUCOM region, many of the species found within the USCENTCOM region are quite dangerous. Several genera that are more commonly found in southeast Asia or Africa occur here, and some of these can be quite deadly to man.

This is a predominately arid region, although it does not contain quite as much sterile desert as does north Africa. This trend towards a drier climate in this region is quite recent, marked changes having occurred within historic times. Overgrazing, deforestation, and other forms of human misuse have contributed to the trend toward more desertification.

As in the USEUCOM region, vipers cause most of the bites in this region. Other types of venomous snakes occur here, but they are usually rare or restricted in range, and inflict few bites.

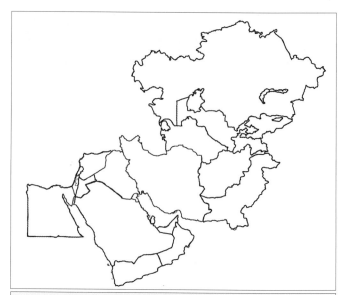

MAP 132. Region 4. United States Central Command, The Middle East and western Asia.

Family - Viperidae

Subfamily - Crotalinae - Pit Vipers

Genus- Gloydius

Asian Moccasins

At least 12 species are recognized. These pit vipers are primarily Asian in origin and they are found mostly in the USPACOM region. They are also found in the USEUCOM region.

These snakes are often called "Asian Moccasins" because they were once included in the genus *Agkistrodon* with the North American Copperheads and Cottonmouths. They are also sometimes known by the name "Mamushi," which is the Japanese name for the *Gloydius* species that is native to Japan (*G. blomhoffi*). The members of this genus are the only pit vipers found in the USCENTCOM region, and thus are readily identified by the presence of a loreal pit.

Definition: Head broad, flattened, very distinct from narrow neck; a sharply distinguished canthus.

Eyes moderate in size, pupils vertically elliptical.

Head scales: 9 large plates on the crown.

Body scales: Dorsal scales keeled in 20-15 rows at midbody.

Haly's Pit Viper,

Gloydius halys

Description and Identification: The presence of a loreal pit distinguishes this genus from all other snakes of the USCENTCOM region.

Color yellowish, tan, reddish, or grayish with many dark brown or gray crossbands alternating with spots on the sides or with cross bands and spots fusing to produce an irregular network; belly cream to yellow with fine black punctuation especially toward the tail; top of head with dark spot above each eye and at nape. Tip of tail yellowish. Average length 22 to 28 inches; maximum about 35 inches.

Distribution, Habitat, and Biology: A snake of the vast Asian steppe where it occurs in grassland and desert; often abundant around rocky bluffs that probably are hibernating dens. This species also occurs in the USEUCOM and USPACOM regions. In the USCENTCOM region it is widespread across most of Kazakhstan, Uzbekistan, and Kyrgyzstan as well as parts of Turkmenistan, Tajikistan, Afghanistan, and Iran.

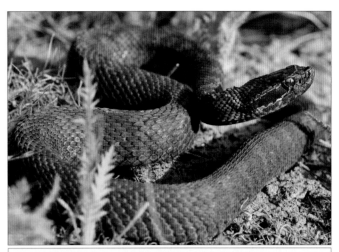

Photo 120. Haly's Pit Viper, *Gloydius halys*

The World Health Organization's website lists a specific antivenom "Agkistrodon halys antivenin" produced by the Shanghai Institute Biological Technology Co., Ltd, Shanghai, China.

Additional Species: The very similar Himalayan Pit Viper (*G. himalayanus*) can be found in the USCENTCOM region in the mountains of northern Pakistan.

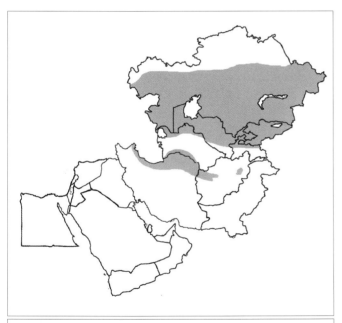

Map 133. Range of the Haly's Pit Viper, *Gloydius halys*, in the USCENTCOM region.

Family - Viperidae

Subfamily - Viperinae - True Vipers

Genus- Vipera

True Adders

The genus *Vipera* contains a minimum of 20 species and some experts recognize up to 23. Most are found in USEUCOM region. Three species can be found in the USCENTCOM region, one of these is endemic to Iran and the other two are wide-ranging species found from Europe to northwestern Asia.

Definition: Head broad; distinct from narrow neck; canthus distinct. Body cylindrical, varying from moderately slender to stout; tail short.

Eyes moderate in size to small; pupils vertically elliptical.

Body scales: Dorsals keeled with apical pits in 19 to 23 nonoblique rows at midbody. Ventrals rounded 114 to 170; subcaudals paired , 18-49. Anal scute undivided.

Most *Vipera* are relatively small snakes and although several species are known to have caused human fatalities, deaths from their bites are not common.

Venom and Bite: Perhaps one of the least dangerous snakes found in the USCENTCOM region, but Clinical Toxinology Resources Website 2012-*www.toxinology.com* states that "lethal potential cannot be excluded". That website also lists procoagulants in the form of prothrobin converters and possibly haemorragins as venom toxins.

Iranian Mountain Steppe Viper,
Vipera ebneri

Description and Identification: These are small snakes that reach a maximum length of only about 18 inches. They are grayish to brown with a classic "zig-zag" mid-dorsal stripe that is dark brown or dark gray. There are a series of small lateral spots on each side that match the color of the mid-dorsal stripe. The top of the head is covered with large plate-like scales. To the trained eye they are rather easily recognized as a "true viper," and are the only species of *Vipera* occurring within their range, making for easier identification.

This species is regarded by some sources as synonymous with *V. eriwanensis* (page 133, Chapter 10).

Distribution, Habitat, and Biology: Endemic to the Elburz Mountains in the country of Iran. Inhabits mountain Steppe terrain from between about 4,000 and 6,000 feet elevation. Like most *Vipera* feeds on both invertebrates and small vertebrates like lizards and mice.

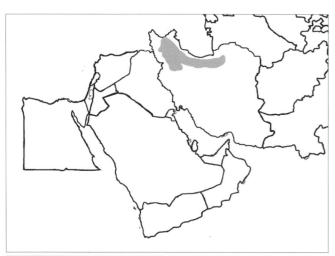

Map 134. Range of the Iranian Mountain Steppe Viper, *Vipera ebneri*.

Venom and Bite: Undoubtably one of the least dangerous venomous snakes in the USCENTCOM region. However, the website Clinical Toxinology Resources (2012) states that untreated bites have caused deaths.

The same website lists as an antivenom Viper Venom Antitoxin European by Institute of Immunology, Inc. in Zagreb, Croatia.

European Viper,
Vipera berus

Though found in the northern portions of the US-CENTCOM region, this species is more widespread in the USEUCOM region. For information on this species see page 125, Chapter 10 (USEUCOM).

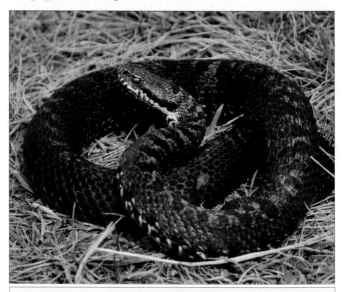

Photo 121. European Viper, *Vipera berus*

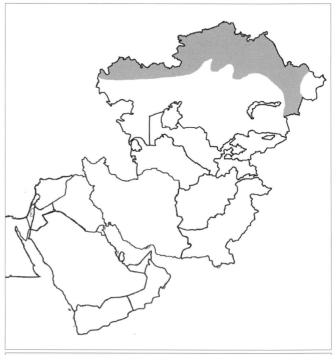

Map 135. Range of the European Viper, *Vipera berus*, in the USCENTCOM region.

Steppe Viper,
Vipera renardi

This species is fairly widespread in both the USCENT-COM region and the USEUCOM region. For information on this species see page 132, Chapter 10 (USEUCOM).

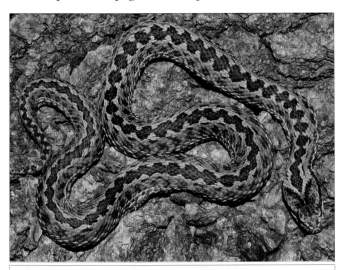

PHOTO 122. Steppe Viper, *Vipera renardi*

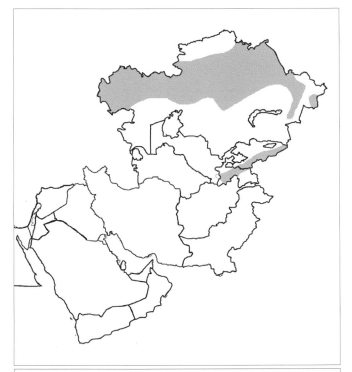

MAP 136. Range of the Steppe Viper, *Vipera renardi*, in the USCENTCOM region.

Family - Viperidae

Subfamily - Viperinae - True Vipers

Genus- Macrovipera

Blunt-headed Vipers

These vipers are found in deserts and mountains both in the middle east and north Africa. They are similar in many respects to both the *Vipera* and *Montivipera,* but they are the largest of these three genera, and one species (*M. lebatina*) is highly dangerous to man. They are also similar to the *Daboia* genus of vipers (another highly dangerous group of Asian / near eastern vipers) and may be most closely related to them. Some specimens can reach 6 feet in length. This is a small genus, with only 4 species. They are found in both the USEU-COM, USAFRICOM and the USCENTCOM regions. This region has but a single species (*M. lebantina*), but it is widespread across the region and it has as many as 5 subspecies.

Definition: Pupil elliptical. Head broad with numerous small scales, snout rounded.

Dorsal scales 23-25, strongly keeled. Ventrals rounded 146 to 177; subcaudals paired , 35-51. Anal scute entire.

Levantine Viper,
Macrovipera lebatina

Description and Identification: A large and heavy bodied viper that can exceed 5.5 feet in length. Typically a stone gray snake with darker gray vertebral blotches, or crossbars. There is also a series of smaller lateral spots one each side that alternate with the vertebral blotches. Blotches may be well defined or obscured, and are sometimes brown or tan. Specimens with obscured markings may be somewhat drab.

Head broad, triangular distinct from neck. Snout blunt; body stout; tail tapers abruptly behind vent. Crown with small keeled scales; nostril lateral; supraocular divided into 3 small shields; usually 3 scale row between eye and upper labials; dorsal body scales keeled, in 23-27 rows at midbody, subcaudals divided.

Distribution, Habitat, and Biology: These snakes can be found from the eastern end of the Mediterranean all the way to northern India. Inhabits barren rocky areas usually at altitudes of 3,000 to 6,000 feet. Very slow to move; seeming almost oblivious to stimuli when encountered by day. More active and alert at night but may strike quickly and savagely at any time. Occasionally climbs into bushes.

Unlike most other vipers which are live-bearers, these snakes are egg layers.

Venom and Bite: Procoagulants. Probably myotoxins. This is a dangerous species and throughout its range it is responsible for a significant percentage of snakebite deaths.

World Health Organization's Venomous Snake Antivenoms Database list of antivenoms for treating bites by this species (www.int/bloodproducts/snakeantivenoms/database-2012):

> Product: Anti-Viperin
> Manufacturer: Institute Pasteur d'Algerie
> Country of Origin: Algeria
> Product: Gamma-Vip
> Manufacturer: Institute Pasteur de Tunis
> Country of Origin: Tunisa
> Product: Polyvalent Snake Antivenom
> Manufacturer: Razi Vaccine & Serum Research Institute
> Country of Origin: Iran

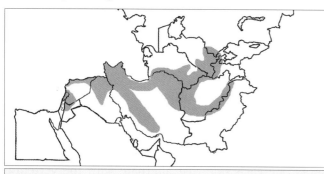

MAP 137. Range of the Levantine Viper, *Macrovipera lebatina*, in the USCENTCOM region.

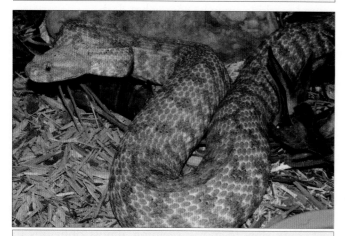

PHOTO 123. Levantine Viper, *Macrovipera lebatina*

Family - Viperidae

Subfamily - Viperinae - True Vipers

Genus- Montivipera

Eurasian Mountain Vipers

This genus consists of a total of 8 species. They are most widespread in the USEUCOM region. Five species are found in USCENTCOM region. Three are endemic to parts of Lebanon, Syria, and Iran, and two are also found in the USEUCOM region. All are rather rare snakes with limited ranges. All are probably dangerous to man, and at least one species, *M. latifi* (Latifi's Viper) is known to have caused fatalities in humans. For more information about this genus see page 133, Chapter 10 (USEUCOM).

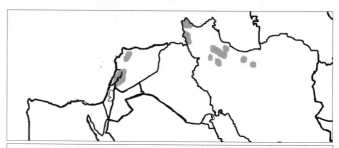

MAP 138. Combined ranges of the five species of, *Montivipera* Vipers found in the USCENTCOM region. For information about these snakes see pages 129-131, Chapter 10 (USEUCOM).

Family - Viperidae

Subfamily - Viperinae - True Vipers

Genus- Bitis

African Vipers

These dangerous vipers are found almost entirely on the African continent. A single species, *B. arietans*, the Puff Adder, can be found in the USCENTCOM region in a small area of the Arabian Peninsula. For information about this species see page 165, Chapter 12 (USAFRICOM).

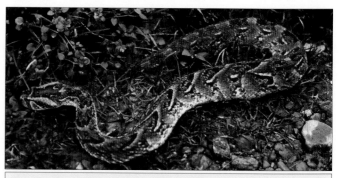

PHOTO 124. Puff Adder, *Bitis arietans*

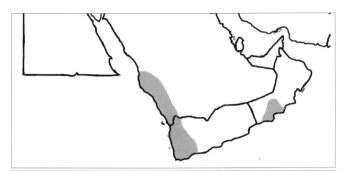

MAP 139. Range of the Puff Adder, *Bitis arietans*, in the USCENTCOM region.

Family - Viperidae

Subfamily - Viperinae - True Vipers

Genus- Daboia

Large Middle Eastern and Asian Vipers

The elongated, oval shaped head is distinctive of this genus. The *Daboia* genus contains only 3 species and all are large and dangerous snakes. They are similar in many respects to the *Macrovipera*. Two species are found in the USCENTCOM region. One (*palaestinae*) is endemic to this region but the other (*russelli*) is also found in the USPACOM region where it is much more widespread.

Definition: Pupil elliptical. Head distinct from the neck, broad; snout blunt or pointed, dorsum of head covered with small scales.

Body scales: Dorsal scales keeled in 24-33 rows at midbody. Ventrals 162-180; subcaudals paired 35-68; anal scute undivided.

Palestine Viper,
Daboia palaestinae

Description and Identification: Can reach a length of nearly 6 feet. Stout and heavy bodied. Ground color usually brownish, tan or grayish with dark brown dorsal blotches that may connect to form an irregular mid-dorsal stripe. Head markings are distinctive. A dark brown sub-ocular stripe is as wide as the eye and extends onto lower labials. There is also a distinct dark brown post-ocular stripe and two dark brown stripes on the head which converge on the snout to form a "V" on the top of the head.

Distribution, Habitat, and Biology: Restricted in range to a small are of the middle east including northern Israel, Lebanon, and parts of Syria and Jordan. Habitat is Mediterranean woodland and scrub, rocky hillsides, and agricultural areas where it may be quite common. Reportedly feeds mostly on rodents. Known to climb trees, an unusual behavior for a middle eastern viperidae.

Venom and Bite: Myotoxins, procoagulants, and haemorragins are known to be present in the venom. Small amounts of neurotoxins may also be present This species can be highly dangerous to man and is often common in areas of human habitation, especially irrigated agricultural areas. The original authors of this volume gave a fatality rate of 5 percent for the Palestine Viper (that was in 1965). It is still an important snakebite hazard within its small range. Though quite capable of killing, deaths today are rare due to an effective antivenom (listed below).

Product: Anti Vipera palestinae
Manufacturer: Felsenstein Medical Research Center
Country of Origin: Israel

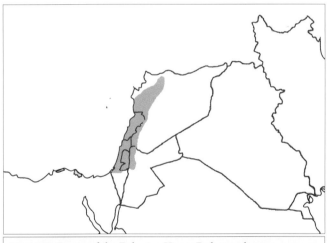

MAP 140. Range of the Palestine Viper, *Daboia palestinae.*

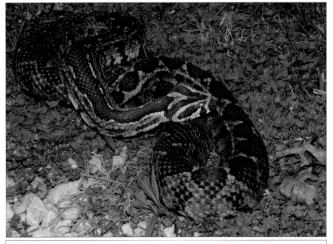

PHOTO 125. Palestine Viper, *Daboia palestinae*

Additional Species: The Western Russell's Viper (*Daboia russelli*) is a very dangerous member of this genus that occurs in the USCENTCOM region in eastern Pakistan. Most of this snake's range is found in the US-PACOM-Part 1 region and information on the Russell's Viper can be found in that chapter (13) on page 229.

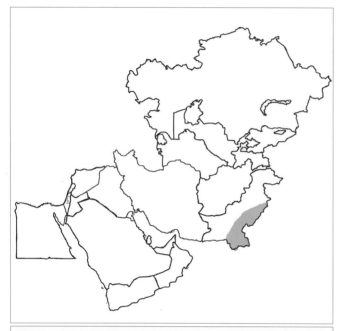

MAP 141. Range of the Western Russell's Viper, *Daboia russelli* in the USCENTCOM region.

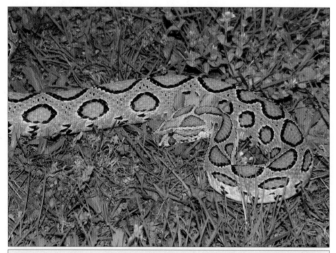

PHOTO 126. Western Russell's Viper, *Daboia russelli*

Family - Viperidae

Subfamily - Viperinae - True Vipers

Genus- Eristocophis

Asian Sand Viper

This genus consists of a single species found in the deserts of southeastern Iran, southern Afghanistan, and western Pakistan. It is a rather small snake, less than 3 feet in length, but is potentially deadly.

Definition: Head broad and flattened, very distinct from neck; snout broad and short, canthus not distinct. Body slightly depressed, moderately to markedly stout; tail short.

Eyes moderate in size; pupils vertically elliptical.

Head scales: Crown covered by small scales; rostral broad, bordered dorsally and laterally by greatly enlarged naso-rostral scales. Laterally, eye separated from labials by 3-4 rows of small scales; nasal separated from rostral by naso-rostral scale.

Body scales: Dorsals keeled, short, in 23-26 vertical rows at midbody. Ventrals with lateral keels, 140-148; subcaudals paired, without keels, 29-36.

MacMahon's Desert Viper,
Eristocophis macmahonii

Description and Identification: Adults average about 16 inches, reaching a maximum of 2.5 feet.

The nearly uniformly sandy brown dorsal color is highlighted by a series of evenly spaced small dark spots along the side, each of which is accompanied by two or more smaller white spots above. The top of the head is

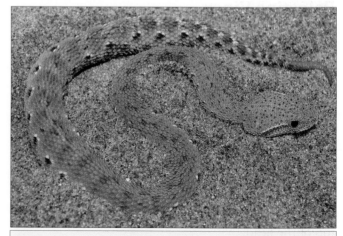

PHOTO 127. MacMahon's Desert Viper, *Eristocophis macmahonii*

uniformly sandy brown and there is a dark post-ocular stripe outlined above by a narrow white line.

Distribution, Habitat, and Biology: These small serpents are pure desert dwellers. They live in sandy regions where they often bury themselves in the sand with just the top of the head and eyes exposed. May use "side-winding" locomotion technique when fleeing danger.

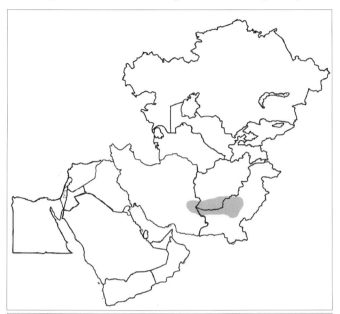

MAP 142. Range of the MacMahon's Desert Viper, *Eristocopis macmahonii.*

Venom and Bite: Reputed to be ill-tempered and quick to strike at an intruder. Clinical Toxinology Resources Website (*www.toxinology.com* - 2012) states that deaths have been recorded and lists procoagulants and neurotoxins possibly present.. Likewise, Tony Phelps' book *Old World Vipers* (2010), mentions several fatalities, and he states "this species has potent venom, equal at least to *Echis.*" Considering that *Echis* is one of the worlds deadliest snake genera, bites by this species are cause for great concern. Apparently, no antivenom exists for this species.

Family - Viperidae

Subfamily - Viperinae - True Vipers

Genus- Echis

Saw-scaled Vipers

In the 1965 edition of *Poisonous Snakes of the World*, two species of Saw-scaled Vipers were known. Today, some experts recognize up to 12 species. Most are remarkably similar to one another and the exact taxonomic status of this group is still confusing and probably subject to future revision.

At least 5 species (maybe 6) are found in the USCENTCOM region in suitable habitats from Egypt to Pakistan and north to Uzbekistan and Tajikistan. One of these species is also found in parts of the USPACOM region and another is also found in parts of the USAFRICOM region. Meanwhile, an additional 6 species are endemic to the USAFRICOM region. Although none attain a length of 3 feet, they possess a highly toxic venom and have been responsible for many deaths. When disturbed they inflate the body and produce a hissing sound by rubbing the saw-edged lateral scales against one another. This same pattern of behavior is shown by the nonvenomous egg-eating snakes *Dasypeltis.*

Definition: Head broad, very distinct from narrow neck; canthus indistinct. Body cylindrical, moderately slender; tail short.

Eyes moderate in size. Pupils vertically elliptical.

Head Scales: A narrow supraocular sometimes present; otherwise crown covered with small scales, which may be smooth or keeled. Rostral and nasals distinct. Laterally, eye separated from labials by 1-4 rows of small scales; nasal in contact with rostral or separated from it by a row of small scales.

Body scales: Dorsals keeled, with apical pits, lateral scales smaller, with serrate keels, in 27-37 oblique rows at midbody. Ventrals rounded, 132-205; subcaudals single, 21-52.

Echis venoms are extremely potent hemotoxins consisting of procoagulants, haemorragins, and probably anticoagulants. Nephrotoxins and necrotoxins may also be present. Because these snakes are widespread and often very common, they cause many snakebites. The death rate is often high, and statistically these are among the world's deadliest snakes.

Sochurek's Saw-scaled Viper,
Echis sochureki

Description and Identification: Head short and wide, snout blunt; body moderately stout; scales on top of head small, keeled; scales on side of body strongly oblique, the keels with minute serrations; subcaudals single.

Color pale buff or tan to olive brown, chestnut or reddish; midline row of whitish spots; side with narrow undulating white line; top of head usually shows light trident or arrowhead mark. Belly white to pinkish brown stippled with dark gray.

Average length 15 to 20 inches; maximum about 32 inches; sexes of about equal size.

Distribution, Habitat, and Biology: Widespread throughout much of the USCENTCOM region and ranges eastward into the USPACOM region as well.

The *Echis* that is endemic to the USCENTCOM region is the species *sochureki*. Most local experts within its range regard it as a separate species from *carinatus*, though some sources list it as a subspecies. The distinction may have important implications for treatment of bites, as *sochureki* is a significant source of snakebite within its range (Harold Harlan, personal communication).

Very adaptable, found from almost barren rocky or sandy desert to dry scrub forest and from seacoast to elevations of about 6,000 feet.

Primarily nocturnal. Will bury its body in the sand with only the top of head and eyes exposed. These are high strung snakes that are quick to strike if disturbed.

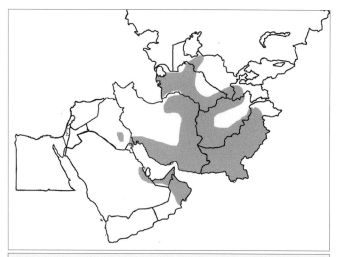

MAP 143. Range of the Sochurek's Saw-scaled Viper, *Echis sochureki* in the USCENTCOM region.

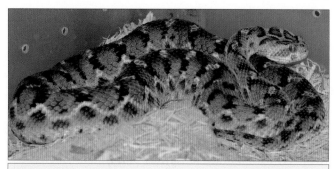

PHOTO 128. Sochurek's Saw-scaled Viper, *Echis sochureki*

Venom and Bite: As with all *Echis* species, this is an extremely dangerous snake. Throughout the region of its range it is a very significant health problem. Bites are not uncommon and the death rate is very high in non-treated or poorly treated bites.

There are several antivenoms listed by the World Health Organization for treating bites by this species.

Product: Polyvalent Antisnake Venom.
Manufacturer: National Institute of Health.
Country of Origin: Pakistan
Product: Polyvalent Snake Antivenom (Asia)
Manufacturer: Biological Limited.
Country of Origin: India
Product: Polyvalent Snake Antivenom.
Manufacturer: Razi Vaccine and Serum Research Institute.
Country of Origin: Iran
Product: Snake antivenin I.P.
Manufacturer: Haffkine Biopharmaceutical Corporation Ltd.
Country of Origin: India

Painted Saw-scaled Viper,
Echis coloratus

Description and Identification: A typical Saw-scaled Viper in overall body form. Tends to be more brightly colored than most species and often shows more vivid markings. Sometimes called the Painted Carpet Viper.

Distribution, Habitat, and Biology: Mostly a species of the Arabian Peninsula but also occurs in Egypt. Lives in rocky habitats rather than sandy desert.

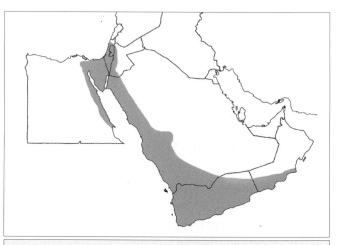

MAP 144. Range of the Painted Saw-scaled Viper, *Echis coloratus*.

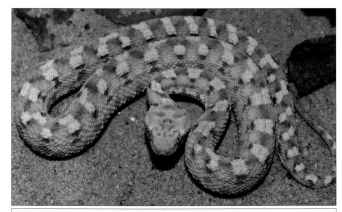

Photo 129. Painted Saw-scaled Viper, *Echis coloratus*

Venom and Bite: Considered as a group and based on the number of people killed, many experts consider the Saw-scaled Vipers to be among the world's deadliest snakes. The venom is strongly haemotoxic and almost entirely inhibits the blood's ability to clot. Antivenom listed by the World Health Organization for *Echis coloratus* is Polyvalent Snake Antivenom

Manufactured by National Antivenom and Vaccine Production Center in Saudi Arabia.

Similar species: Four additional species of Saw-scaled Vipers occur in the USCENTCOM region. In appearance and biology, they are all much the same. They are *E. khosatzkii* (Dhofar Saw-scaled Viper), *E. omanensis* (Oman Saw-scaled Viper), *E. borkini* (Arabian Saw-scaled Viper), and *E. pyramidum* (Egyptian Saw-scaled Viper). Range maps for these other species follows. For information on the Egyptian Saw-scaled Viper (*E. pyramidum*) see page 181 in Chapter 12 (USAFRICOM).

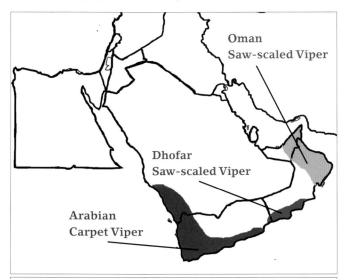

Oman
Saw-scaled Viper

Dhofar
Saw-scaled Viper

Arabian
Carpet Viper

Map 145. Range of the Oman Saw-scaled Viper, *E. omanensis*, the Arabian Carpet Viper, *E. borkini*, and the Dhofar Saw-scaled Viper, *E. khosatzkii*.

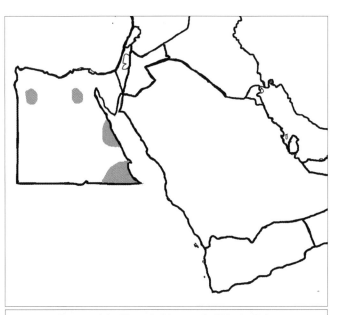

Map 146. Range of the Egyptian Saw-scaled Viper, *Echis pyramidum* in the USCENTCOM region.

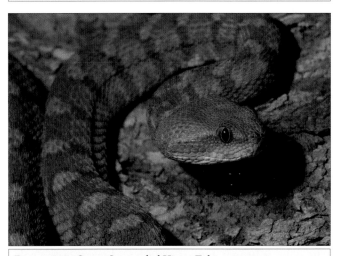

Photo 130. Oman Saw-scaled Viper, *Echis omanensis*

Family - Viperidae

Subfamily - Viperinae - True Vipers

Genus- Cerastes

Horned Vipers

Four species are recognized and 3 occur in the US-CENTCOM region (although 2 are mainly North African in distribution). None are large snakes, but the venom of some specimens appears to be highly toxic. Their name is derived from the presence in many specimens of an elongated "horn" above each eye. In some individuals the horn is reduced or lacking, and one species (*C. vipera*) is totally hornless.

As with the Saw-scaled Vipers, these snakes may rub the sides of their body coils together to produce a hissing sound when threatened. Highly adapted to life in the desert, these snakes are capable of "sidewinding" means of locomotion across loose sands.

Definition: Head broad, flattened, very distinct from neck; snout very short and broad, canthus indistinct. Body depressed, tapered, moderately slender to stout; tail short.

Eyes small to moderate in size; pupils vertically elliptical.

Head scales: Head covered with small irregular, tubercularly-keeled scales.

Body scales: Dorsals with apical pits, large and heavily keeled on back, smaller laterally, oblique, with serrated keels, in 23-27 rows at midbody. Ventrals with lateral keel, 102-165; subcaudals keeled posteriorly, all paired, 18-42.

Arabian Horned Viper,
Cerastes gasperettii

Description and Identification: Most individuals of this species possess horns, although the subspecies which occurs in Jordan and Israel always lacks horns. The "horn," when present is a long, spike-like protuberance above the eye. It is believed this spike helps prevent a build up of sand around the eye when the snake buries its body in the sand with just the top of the head exposed.

The color is brown, tan, or grayish and matches the color of the sand in the snake's habitat. There is a pattern of dark markings on the back that are more or less transverse bars except anteriorly where they may appear as paired spots. There is a fairly distinct dark postocular stripe.

Distribution, Habitat, and Biology: This snake ranges throughout most of the Arabian Peninsula where it lives in true desert. Inhabits both sandy desert and rocky desert up to 4,500 feet in elevation.

As with other members of its genus this is primarily a nocturnal or crepuscular snake. Although it may bask in early morning, it seeks refuge during the day from the desert heat, either in small animal burrows or by burying itself in the sand. Capable of "sidewinding" locomotion in loose sands.

Venom and Bite: Bites by this species are fairly rare due to its habitat being harsh desert. It is regarded as

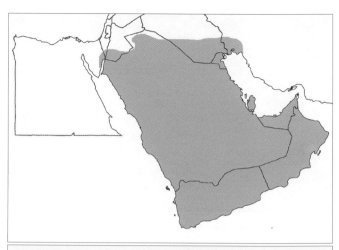

MAP 147. Range of the Arabian Horned Viper, *Cerastes gaperettii.*

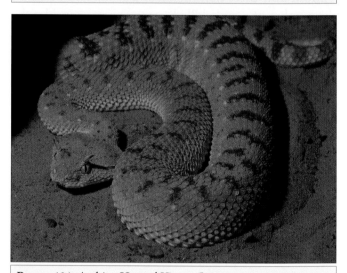

PHOTO 131. Arabian Horned Viper, *Cerastes gasperettii*

less dangerous than many of the region's snakes, but it is possibly capable of killing a human.

World Health Organization's Venomous Snake Antivenoms Database list of antivenoms for treating bites by this species: (www.int/bloodproducts/snakeantivenoms/database-2012).

Product: Polyvalent Snake Antivenom
Manufacturer: National Antivenom & Vaccine Production Center (NAVPC).
Country of Origin: Saudi Arabia.

Additional species: Two other species of *Cerastes* that are mainly North African also range into the USCENTCOM region in Egypt, the Sinai Peninsula, and the southwestern tip of the Arabian Peninsula. For information on these two snakes (*C. cerastes*, the Sahara Horned Viper and *C. vipera*, the Sahara Sand Viper, see page 183, Chapter 12 (USAFRICOM). The ranges of these two other *Cerastes* species within the USCENTCOM region is shown on the opposite page.

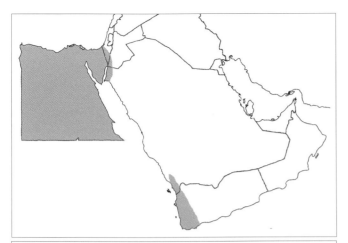

Map 148. Range of the Sahara Horned Viper, *Cerastes cerastes* within the USCENTCOM region.

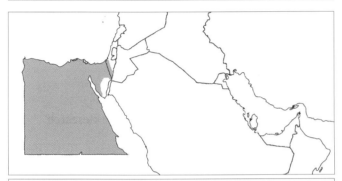

Map 149. Range of the Sahara Sand Viper, *Cerastes vipera* within the USCENTCOM region.

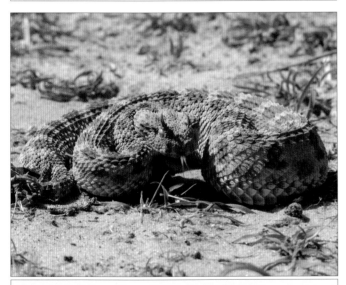

Photo 132. Sahara Horned Viper, *Cerastes cerastes*

Family - Viperidae

Subfamily - Viperinae - True Vipers

Genus- Pseudocerastes

False Horned Vipers

Three species are recognized. All are endemic to the US-CENTCOM region. They all have raised scales above the eye that form a short horn-like protuberance. The "horns" of these snakes, however, are not much more than slightly raised "eyebrow" scales. Although they are similar in appearance to the Horned Vipers, they are not closely related to them and the similarities are the result of adaptations for a desert lifestyle and are a classic example of convergent evolution. Their adaptive traits extend beyond morphological characters and include behavioral adaptation such as sidewinding locomotion and burying into sand. In this respect they and the Horned Vipers are analogous to the North American Rattlesnakes known as the Sidewinders. Again, they are all unrelated, but all share identical adaptations and behaviors for a desert existence.

Two of the 3 species are very similar in appearance and biology, and the third is so rare that only two specimens have ever been found.

Definition: The head is broad and very distinct from the neck. Snout short and broadly rounded; nostrils dorsolateral, valves present in nostrils.

Eyes small to moderate, pupils vertically elliptical.

Head scales: Head covered with small, imbricate scales; an erect hornlike projection covered with imbricate scales above the eye. Laterally, nasals separated from rostral by small scales; eye separated from labials by 3-4 rows of small scales.

Body scales: Dorsals keeled, in 21-25 nonoblique rows at midbody. Ventrals 134-163, subcaudals paired, 35-50.

Western False Horned Viper,
Pseudocerastes fieldi

Description and Identification: Differs from the Horned Vipers in the absence of keels on the ventrals and in the nature of the horn which is composed of several small scales in this species rather than a single spine-like scale in *Cerastes.* From other vipers within its range, it differs in the dorsolateral position of the nostril.

Color pale gray or bluish gray to khaki with dark blotches or crossbands; dark band on side of head; belly white. Some specimens from areas of lava deposits are quite dark (see photo 134).

Record size 43 inches. Average about 30 inches.

Distribution, Habitat, and Biology: Endemic to the USCENTCOM region where it is found in desert areas in portions of Saudi Arabia and Syria and most of Jordan, Israel, and the Sinai Peninsula .

Primarily nocturnal in habits but may be seen sunning or crawling about by day in the early spring.

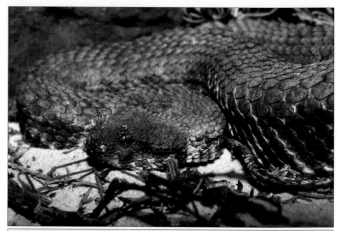

Photo 134. Western False Horned Viper (dark), *Pseudocerastes persicus*

World Health Organization's Venomous Snake Antivenoms Database (www.int/bloodproducts/snakeantivenoms/database-2012) lists the following antivenom for treating bites by this species:

Product: Polyvalent Snake Antivenom

Manufacturer: Razi Vaccine & Serum Research Institute

Country of Origin: Iran

Additonal Species: The Eastern False Horned Viper, *P. persicus*, is nearly identical. Its range appears below.

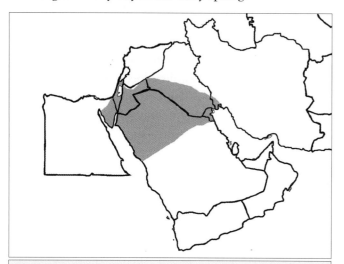

Map 150. Range of the Western False Horned Viper, *Pseudocerastes fieldi.*

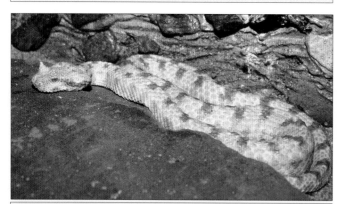

Photo 133. Western False Horned Viper (light), *Pseudocerastes fieldi*

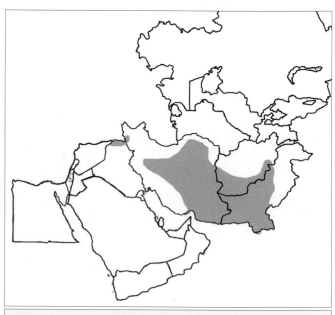

Map 151. Range of the Eastern False Horned Viper, *Pseudocerastes persicus.*

Venom and Bite: The venom of this species is reported to be a potent haemotoxin, but its significance as a threat to humans is mitigated by the fact that it prefers areas uninhabited by man (Phelps 2010). Clinical Toxinology Resources Website (*www.toxinology.com* - 2012) states bites "unlikely to prove fatal."

Family - Lamprophiidae:

Genus - Atractaspis

Mole Vipers

Nineteen species are currently recognized. Most are African, but two species occur in the USCENTCOM region in the Arabian Peninsula. All Mole Vipers are small snakes, less than 3 feet in length. However, they have large fangs (which look enormous in their small mouths) and are capable of inflicting serious bites to those picking them up or stepping on them with bare feet.

Definition: Head short and conical, not distinct from neck, no canthus; snout broad, flattened, often pointed. Body cylindrical, slender in small individuals, stout in large ones; tail short, ending in a distinct spine.

Eyes very small; pupils round.

Head scales: The usual 9 crown scales, rostral enlarged, extending between internasals to some degree, often pointed; frontal large and broad, supraoculars small. Laterally, nasal in contact with single pre-ocular (no loreal), usually one postocular.

Body scales: Dorsals smooth without apical pits, in 19-37 oblique rows at midbody. Ventrals 178-370; anal plate entire or divided. Subcaudals single or paired, 18-39.

Two species of Mole Vipers are found in the USCENTCOM region; the Arabian Mole Viper (*A. andersonii*) and the Israeli Mole Viper (*A. engadennsis*) both in the Arabian Peninsula. The ranges of these two snakes are shown below. For photographs and information about similar Mole Vipers see page 204, Chapter 12 (USAFRICOM).

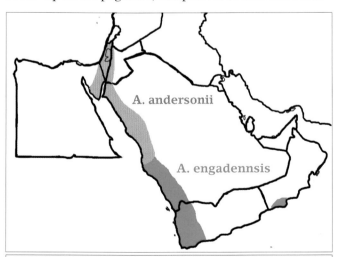

MAP 152. Range of the two Mole Vipers, (*A. andersonii and A. engadennsis*) found in the USCENTCOM region.

Family - Elapidae

Genus - Walterinnesia

Desert Cobras

This genus is endemic to the USCENTCOM region, and contains only two species. They are relatively large, 3 to 4 feet, and are probably dangerous species.

Definition: Head relatively broad; flattened, distinct from neck; snout broad, a distinct canthus. Body cylindrical and tapered, moderately slender; tail short.

Eyes moderate in size; pupils round.

Head scales: Dorsals smooth at midbody, feebly keeled posteriorly, in 24rows at midbody, more (27) anteriorly. Ventrals 189-197; anal plate divided; subcaudals 45-48, first 2-8 single, remainder paired.

Maxillary teeth: Two large tubular fangs with external grooves followed after an interspace, by 0-2 small teeth.

Unlike the true Cobras (genus *Naja*), these snakes do not hood when threatened.

Black Desert Cobra,
Walterinnesia aegyptia

Description and Identification: A moderately stout snake with short tail and small head not distinct from neck; crown with large shields. The following combination of scale characters is useful in distinguishing this species from non-venomous snakes and "true" cobras. 1. Loreal plate absent; 2. Dorsal scales smooth anteriorly, keeled posteriorly; 3. Anal plate divided; 4. Some single subcaudals, although most are paired.

Adults are uniformly black or very dark brown or gray above, a little paler ventrally. Average length 3 to 3.5 feet; maximum about 54 inches.

Distribution, Habitat, and Biology: Found throughout the Sinai Peninsula and adjacent regions of northeast Egypt and Israel, also in southwest Jordan and northeast Saudi Arabia. Found in both remote desert and irrigated agricultural areas; also includes rocky foothills. Absent from barren, sandy desert. A terrestrial species that is nocturnal in habits. Feeds on a wide variety of prey but mostly eats lizards and other snakes. Also known to feed on carrion.

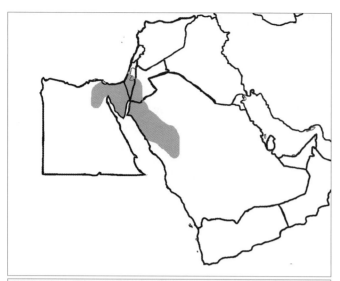

Map 153. Range of the Black Desert Cobra, *Walterinnesia aegyptia*.

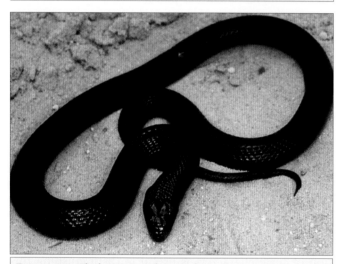

Photo 135. Black Desert Cobra, *Walterinnesia aegyptia*

Venom and Bite: Toxicity of the venom for experimental animals is about the same as that of the Indian Cobra but quantity is considerably less (about 20 mg. vs. 50 to 100 mg.).

World Health Organization's Venomous Snake Antivenoms Database list of antivenoms for treating bites by this species: (www.int/bloodproducts/snakeantivenoms/database-2012):

> Product: Bivalent Naja/Walterinnesia Snake AV
>
> Manufacturer: National Antivenom and Vaccine Production Center (NAVPC)
>
> Country of Origin: Saudi Arabia
>
> Product: Polyvalent Snake Antivenom
>
> Manufacturer: National Antivenom and Vaccine Production Center (NAVPC)
>
> Country of Origin: Saudi Arabia

Additional Species: One other *Walterinnesia* species, the Morgan's Desert Cobra (*W. morgani*) is widespread and fairly common in the USCENTCOM region.

In both appearance and biology it is very similar to the Black Desert Cobra, but has a larger range (see map below). The venom of this species is presumed to be similar to *W. aegyptia* and the antivenoms recommended for treating bites are the same.

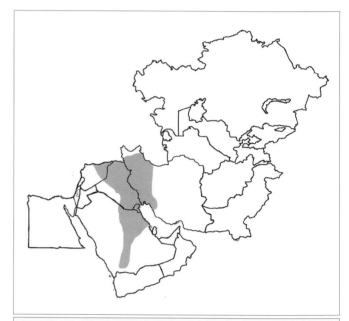

Map 154. Range of the Morgan's Desert Cobra, *Walterinnesia morgani* in the USCENTCOM region.

Family - Elapidae: Genus - Naja

True Cobras

As many as 28 species are recognized. These snakes are mostly African or Asian, but there are some species in the Pacific region of Indonesia and the Philippines. Five are found in the USCENTCOM region. This genus has seen much revision since the book *Poisonous Snakes of the World* was first published in 1965 and additional taxonomic changes are possible in the future. *Naja* cobras are moderate to large in size (4 to 8 feet as adults). They have large fangs and toxic venom. Some species are capable of "spitting" venom into the eyes of an aggressor.

Definition: Head rather broad, flattened, only slightly distinct from the neck. Snout rounded, a distinct canthus. Body moderately slender, slightly depressed, tapered, neck capable of expansion into a hood. Tail of moderate length.

Eyes moderate in size; pupils round.

Head Scales: The usual 9 on the crown; frontal short; rostral rounded. Laterally, nasal in contact with the one or two preoculars.

Body scales: Dorsals smooth in 17-25 oblique rows at midbody, usually mor on the neck, fewer posteriorly. Ventrals 159-232, subcaudals 42-88, mostly paired.

Central Asian Cobra,
Naja oxiana

Description and Identification: Adults brown, sometimes with traces of wide dark crossbands; hood mark never present; belly pale with dark bars on neck. Young tan or buff with regular dark crossbands; no hood mark. The smooth dorsal scales are strongly oblique in this species and the hood is noticeably narrower than in many other *Naja*.

Length can reach 6 feet.

Distribution, Habitat, and Biology: This species ranges from northern India to the Caspian Sea, but there is a wide gap in the range in northeastern Afghanistan which separates the range into two disjunct populations.

Although primarily a terrestrial species these snakes are good climbers. They are mainly crepuscular or diurnal but can be nocturnal during hot weather.

Like many cobras, their diet is catholic and they will eat a wide variety of vertebrate prey.

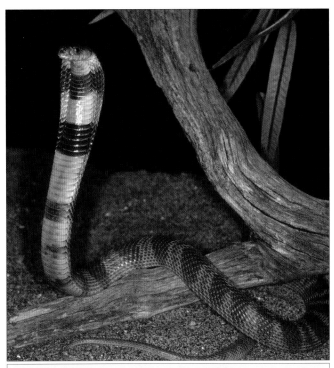

PHOTO 136. Central Asian Cobra, *Naja oxiana*

Venom and Bite: Post-synaptic neurotoxins and possible cardiotoxins. Some studies using subcutaneous LD50's in mice suggest this species has an extremely toxic venom. Fortunately, these snakes are usually not easily provoked, but their bite is undoubtably highly dangerous to man. Despite their apparent potential for lethality, there does not seem to be a specific antivenom available and the only reference found for antivenom for this species at the time of this writing was a single listing (shown below).

> Product: Polyvalent Snake Antivenom
> Manufacturer: Razi Vaccine and Serum Research Institute
> Country of Origin: Iran

It should be noted that *N. oxiana* was long considered as a subspecies of the Spectacled Cobra (*N. naja*), and a number of antivenoms are produced for that species. See page 214, Chapter 13 (USPACCOM). The effectiveness of *N. naja* antivenoms against this species may not be high.

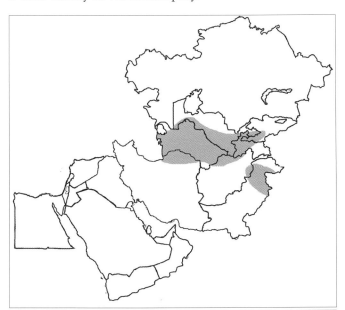

MAP 155. Range of the Central Asian Cobra, *Naja oxiana* in the UCENTCOM region.

Arabian Cobra,
Naja arabica

Description and Identification: A large cobra that can reach a length of 8 feet. Neck ribs expandable into a hood. The head is broad and slightly distinct from the neck and there is a distinct canthus.

Color is brown with light brown or yellowish highlights on the dorsal scales. Darker anteriorly and the head is usually a dark brown.

Distribution, Habitat, and Biology: Mainly a diurnal species that inhabits brushy areas near water in otherwise arid desert. These cobras are capable of "spitting" their venom into the eyes of an antagonist.

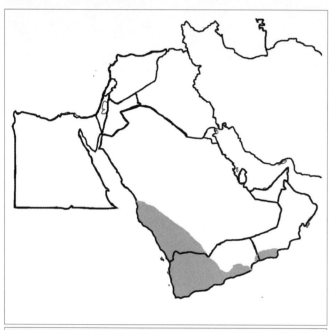

MAP 156. Range of the Arabian Cobra, *Naja arabica*

Venom and Bite: A deadly species that is known to have caused human fatalities.

World Health Organization's Venomous Snake Antivenoms Database list of antivenoms for treating bites by this species: (www.int/bloodproducts/snakeantivenoms/database-2012)

Product: Bivalent Naja/Walterinnesia Snake Antivenom

Manufacturer: National Antivenom & Vaccine Production Center (NAVPC)

Country of Origin: Saudi Arabia

Product: Polyvalent Snake Antivenom

Manufacturer: National Antivenom & Vaccine Production Center (NAVPC)

Country of Origin: Saudi Arabia

Additional Species: The Egyptian Cobra (*N. haje*), and the Nubian Spitting Cobra (*N. nubiae*), are two African species having ranges which invade the USCENTCOM region in parts of Egypt. For information on those species see page 188, Chapter 12, (USAFRICOM).

Also, the Common Cobra (*N. naja*), frequently called the Spectacled Cobra, extends its range westward from India into the USCENTCOM region in Pakistan. For information about the Common Cobra see page 211 Chapter 13 (USPACOM).

The ranges of these additional *Naja* species within the USCENTCOM region appears below.

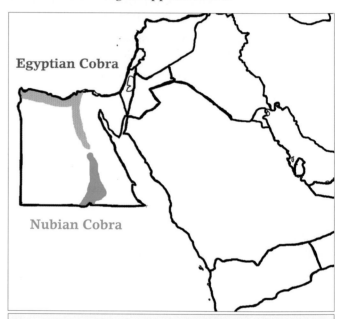

MAP 157. Range of the Egyptian Cobra, *Naja haje*, the Nubian Spitting Cobra and *Naja nubiae*, the Nubian Cobra within the USCENTCOM region.

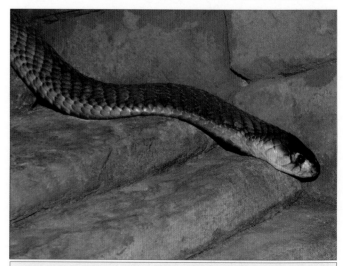

PHOTO 137. Egyptian Cobra, *Naja haje*. For information on this snake see page 188, Chapter 12, (USAFRICOM region).

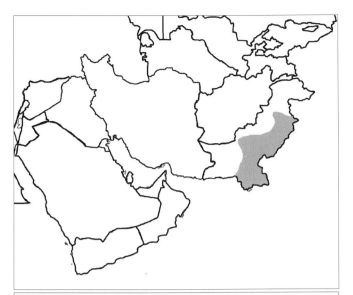

Map 158. Range of the Common Cobra, *Naja naja* within the USCENTCOM region.

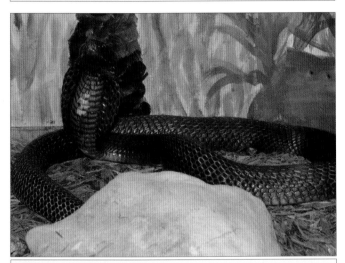

Photo 138. Common Cobra, *Naja naja*. This color phase of the Common Cobra is known as the "Pakistani Black Cobra."

Family - Elapidae: Genus - Bungarus

Kraits

Thirteen species are recognized; all inhabit Asia and most are found in southeastern Asia. Two species range into the USCENTCOM region in eastern Pakistan and eastern Afghanistan. Kraits are innocuous looking snakes and are usually hesitant to bite but their venom is a potent neurotoxin. Most species are of moderate (4 to 5 feet) length, but all are considered extremely dangerous. A few individuals reach lengths approaching 7 feet.

Definition: Head small, flattened, slightly distinct from neck; no distinct canthus. Body moderately slender, cylindrical; tail short.

Eyes small; pupils round or vertically sub-elliptical.

Head scales: The usual 9 on the crown; frontal broad. Laterally, nasal in broad contact with single preocular.

Body scales: Dorsals smooth, vertebral row enlarged and hexagonal (strongly so except in B. lividus), in 13-17 oblique rows at midbody. Ventrals 193-237; anal plate entire; subcaudals single or paired, 23-56.

Common Krait,
Bungarus caeruleus

Description and Identification: Body cylindrical with slight even taper; tail with pointed tip. All subcaudals undivided.

Black to dark brown or blueish with a series of narrow white or yellow crossbands that tend to be in pairs and often fade out or break up on the anterior quarter of the body. Upper lip white or yellow; belly an immaculate white. Average adult length 3-4 feet, maximum slightly over 5 feet.

Distribution, Habitat, and Biology: In the USCENTCOM area, found only in Pakistan and eastern Afghanistan. Widespread across nearly all of India and as far east as Bangladesh and Myanmar. Also frequently called the Indian Krait. A nocturnal snake that is typically docile during daylight, but much more alert and apt to bite after dark. Often found near human habitations and frequently enters poorly constructed or dilapidated buildings.

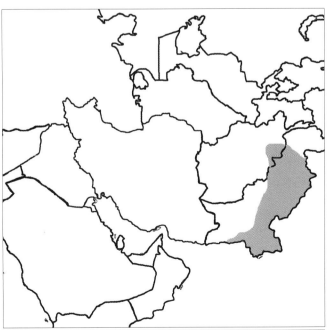

Map 159. Range of the Common Krait, *Bungarus caeruleus* in the USCENTCOM region.

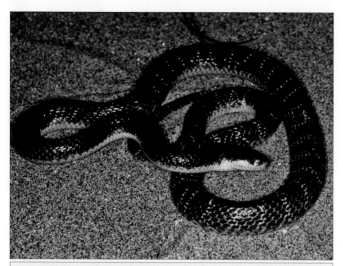

PHOTO 139. Common Krait, *Bungarus caeruleus*, See also page 222 Chapter 13 USPACOM

Venom and Bite: Both pre-synaptic and post-synaptic neurotoxins in venom. This is perhaps the most dangerous of the Kraits for it has a venom of very high toxicity for man. The lethal dose is estimated to be between 2.5 and 4 mg., a tiny amount considering a large specimen may possess as much as 30 mg. of venom. Bites are uncommon but deaths from untreated bites may be as high as 80 percent. One of the world's most deadly snakes.

World Health Organization's Venomous Snake Antivenoms Database list of antivenoms for treating bites by this species: (www.int/bloodproducts/snakeantivenoms/database-2012)

> Product: Polyvalent Antisnake Venom
> Manufacturer: National Institute of Health
> Country of Origin: Pakistan
> Product: Polyvalent Snake Antivenom (Asia)
> Manufacturer: Bharat Serums and Vaccines
> Country of Origin: India
> Product: Snake Antivenom IP (Asia)
> Manufacturer: Haffkine Biopharmaceutical Corporation, Ltd.
> Country of Origin: India
> Product: Snake Antivenom Antiserum I.P. (Asia)
> Manufacturer: VINS Bioproducts Ltd.
> Country of Origin: India

Additional Species: One other Krait species, the Sind Krait (*B. sindanus*) is also found in the USCENTCOM region. It is a rare snake that occurs in a small area of Pakistan (though it is more common in India). Nearly identical to the Common Krait in appearance, it is no doubt a highly dangerous species.

NOTES

Current References

Books

David, Patrick & Gernot Vogel. 2010. *Venomous Snakes of Europe, Northern, Central, and Western Asia.* TERRALOG Vol 16. Edition Chimaira, Frankfort, Germany.v.

Dobiey, Maik & Gernot Vogel. 2007. *Venomous Snakes of Africa.* TERRALOG Vol. 15. Edition Chimaira, Frankfort, Germany.

Dowling, Herndon G., Sherman A. Minton, and Findlay E. Russell. 1965. *Poisonous Snakes of the World.* Department of the Navy Bureau of Medicine and Surgery. Washington, DC.

Phelps, Tony. 2010. *Old World Vipers, A Natural History of the Azemoipinae and Viperinae.* Edition Chimaira. Frankfort, Germany.

Journals

Stumpel N., Joger U (2009) "Recent advances in phylogeny and taxonomy of Near and Middle Eastern vipers an update". ZooKeys 31: 179-191.

Web References

World Health Organization - www.who.int/bloodproducts/snakeantivenoms/database

The Reptile Database - http//www.reptiledata-base.org

Armed Forces Pest Management Board - www.afpmb.org/content/living-hazards-database

University of Adelaide, Clinical Toxinoogy Resources Wesbsite (2012) - *www.toxinology.com*

www.venomousreptiles.org

Munich Antivenom Index (MAVIN) - www.toxinfo.org/antivenoms

www.iucnredlist.org

Original References

ANDERSON, Steven C. 1963. Amphibians and Reptiles from Iran. Proc. Calif. Acad. Sci., vol. 31, pp. 417–498, figs. 1–15.

KHALAF, Kamal T. 1959. Reptiles of Iraq with Some Notes on the Amphibians. Ministry of Education: Baghdad, 96 pp., 40 figs.

MENDELSSOHN, H. 1963. On the Biology of the Venomous Snakes of Israel. Part I. Israel Jour. Zool., vol. 12, pp. 143–170, figs. 1–9. 1965. Part II, *ibid*, vol. 14, pp. 185–212.

MERTENS, Robert. 1952. Amphibien und Reptilien aus der Tuerkei. Rev. Fac. Sci. Univ. Istanbul, ser. B, no. 1, pp. 41–75.

MERTENS, Robert. 1965. Wenig bekannte "Seitenwinder" unter den Wüstenottern Asiens. Nat. u. Mus. vol. 95, pp. 346–352, figs. 1–5.

NIKOLSKY, A. M. 1916. Faune de la Russie. Reptiles. Petrograd. vol. 2, 349 pp., 8 pls.

SHAW, C. J. 1925. Notes on the Effect of the Bite of Mc Mahon's Viper (*E. macmahonii*). J. Bombay Nat. Hist. Soc., vol. 30: 485–486.

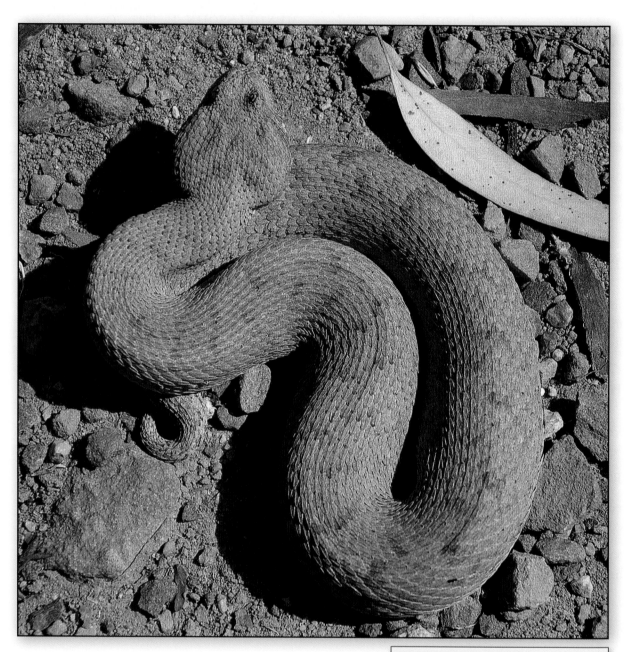

Red Adder, *Bitis rubida*

CHAPTER **12**

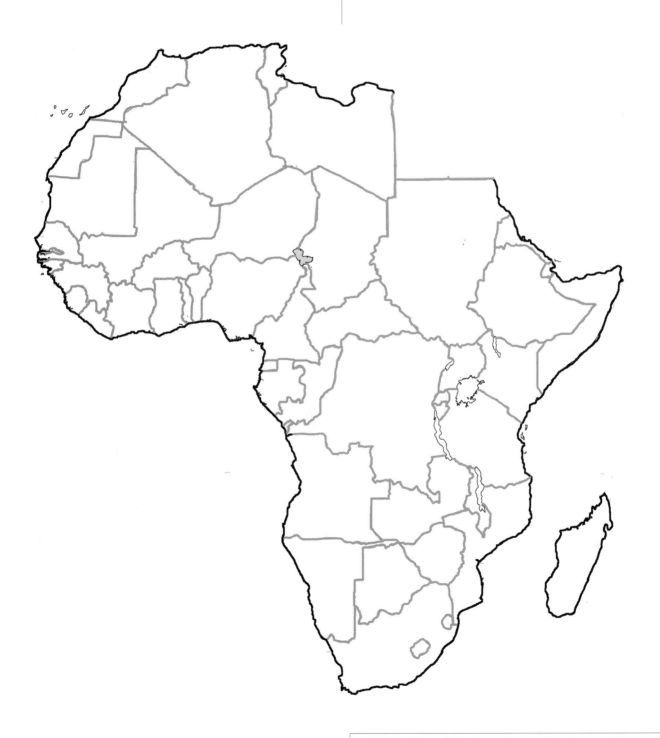

Map 160. Region 5, The United States Africa Command.

Introduction

This region ranks third among the six regions in this book for the actual number of venomous snake species (92), but it equals or exceeds every other region in diversity of species. There are 4 families of venomous snakes native to the region and a total of 22 genera.

The most well represented are the Viperidae (true vipers) with 11 genera totaling 50 species. Five of these genera are endemic to the region and a sixth has 16 of its 17 species found only on the continent of Africa. Some members of this family are so poorly understood that virtually nothing is known about the effects of their venom on humans, but several species are known to be quite deadly. The most notable of these are the larger members of the *Bitis* genus, some of which are frightfully dangerous. The Gaboon Vipers (*B. gabonica* and *B. rhinoceros*) are both huge snakes with fangs up to 2 inches in length and enormous venom glands. Meanwhile the closely related Puff Adder (*B. arietans*) has the distinction of killing more humans than any other snake on the African continent.

The second most diverse family here are the Elapidae (cobra family) with a total of 8 genera. Some of these genera, however, the African Garter Snakes (*Elapsoidea*) and the Harlequin Snakes, (*Homorselaps*) are considered to be mildly venomous are not generally regarded as dangerous to man. Thus, these snakes are not included in this book. Excluding those mildly venomous snakes there are at least 23 members of the Cobra family in the region that are dangerous to man, and some are among the world's deadliest snakes. In fact one species, the Black Mamba (*Dendroaspis polylepsis*), is regarded by many as the world's most deadly serpent.

The unusual family Lamprohiidae includes several species of small to medium sized, mildly venomous snakes endemic to the region that are widespread but pose little threat to man. Among these are Purple Glossed Snakes (*Amblyodipsas*) Centipede Eaters (*Aparpallactus*), Two-headed Snakes (*Chilorhinophis*) Snake Eater Snakes (*Polemon*), Quill-snouted Snakes (*Xenocalamus*), and the monotypic genera *Hyoptophis* and Elapotinus. There is one genus of the Lamprohiidae however that is dangerous to man and that genus (*Atractaspis*) is widespread, common, and highly diverse with USAFRICOM region.

Commonly known as Mole Vipers, there are at least 19 species, 17 of which are endemic to the region.

Finally, the worldwide family Colubridae, which contains most of the world's harmless snake species has 2 genera native to this region that are deadly to man. The Twig Snakes (*Thelotornis*), with 4 species and the Boomslang (*Dispholidus*), with a single species, are rear-fanged snakes that have killed humans.

The significance of snakebite death and injury in this region is notable, and only surpassed by the number of people killed and injured in the USPACOM region. The problem of snakebite on the African continent is complicated by the fact that medical treatment for many indigenous peoples is remote, and antivenom is often not readily available.

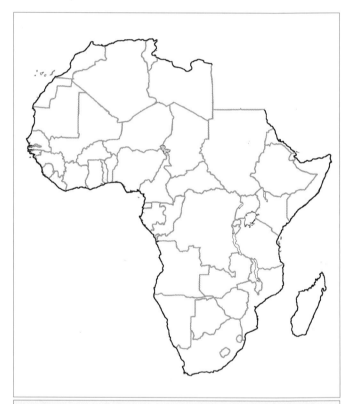

MAP 161. Region 5, United States Africa, Command. The African continent excluding Egypt.

Generic And Species Descriptions

Family - Viperidae

Subfamily - Viperinae - True Vipers

Genus- Bitis

African Vipers

This genus totals 17 species. All are indigenous to the African continent and all but one are endemic. They range in size from the world's smallest viper, the Namaqua Dwarf Viper (less than foot), to the world's largest, the East African Gaboon Viper (over seven feet and extremely heavy bodied, weighing up to thirty-five pounds!). All of the larger species are dangerous to man and some are extremely deadly snakes. One species, the common and widespread Puff Adder (*B. arietans*) holds the distinction of having killed more people than any snake species in Africa. By contrast some of the smaller species may lack the ability to kill a healthy adult human.

Definition: Head broad, flat on top, triangular in shape and very distinct from neck. Stout bodied, larger species are extremely stout. Snout short and rounded, canthus distinct. Body somewhat dorso-ventrally flattened. Tail short.

Eyes small, pupils vertically elliptical.

Head scales: Top of head covered with small scales. Several smaller species may have raised scales above the eye and some of the larger species have elongated, rhinoceros horn-like scales on the top of the snout.

Body Scales: Dorsal scales keeled in 21-46 rows at midbody. Ventrals 112-160. Subcaudals 16-37. Anal scute entire.

All *Bitis* are ambush predators that typically sit and wait for prey to come within striking distance. All are cryptically colored and some are extremely intricate in color and pattern. Though quite beautiful, some appear almost gaudy when removed from their natural habitats.

These snakes are found for the most part in sub-saharan Africa and several species have extremely restrictive ranges. In contrast, one species, the Puff Adder (*B. arietans*) can be found throughout most of the continent of Africa as well as on the Arabian Peninsula.

Puff Adder,

Bitis arietans

Description and Identification: The rough-scaled appearance and pattern of dark and light chevron-shaped markings are characteristic. Head lanceolate; nostrils face more directly upward than in other African vipers. Adults average 3-4 feet; occasional individuals attain a length of6 feet.

A light band crosses the head between the eyes and is continued as a diagonal band from the eye to the rear of the mouth. Ground color varies from light grayish tan or yellow to dark brown; either the light or the dark chevron series may be emphasized, depending on the density of the ground color.

Dorsal in 29-41 rows at midbody. Ventrals 124-147; sucaudals 16-37.

Distribution, Habitat, and Biology: Widespread and common throughout sub-saharan Africa except for the rainforest in the west central regions of the continent. It can be found from sea level to 9,000 feet. A disjunct population occurs in southern Morocco and northernmost Western Sahara. A second disjunct population is found on the Arabian Peninsula.

Occupies a variety of habitats and in fact can be found nearly anywhere except the sand desert of the Sahara and dense tropical forests.

Due to its wide distribution, common occurrence and highly toxic venom, the Puff Adder kills more people than any other African Snake. The abundance of this snake throughout its range may be attributed to its extremely high reproductive capabilities. Litters of over 150 babies have been recorded and the average litter size is usually more than two dozen.

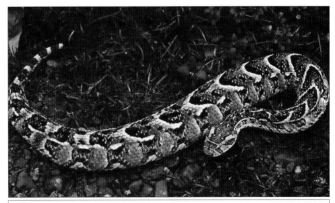

Photo 140. Puff Adder, *Bitis arietans*

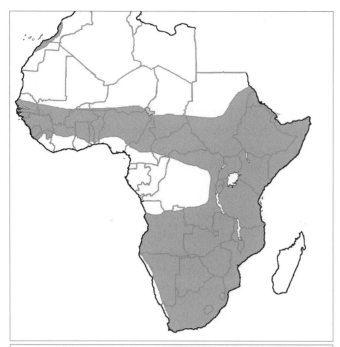

MAP 162. Range of the Puff Adder, *Bitis arietans*, in the USAFRICOM region.

Venom and Bite: Puff Adder venom contains both powerful haemotoxins and powerful cytotoxins.

Bites often result in extreme necrosis and those who survive its bite may bear the scars for life. Amputations of bitten limbs are common in those for whom treatment is delayed. These are large snakes with large fangs and large amounts of highly toxic venom. They are also widespread and common and in terms of the number of fatal bites they are the deadliest snake on the African continent.

World Health Organization list of Antivenoms:

> Product: FAV-Afrique
>
> Manufacturer: Sanofi-Pastuer
>
> Country of Origin: France
>
> Product: Favirept
>
> Manufacturer: Sanofi-Pastuer
>
> Country of Origin: France
>
> Product: Polyvalent Snake Antivenom
>
> Manufacturer: National Antivenom and Vaccine Production Center (NAVPC)
>
> Country of Origin: Saudi Arabia
>
> Product: SAIMR Polyvalent Snake Antivenom
>
> Manufacturer: South African Vaccine Producers (SAVP).
>
> Country of Origin: South Africa

From www.who.int/bloodproducts/snakeantivenoms/database (2012).

East African Gaboon Viper,
Bitis gabonica

Description and Identification: A very large and extremely heavy bodied viper with an intricate dorsal pattern of colors and shapes that defies written description but which has a remarkable cryptic effect when in natural environs. Very similar to the West African Gaboon Viper, but lacks the presence of nasal "horns" seen on that species. The head is quite broad and flat, very distinct from the neck and uniformly tan above with a narrow, dark brown medial stripe and a large somewhat triangular, dark brown postocular blotch. The postocular blotch is divided by a light line which runs at a slight angle from the bottom of the eye to the mouth. This character along with the lack of nasal horns distinguishes this species from the very similar West African Gaboon Viper. Can reach over 5 feet in length.

Distribution, Habitat, and Biology: Primarily a forest species that occupies a large range in central Africa including most of the Congo River basin. Also inhabits coastal areas west to southern Nigeria. In addition to forest it can also be found in areas of human disturbance (agricultural areas or secondary growth). These are huge snakes with remarkable girth and enormous heads and they can swallow animals up to the size of a small antelope. Large ground dwelling birds like Guinea Fowl are also eaten, along with a variety of small mammals.

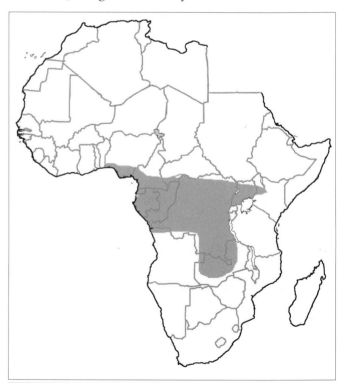

MAP 163. Range of the East African Gaboon Viper, *Bitis gabonica*.

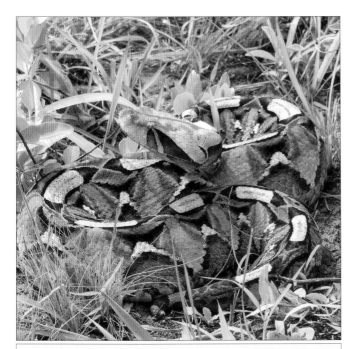

Photo 141. East African Gaboon Viper, *Bitis gabonica*

Venom and Bite: Procoagulants, haemorragins, cardiotoxins, and possibly anticoagulants. These snakes have huge venom glands and the venom is quite toxic. In addition, they boast some of the largest fangs in the snake world, being over 2 inches in length in the largest specimens. Fortunately, they are reportedly not quick to strike and bites are not common. They are however extremely dangerous animals and the probability of survival for untreated bites is low.

World Health Organization list of Antivenoms:

Product: FAV-Afrique

Manufacturer: Sanofi-Pastuer

Country of Origin: France

Product: SAIMR Polyvalent Snake Antivenom

Manufacturer: South African Vaccine Producers (SAVP)

Country of Origin: South Africa

From www.who.int/bloodproducts/snakeantivenoms/database (2012).

In addition, the Clinical Toxinology Resources Website (2012) - www.toxinology.com, also lists the above antivenoms as well the one shown below:

Product: Antivipmyn Africa

Manufacturer: Instituto Bioclone

Country of origin: Mexico

West African Gaboon Viper,
Bitis rhinoceros

Description and Identification: Very similar to the preceding species. A very large and extremely heavy bodied viper with an intricate dorsal pattern of colors and shapes that defies written description but which has a remarkable cryptic effect when in natural environs. Very similar to the East African Gaboon Viper from which it may be distinguished by the presence of nasal "horns" and by the absence of a light line running through the dark brown postocular patch (from the bottom of the eye to the mouth). The head is quite broad and flat, very distinct from the neck and uniformly tan above with a narrow, dark brown medial stripe and a large somewhat triangular, dark brown postocular blotch. Maximum size is even larger than for the East African Gaboon Viper with a record length of well over 7 feet.

Distribution, Habitat, and Biology: This species has a much smaller range than the East African Gaboon, being found in the tropical forests from Ghana westward to Guinea. Its range includes all of Sierra Leone and Liberia, but only the southernmost portions of Ghana, Ivory Coast, and Guinea.

In biology and habitats it is similar to the previous species and until recently was considered to be a subspecies of *B. gabonica*.

Venom and Bite: Very similar to the preceding species, but if anything this species is probably even more dangerous than the East African Gaboon, due simply to its larger size.

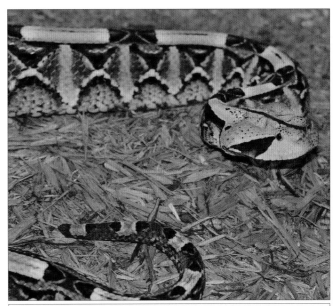

Photo 142. West African Gaboon Viper, *Bitis rhinoceros*

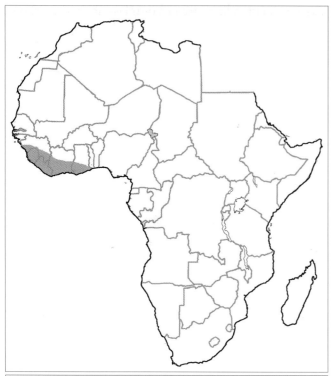

MAP 164. Range of the West African Gaboon Viper, *Bitis rhinoceros*.

Although the World Health Organization's website listing gives no specific Antivenom for this species, the Antivenoms listed for the East African Gaboon (*B. gabonica*) should be effective in treating bites by this species. Those antivenoms are as follows:

Product: FAV-Afrique

Manufacturer: Sanofi-Pastuer

Country of Origin: France

Product: SAIMR Polyvalent Snake Antivenom

Manufacturer: South African Vaccine Producers (SAVP)

Country of Origin: South Africa

From www.who.int/bloodproducts/snakeantivenoms/database (viewed 2012).

In addition, the Clinical Toxinology Resources website, www.toxinology.com (viewed 2012), also lists the above antivenoms as well the one shown below:

Product: Antivipmyn Africa

Manufacturer: Instituto Bioclone

Country of origin: Mexico

Nose-horned Viper,
Bitis nasicornis

Description and Identification: Intricately patterned with brownish, reddish, or purplish ground color highlighted by black, yellow, blue, and cream colored geometric markings. Scales are very heavily keeled and produce a velvety appearance to the skin.

The top of the head has a large dark "arrowhead" marking. The top of the back has a series of blueish green "butterfly wing" markings that are quite pronounced. The most diagnostic feature are the two elongated "nasal horns" that are yellowish in color and up to 2 inches long. Anterior to the two large horns are two or more smaller horns. The side of the face is distinctly marked with dark-edged white lines or patches. Despite its colorful pattern, this snake is extremely cryptic in its natural habitat of the forest floor.

Another very heavy bodied viper with a short tail and an overall "fat" appearance. Average length about 2.5 - 3 feet, maximum of about 3.5 feet.

Distribution, Habitat, and Biology: Habitat is forests and plantations. More aquatic than most vipers and is often found along rivers and streams as well as swamps and marshes. Range closely coincides with that of the Gaboon Vipers (see maps165, & 166).

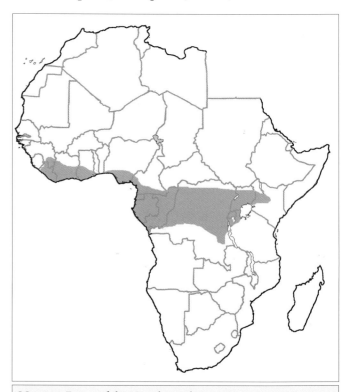

MAP 165. Range of the Nose-horned Viper, *Bitis nasicornis*.

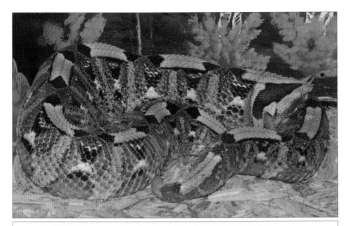

Photo 143. Nose-horned Viper, *Bitis nasicornis*

Venom and Bite: Little is known about the venom. Although bites by this species are apparently not very common, it is a highly dangerous snake and deaths from its bite are known to have occurred.

Although the World Health Organization's website listing gives no specific Antivenom for this species, the Antivenoms listed for the East African Gaboon (*B. gabonica*) may be effective in treating its bite. Those antivenoms are as follows:

Product: FAV-Afrique

Manufacturer: Sanofi-Pastuer

Country of Origin: France

Product: SAIMR Polyvalent Snake Antivenom

Manufacturer: South African Vaccine Producers (SAVP)

Country of Origin: South Africa

From www.who.int/bloodproducts/snakeantivenoms/database (2012).

In addition, the Clinical Toxinology Resources Website (2012) - www.toxinology.com, also lists the above antivenoms as well the one shown below:

Product: Antivipmyn Africa

Manufacturer: Instituto Bioclone

Country of origin: Mexico

Ethiopian Mountain Viper,
Bitis parviocula

Description and Identification: Another large and very heavy bodied *Bitis* that in appearance is similar to the preceding species. This species however lacks the "nasal horns" and is less intricately patterned. The dorsal ground color is greenish to olive brown. There are a series of light yellow green hourglass shaped markings along the spine that are separated by black blotches that are often diamond shaped. Smaller black blotches also occur laterally on each side of the light hourglass markings. There is usually a dark spear point marking atop the head between the eyes. The scales are heavily keeled and create a rough, textured appearance.

Distribution, Habitat, and Biology: Very little is known about the natural history of this snake except that it is a montane species, living at altitudes of up to 6,000 feet in the Ethiopian Highlands.

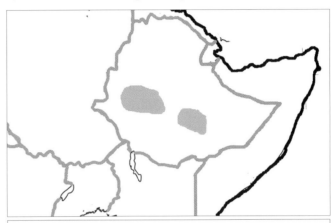

Map 166. Range of the Ethiopian Mountain Viper, *Bitis parviocula.*

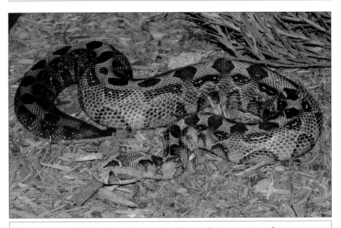

Photo 144. Ethiopian Mountain Viper, *Bitis parviocula*

Venom and Bite: Virtually nothing is known about the venom or effects of the bite of the Ethiopian Mountain Viper. As a large member of the *Bitis* genus, however, it must be assumed to be a dangerously venomous snake.

There is apparently no specific antivenom available for the Ethiopian Mountain Viper. It is possible that antivenoms produced for the Gaboon Vipers and or Puff Adder (see pages 165) could effectively be used to treat bites by this species.

Horned Adder,

Bitis caudalis

Description and Identification: This is a small species that attains a maximum length of 20 inches. In general appearance and in habits this *Bitis* species is similar to the Desert Horned Vipers (genus *Cerastes*). There is a single horn above each eye that is distinctive. In color they are drab in comparison to the larger members of this genus, exhibiting a ground color of gray or brown with a series of alternating dark and light blotches vertebrally. The dorsal blotches are usually non-contrasting lighter/darker shades of the ground color, but on some specimens the dark blotches may be almost black and contrast rather sharply.

Distribution, Habitat, and Biology: Raised horns above the eye in snakes is usually an adaptation for living a lifestyle that involves sandy deserts and the habit of hiding beneath the sand with just the top of the head exposed. Several very diverse snake species from different deserts of the world exhibit this trait which is a classic example of convergent evolution. The Horned Adder lives in deserts in southern Africa, but exhibits many of the same behaviors and physical traits as seen in the vipers of north Africa and the Sidewinder Rattlesnakes of the southwestern United States. These small snakes feed mostly on lizards and like many desert species are mainly nocturnal except during cooler weather when they may be found basking during the day.

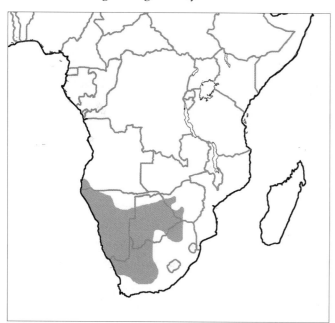

MAP 167. Range of the Horned Adder, *Bitis caudalis*.

Venom and Bite: There are apparently no known fatalities from the bite of this species and no antivenom is produced for treating bites. Local symptoms such as swelling, local necrosis, and pronounced pain have been reported from its bite. Severe envenomations may require the use of a polyvalent antivenom.

The Clinical Toxinology Resources website-www.toxinology.com (2012) recommends among others the following antivenom:

Product: SAIMR Polyvalent Antivenom

Manufacturer: South African Vaccine Producers (SAVP)

Country of Origin: South Africa

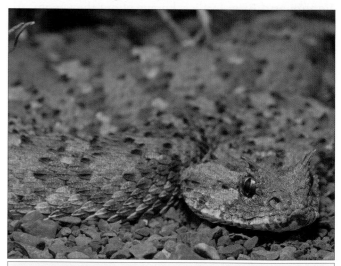

PHOTO 145. Horned Adder, *Bitis caudalis*

Berg Adder,

Bitis atropos'

Description and Identification: A small *Bitis* that can reach a length of up to 2 feet but averages about 18 inches. Highly variable. Ground color may be gray, brown, or reddish. Pattern consists of two rows of paired dorsolateral blotches that are darker than the ground color and may be indistinct or distinct. Blotches are usually edged in a light color and there is often a light patch separating the paired dark blotches. On most specimens the top of the head has an arrowhead shaped marking.

Distribution, Habitat, and Biology: Occurs in a half dozen or so disjunct populations that extend from the coast of South Africa northeast to the Zimbabwe-Mozambique border. Habitat is described by Phelps (2010) as "rocky grass slopes and montane fynbos from sea level to 3,000 meters" (over 6,000 feet).

Venom and Bite: Venom contains neurotoxins and this species has been responsible for human deaths. No specific antivenom is produced, but the Clinical Toxinology Resources website (www.toxinology.com viewed 2012) recommends, among others, the following antivenom for this species.

Product: SAIMR Polyvalent Antivenom

Manufacturer: South African Vaccine Producers (SAVP)

Country of Origin: South Africa

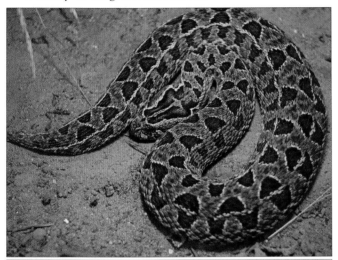

PHOTO 146. Berg Adder, *Bitis atropos*

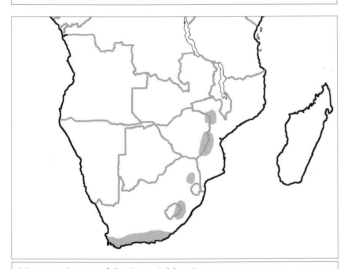

MAP 168. Range of the Berg Adder, *Bitis atropos*.

Southern Adder,
Bitis armata

Description and Identification: A small viper with a maximum length of just over 16 inches. A grey snake with paired darker gray dorsal blotches.

Raised scales above the eye create the appearance of a "tufted" eyebrow.

Distribution, Habitat, and Biology: Range is restricted to two tiny areas along the southwestern coast of South Africa (see map 169).

Venom and Bite: Nothing is known about the venom of these snakes and no antivenom is produced for this species.

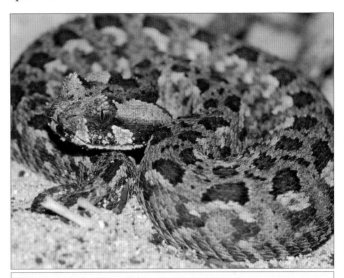

PHOTO 147. Southern Adder, *Bitis armata*

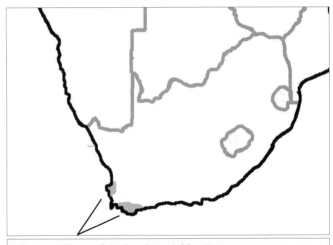

MAP 169. Range of the Southern Adder, *Bitis armata*.

Many-horned Adder,
Bitis cornuta

Description and Identification: A group of three or more raised scales above the eye is this snake's most distinctive character. The top of the head shows a distinct dark arrowhead edged in white. Ground color gray with dark gray dorsal blotches.

Distribution, Habitat, and Biology: Found along the coastal regions of southwest Namibia and western South Africa.

Venom and Bite: Little information is available regarding the venom and bite of this species. There is no antivenom produced because it is probably not deadly to a healthy adult.

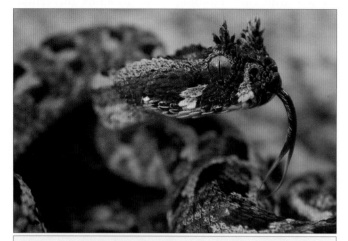

PHOTO 148. Many-horned Adder, *Bitis cornuta*

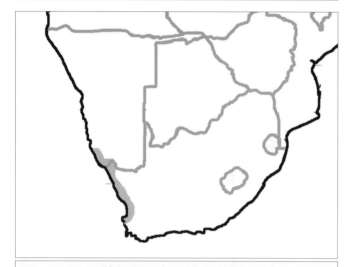

MAP 170. Range of the Many-horned Adder, *Bitis cornuta*.

Red Adder,
Bitis rubida

Description and Identification: Most specimens exhibit a decidedly reddish hue in both the ground color and in the faint dorsal markings. Some specimens tend to be more brownish or grayish with more distinct dorsal blotches. These are small vipers that may reach at most a foot and a half in length. Like many other small members of the *Bitis* genus, these snakes have raised, tuft-like scales above the eye.

Distribution, Habitat, and Biology: Endemic to Cape of South Africa where it lives in the uniquely South African habitat known as "Fynbos." Reported to feed on lizards and mice (Phelps 2010).

Venom and Bite: Little information is available regarding the venom and bite of this species and there is no antivenom produced for its bite. It is possible that antivenoms produced for the larger and more dangerous members of this genus (Puff Adder, Gaboon Viper, etc.) could be used effectively to treat bite by this and other small *Bitis* species.

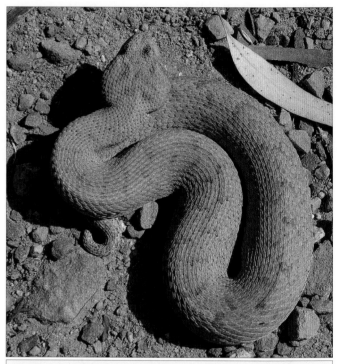

PHOTO 149. Red Adder, *Bitis rubida*

Additional Bitis species: In addition to the 10 species just described, there are 7 more members of this genus found in the USAFRICOM region. All are small snakes that are either quite rare or occur in very small areas and thus are not a significant threat for snakebite. Most are so small that even if they do bite humans the bite is probably not capable of killing. However, it should be noted that very little is known about the venom of some of these snakes and it would be unwise to regard them carelessly.

The list of additional *Bitis* species is as follows:

Kenyan Horned Adder - *Bitis worthingtoni*
Desert Mountain Adder - *Bitis xerophaga*
Albany Viper - *Bitis albanica*
Angolan Adder - *Bitis heraldica*
Plain Mountain Adder - *Bitis inornata*
Namaqua Dwarf Adder - *Bitis schneideri*
Peringuey's Adder *Bitis peringueyi*

The following set of range maps depict the approximate range of the above 7 species.

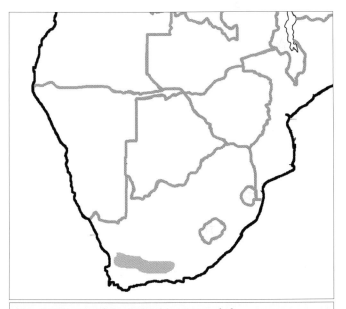

Map 171. Range of the Red Adder, *Bitis rubida*.

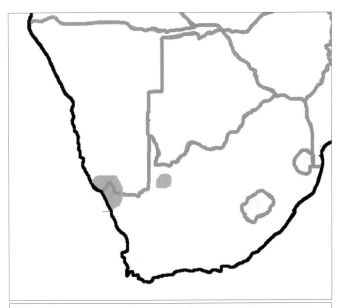

Map 173. Range of the Desert Mountain Adder, *Bitis xerophaga*.

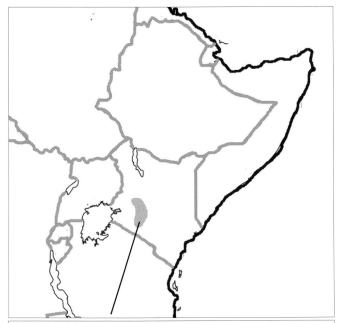

Map 172. Range of the Kenyan Horned Adder, *Bitis worthingtoni*.

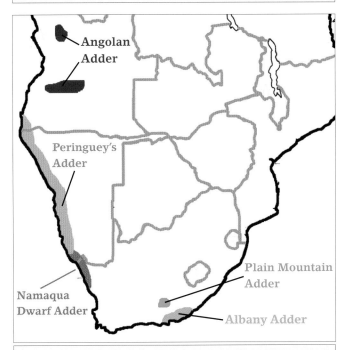

Map 174. Combined ranges of the Albany Adder, *Bitis albanica*, Angolan Adder, *Bitis heraldica*, Plain Mountain Adder, *Bitis inornata*, Namaqua Dwarf Adder, *Bitis schneideri,* and Peringuey's Adder, *Bitis peringueyi.*

Family - Viperidae

Subfamily - Viperinae - True Vipers

Genus- Macrovipera

Blunt-headed Vipers

The blunt, oval shaped head is distinctive of this genus. The *Macrovipera* genus contains only 4 species, but all are large and dangerous snakes. They are similar in many respects to the *Daboia* and two species (*mauritanica & deserti*) were once assigned to that genus by some experts. Two species are found in the USAFRICOM region and two more are within the USCENTCOM region.

Definition: Pupil elliptical. Head distinct from the neck, snout blunt or pointed, dorsum of head covered with small scales.

Body scales: Dorsal scales keeled in 24-33 rows at midbody. Ventrals 162-180; subcaudals paired 35-68; anal scute undivided.

Moorish Viper,
Macrovipera mauritanica

Description and Identification: A large, heavy bodied viper that can reach a length of 6 feet. Ground color light brown with a series of dark chocolate dorsal blotches that are somewhat rounded and often fuse together to create broad, wavy dorsal stripe. The head is distinct from the neck and the snout is rounded. Occurs with two species of much smaller *Vipera* species in Morocco and northern Algeria, but adults can be told from those snakes by size alone. Also is sympatric with the Puff Adder in southwestern Morocco, but that snake is a much stouter bodied species and has a much wider head.

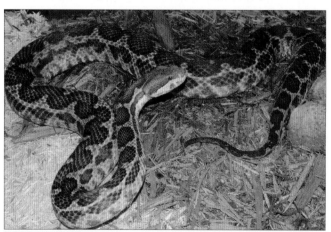

PHOTO 150. Moorish Viper, *Macrovipera mauritanica*

Distribution, Habitat, and Biology: Found in northern Tunisia, northern Algeria, and most of Morocco. Feeds on small mammals mostly. Primarily nocturnal.

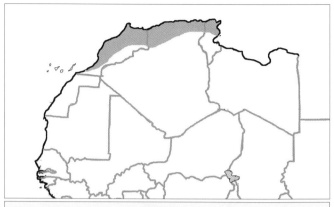

MAP 175. Range of the Moorish Viper, *Macrovipera mauritanica.*

Venom and Bite: Venom toxins include procoagulants, haemorragins, probably myotoxins, and possibly necrotoxins. These large snakes have a highly toxic venom and deaths from their bite is not uncommon.

Both www.toxinology.com and the MAVIN Antivenom Index (www.toxinfo.org/antivenoms) list the following Antivenom:

Product: Antiviperin Sera

Manufacturer: Institut Pasteur de Tunis

Country of Origin: Tunisia

Additional Species: One other very similar species, the Blunt-nosed Desert Viper, *Macrovipera deserti* can be found in a small area of northeast Libya and Tunisia. Some sources list this as a subspecies of the Moorish Viper. In all respects except color it is identical to the Moorish Viper. In color, however, it is a grayish snake with a faded, nearly indistinct dorsal pattern. See photo 151.

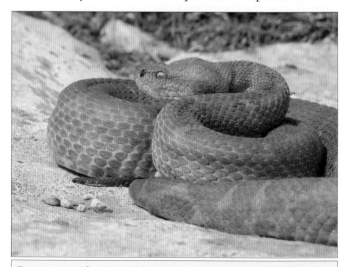

PHOTO 151. Blunt-nosed Desert Viper, *Macrovipera deserti*

Family - Viperidae

Subfamily - Viperinae - True Vipers

Genus- Vipera

True Adders

The genus *Vipera* contains a minimum of 20 species and some experts recognize up to 23. Most (18 species) are found in USEUCOM region. These are the "True Adders" of Europe, western Russia, and the Mediterranean region. With the exception of a few species they are restricted to those regions. However, two species range into the USAFRICOM region in north Africa.

For more information regarding this genus see page 125, Chapter 10 (USEUCOM region).

Snub-nosed Viper and Dwarf Atlas Mountain Viper,

Vipera latastei & Vipera monticola

These two species probably have their origins in southern Europe and made the crossing into northern Africa at a time in the geologic past when the two continents were connected via what is now the Strait of Gibraltar. The Snub-nosed Viper is found throughout the Iberian Peninsula as well as northern Morocco. Meanwhile the Dwarf Atlas Mountain Viper is endemic to the Atlas Mountains in Morocco.

Information on the Snub-nosed Viper can be found on page 128, Chapter 10 (USEUCOM region).

The Dwarf Atlas Viper is a small, rare species that occurs at high elevations (to 8,0000 feet) in the Haut Atlas Mountains.

Both species are readily recognized as being members of the *Vipera* genus, having the typical dark zig-zag dorsal markings on a greyish background. See range map below.

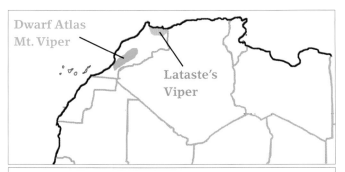

MAP 176. Ranges of the Snub-nosed Viper (*V. latastei*) and Dwarf Atlas Mountain Viper (*V. monticola*).

Venom and Bite: Both these species are capable of producing serious envenomations, but deaths are probably rare. There are no specific antivenoms produced for these snakes but the antivenoms listed below may have some cross reactivity and thus be effective in treating bites.

Product: Viper Venom Antitoxin (polyvalent).

Manufacturer: Institute of Virology, Vaccine and Sera TORLAK.

Country of Origin: Serbia

Product: Viper venom antitoxin European (polyvalent)

Manufacturer: Immunoloski Zavod

Country of Origin: Croatia

Product: Viperfav (polyvalent)

Manufacturer: Sanofi-Pastuer

Country of Origin: France

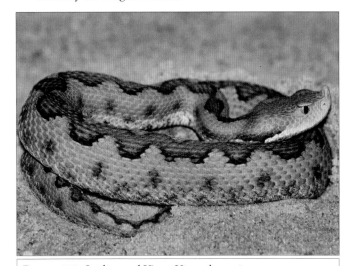

PHOTO 152. Snub-nosed Viper, *Vipera latastei*

Family - Viperidae

Subfamily - Viperinae - True Vipers

Genus- Atheris

Bush Vipers

This genus of small to medium sized vipers are mainly arboreal forest species. All have prehensile tails and very rough, heavily *keeled scales.* On some species the tips of the dorsal scales extend outward from the body and give the snake an almost hairy appearance. All are endemic to the African continent and all are tropical in their distribution. Two species have extensive ranges but most are found only in very small, isolated pockets. There are a total of 13 species.

Definition: Head very distinct from neck. Eyes large and situated forward, pupils elliptical. Body slender to moderately stout. Snout short and rounded.

Body scales: Heavily keeled and often imbricate, serrated on some species. Ventrals 133-175. Subcaudals 38-67, anal scute undivided.

Western Bush Viper,
Atheris chlorechis

Description and Identification: Dorsal coloration bright green with a variable amount of yellow along the back. Rarely this color pattern is reversed creating a pale yellow snake with a variable amount of green blotching. The belly is pale yellow and the throat is white. Adult length about 20 inches. Maximum 28 inches.

Distribution, Habitat, and Biology: Found in western Africa from Senegal south and east to Ghana and inland to Mali and Burkina Faso. Lives in tropical forest where it is arboreal in low bushes.

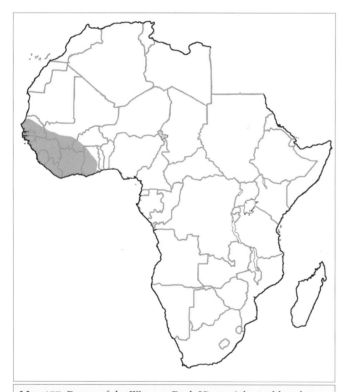

Map 177. Range of the Western Bush Viper, *Atheris chlorechis.*

Venom and Bite: There is little information available on the venom and bite of this species. Phelps (2010) gives an account of a bite that caused very serious systemic poisoning, including renal failure. This is probably a dangerous snake that may be capable of killing a human.

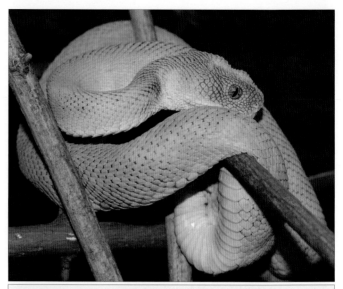

Photo 153. Western Bush Viper, *Atheris chlorechis.*

There is no specific antivenom for this species but Tony Phelps' book *Old World Vipers* recommends the following antivenoms for treating bites by members of this genus.

Product: SAIMR Polyvalent Antivenom
Manufacturer: South African Vaccine Producers (SAVP)
Country of Origin: South Africa
Product: FAV-Afrique
Manufacturer: Sanofi-Pastuer
Country of Origin: France

Green Bush Viper,
Atheris squamigera

Description and Identification: Despite the name this species is not always green. In fact it is a highly variable snake that may be various shades of green, orange, yellow, brown, or purplish. Although usually a uniform color, some individuals show a pattern of dark markings or crossbars. The tips of the scales tend to flare outward, creating a bristly appearance to the skin, especially on the head and neck. The eyes are quite large and situated well forward on the face. This is the largest of the Bush Vipers and may reach a length of 32 inches.

Distribution, Habitat, and Biology: Unlike many Bush Viper species which are quite rare and have very small ranges, the Green Bush Viper is widespread and common. Found throughout the tropical forests of central Africa. Its range overlaps that of several other rarer *Atheris* species. Those species may have different, specialized habitat requirements that keep the species apart.

As with other *Atheris* species the Green Bush Viper is mainly arboreal in low bushes but it will ascend at least as high as 20 feet. Its strongly keeled, bristly body scales may aid in climbing. It is also terrestrial at times and is regularly seen on the ground. Feeds on small vertebrates of all kinds. Some experts believe that this highly variable and widespread snake may in fact constitute more than just a single species.

Venom and Bite: This species has been known to cause human deaths. There is no specific antivenom but Tony Phelps' book *Old World Vipers* recommends the following antivenoms for treating bites by members of this genus.

Product: SAIMR Polyvalent Antivenom

Manufacturer: South African Vaccine Producers (SAVP)

Country of Origin: South Africa

Product: FAV-Afrique

Manufacturer: Sanofi-Pastuer

Country of Origin: France

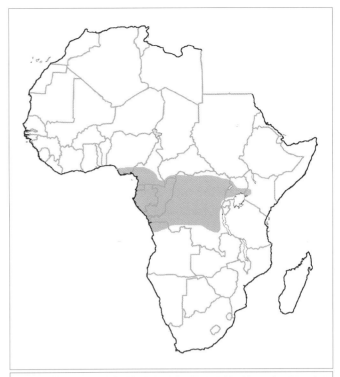

Map 178. Range of the Green Bush Viper, *Atheris squamigera.*

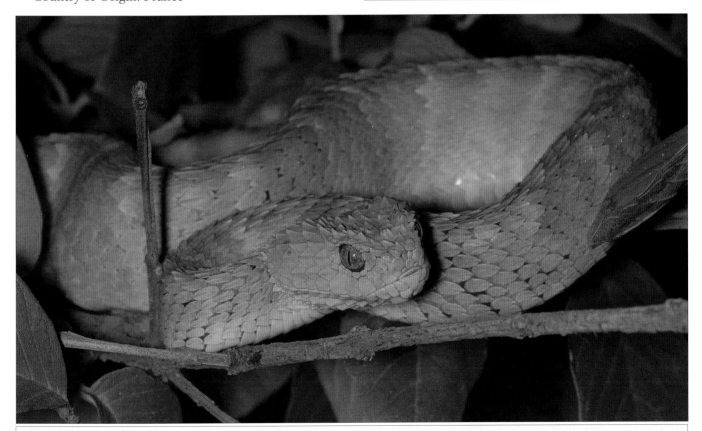

Photo 154. Green Bush Viper, *Atheris squamigera*

Sedge Bush Viper,
Atheris nitschei

Description and Identification: The record length is 28 inches but most are smaller. The ground color is light green and the skin between the scales is black. There is a black triangle on the top of the head and an irregular black line down the center of the back which may be broken into a series of blotches.

Distribution, Habitat, and Biology: This species is indigenous to the great lakes region of east Africa.

In fact it is sometimes called the Great Lakes Bush Viper. It lives in lowland sedge swamps and mountain forests.

Venom and Bite: There is no information available on the venom of this viper, but other members of the *Atheris* genus are known to have caused deaths. Thus this snake should be treated with caution. No specific antivenom is available.

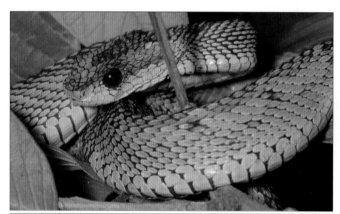

Photo 155. Sedge Bush Viper, *Atheris nitschei*

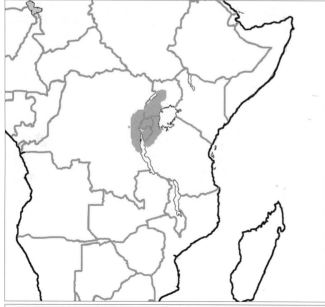

Map 179. Range of the Sedge Bush Viper, *Atheris nitschei*.

Mount Kenya Bush Viper,
Atheris desaixi

Description and Identification: This is a heavy bodied bush viper that reaches about 28 inches maximum length. The color is distinctive. Black with cream speckling on the tip of each dorsal scale (including each head scale).

Distribution, Habitat, and Biology: Range restricted to the vicinity of Mount Kenya in the country of Kenya.

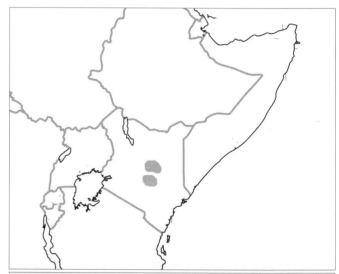

Map 180. Range of the Mt. Kenya Bush Viper, *Atheris desaixi*.

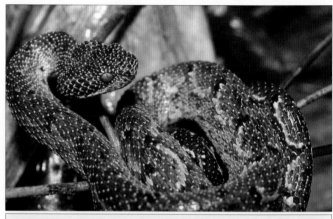

Photo 156. Mount Kenya Bush Viper, *Atheris desaixi*

Additional Species: There are a total of 9 other members of this genus. All are uncommon and have very small, restrictive ranges in central Africa. Some species (*A. acuminata, A. katangensis* and *A. hirsuta*) are known from just a handful of specimens. Little information is available on many of these snakes as they often inhabit remote and inhospitable jungle. There is little known about their venom and bite, although most pose little threat of snakebite. All species should be treated with caution and any bite regarded as potentially serious.

The 9 other species are as follows:

    Acuminate Bush Viper - *Atheris acuminata*

    Mayombe Bush Viper - *Atheris anisolepis*

    Broadley's Bush Viper - *Atheris broadleyi*

    Horned Bush Viper - *Atheris ceratophora*

    Tai Hairy Bush Viper- *Atheris hirsuta*

    Rough-scaled Bush Viper - *Atheris hispida*

    Shaba Bush Viper - *Atheris katangensis*

    Mount Mabu Forest Bush Viper- *Atheris mabuensis*

    Rungwe Bush Viper - *Atheris rungweensis*

The map below shows the combined ranges of these 9 other species.

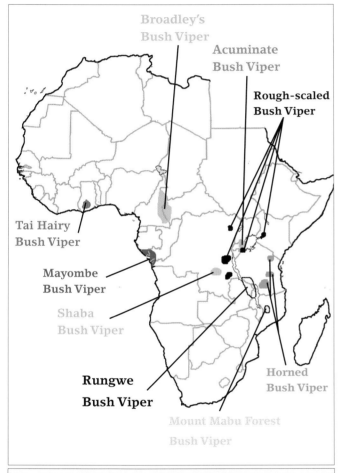

MAP 181. Combined ranges of *Atheris* species.

Family - Viperidae

Subfamily - Viperinae - True Vipers

Genus- Montatheris

Kenyan Mountain Viper

This genus contains only a single, rare species that is found only in two small areas in the African country of Kenya. It is closely related to the previous genus of Bush Vipers (*Atheris*) .

Definition: Head distinct from neck, body moderately slender.

Eyes moderately large, pupils elliptical.

Body scales keeled in 24-27 rows.

Kenyan Mountain Viper,
Montatheris hindii

Description and Identification: A very small viper with a record length of only 14 inches. Ground color brown with darker brown, more or less triangular blotches on each side of the back. Dark V-shaped marking on the top of the head.

Distribution, Habitat, and Biology: Lives in grassland habitats at high elevations.

Venom and Bite: Essentially nothing is known about the venom of this species. Although there is no antivenom cover, it is to rare to be considered much of a snakebite threat.

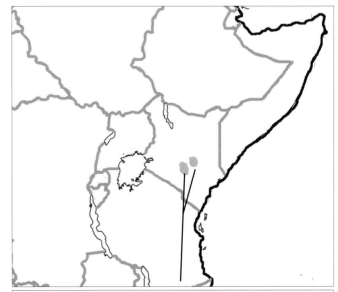

MAP 182. Range of the Kenyan Mountain Viper, *Montatheris hindii.*

Family - Viperidae

Subfamily - Viperinae - True Vipers

Genus- Proatheris

Swamp Viper

Another genus containing only a single species.

Definition: Head only slightly distinct from neck, elongate, snout rounded. Body moderately stout.

Eyes medium in size, pupils elliptical.

Body scales heavily keeled in 27-29 rows. Ventrals 131-159, subcaudals 32-45.

Swamp Viper,
Proatheris superciliaris

Description and Identification: Ground color tan or gray brown with large squarish vertebral blotches that are chocolate brown in color. There is a series of lateral blotches as well that are more or less the same size and shape of the dorsal blotches. There are two distinct, broad white lines on the side of the face and another down the center of the rostrum that continues onto the chin. Each of these are bordered by a broad, very dark (nearly black) band. These are relatively small snakes, less than 2 feet as adults.

Distribution, Habitat, and Biology: Occurs in a series of disjunct populations scattered throughout southeastern Africa. Found in portions of Tanzania, Malawi, and Mozambique. Inhabits grassland habitats in low-lying regions.

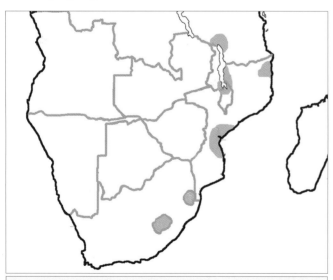

MAP 183. Range of the Swamp Viper, *Proatheris superciliaris.*

Venom and Bite: Two bites described by Phelps (2010), one of which was to himself, indicate this is probably not a deadly species.

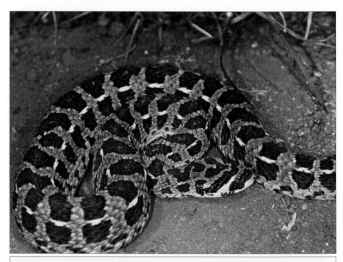

PHOTO 157. Swamp Viper, *Proatheris superciliaris*

Family - Viperidae

Subfamily - Viperinae - True Vipers

Genus- Echis

Saw-scaled Vipers

In the 1965 edition of *Poisonous Snakes of the World* two species of Saw-scaled Vipers were known. Today as many as 12 species are recognized. They are sometimes referred to as Carpet Vipers. Most species are remarkably similar to one another and the exact taxonomic status of this group is still confusing and probably subject to future revision. Six species are found in the USAFRICOM region. Altogether these 6 species range across much of Africa north of the equator. One of these 6 is also found in the USCENTCOM region and at least 5 other species are endemic to parts of the USPACOM and USCENTCOM regions. Although none attain a length of 3 feet, they possess a highly toxic venom and have been responsible for many deaths. In fact in terms of snakebite incidence and human mortality they are among the most dangerous snakes in the world. When disturbed they inflate the body and produce a hissing sound by rubbing the saw-edged lateral scales against one another. This same pattern of behavior is shown by the nonvenomous egg-eating snakes Dasypeltis.

Definition: Head broad, very distinct from narrow neck; canthus indistinct. Body cylindrical, moderately slender; tail short.

Eyes moderate in size. Pupils vertically elliptical.

Head Scales: A narrow supraocular sometimes present; otherwise crown covered with small scales, which may be smooth or keeled. Rostral and nasals distinct. Laterally, eye separated from labials by 1-4 rows of small scales; nasal in contact with rostral or separated from it by a row of small scales.

Body scales: Dorsals keeled, with apical pits, lateral scales smaller, with serrate keels, in 27-37 oblique rows at midbody. Ventrals rounded, 132-205; subcaudals single, 21-52.

Echis venoms are extremely potent hemotoxins consisting of procoagulants, haemorragins, and probably anticoagulants. Nephrotoxins and necrotoxins may also be present. Because these snakes are widespread and often very common, they cause many snakebites. The death rate is often high, and statistically these are among the world's deadliest snakes.

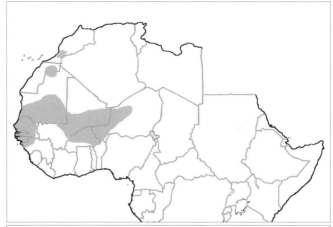

MAP 184. Range of the White-bellied Saw-scaled Viper, *Echis leucogaster.*

White-bellied Saw-scaled Viper,
Echis leucogaster

Description and Identification: This species' most distinguishing characteristic is its immaculately white belly. Locality is the best clue to identification, as throughout most of its range this is the only Saw-scaled Viper. Identification to species level may not be too important when treating bites, as all *Echis* are considered deadly and require aggressive treatment. With a record length of nearly 3 feet this is the largest of the Saw-scaled Vipers.

Distribution, Habitat and Biology: Habitat is listed as "Sahal," which is a semi-desert region that runs in a narrow band across northern Africa south of the more arid Sahara Desert. See range map 184.

Venom and Bite: Antivenom, FAV-Afrique by Sanofi-Pastuer in France.

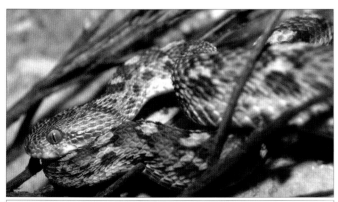

PHOTO 158. White-bellied Saw scaled Viper, *Echis leucogaster*

Egyptian Saw-scaled Viper,
Echis pyramidum

Description and Identification: Reaches a maximum length of about 2 feet but typically smaller. The dorsal pattern consists of well defined white spots or narrow white bands separated by larger, less well defined dark vertebral blotches. There are white crescent shaped markings on the sides that may connect to the white dorsal markings, and below each white crescent is a small dark blotch. The ground color is brownish, grayish, or reddish. Readily identified as an *Echis* species, but difficult to distinguish from other *Echis* when the locality of the specimen is unknown.

Distribution, Habitat, and Biology: Despite the name "Egyptian" Saw-scaled Viper, most of this snake's range is in Somalia, Eritrea, and Ethiopia. They are also found in parts of Libya and Algeria. Found in a variety of habitats within its range and is often a very common snake.

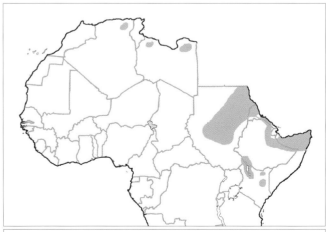

MAP 185. Range of the Egyptian Saw-scaled Viper, *Echis pyramidum*, in the USAFRICOM region.

Venom and Bite: The diminutive Saw-scaled Vipers are deadly far beyond what would be expected from such small vipers. The World Health Organization's website (www.who.int/bloodprducts/antivenoms, 2012) recommends the following antivenom for treating bites by this species.

Product: Polyvalent Anti-viper Venom

Manufacturer: VACSERA

Country of Origin: Egypt

Product: SAIMR Echis Antivenom

Manufacturer: South African Vaccine Producers

Country of Origin: South Africa

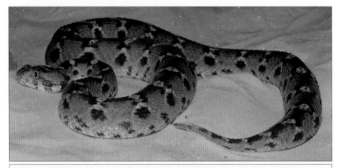

PHOTO 159. Egyptian Saw-scaled Viper, *Echis pyramidum*

West African Saw-scaled Viper,
Echis ocellatus

Description and Identification: Similar to other members of its genus, but has a row of distinct small white spots (ocelli) along each side of the back. Averages about 16 inches in length.

Distribution, Habitat, and Biology: Found in a wide swath of western Africa from the coasts of Senegal, Gambia, and Guinea-Bissau eastward to Cameroon. Like most *Echis* will eat almost anything from invertebrates to small mammals.

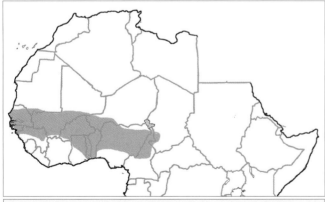

MAP 186. Range of the West African, Saw-scaled Viper, *Echis ocellatus*.

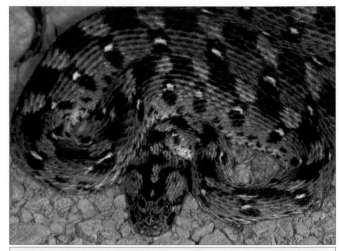

PHOTO 160. West African Saw-scaled Viper, *Echis ocellatus*

Venom and Bite: As with other members of the *Echis* genus, this is a highly dangerous snake.

World Health Organization recommends the following antivenoms:

Product: FAV-Afrique

Manufacturer: Sanofi-Pastuer

Country of Origin: France

Product: SAIMR *Echis* Antivenom

Manufacturer: South African Vaccine Producers (SAVP)

Country of Origin: South Africa

Additional Species: Three additional species of Saw-scaled Vipers are found in the USAFRICOM region. Three have very resticted ranges. *E. hughesi* (Somali Carpet Viper), *E. jogeri* (Mali Carpet Viper), and *E. megalocephalus* (Big Headed Carpet Viper) are only locally important as a snakebite threat. The ranges of these other *Echis* species is shown below.

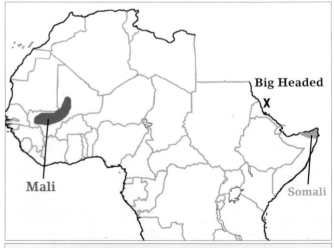

MAP 187. Range of Saw-scaled Vipers, *E. hughesi*, (Somali) *E. megalocephalus* (Big Headed), and *E. jogeri* (Mali).

Family - Viperidae

Subfamily - Viperinae - True Vipers

Genus- Cerastes

Horned Vipers

Four species are recognized and three occur in the US-AFRICOM region (one lives on the Arabian Peninsula). None are large snakes but the venom of some specimens appears to be highly toxic. Their name is derived from the presence in many specimens of an elongated "horn" above each eye. In some individuals the horn is reduced or lacking, and one species (*C. vipera*) is totally hornless.

As with the Saw-scaled Vipers, these snakes may rub the sides of their body coils together to produce a hissing sound when threatened.

As with a few other snake species from around the world that are highly adapted to life in the desert, these snakes are capable of utilizing "sidewinding" locomotion when traversing loose sand.

Definition: Head broad, flattened, very distinct from neck; snout very short and broad, canthus indistinct. Body depressed, tapered, moderately slender to stout; tail short.

Eyes small to moderate in size; pupils vertically elliptical.

Head scales: Head covered with small irregular, tubercularly-keeled scales.

Body scales: Dorsals with apical pits, large and heavily keeled on back, smaller laterally, oblique, with serrated keels, in 23-27 rows at midbody. Ventrals with lateral keel, 102-165; subcaudals keeled posteriorly, all paired, 18-42.

Sahara Horned Viper,
Cerastes cerastes

Description and Identification: Though not very long (about 2 feet in length), these snakes are rather heavy bodied and have a short, very broad head. The snout is somewhat rounded. In some specimens there is a single long horn above each eye. In others the horn may be reduced to a raised scale or be absent. Ground color is sandy-beige or tan with a series of darker brown blotches on the top of the back. Smaller dark brown lateral blotches alternate with the dorsal markings.

Distribution, Habitat, and Biology: The common name Sahara Horned Viper is appropriate for this snake

as it is found throughout the entire Sahara Desert region. In addition to its range in the USAFRICOM region this snake is also found in the USCENTCOM region in Egypt and the Sinai Peninsula. As with other desert adapted species these snakes often bury themselves into the sand with just the top of the head above ground. From this position they ambush small vertebrates.

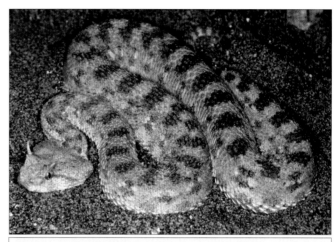

Photo 161. Sahara Horned Viper, *Cerastes cerastes*

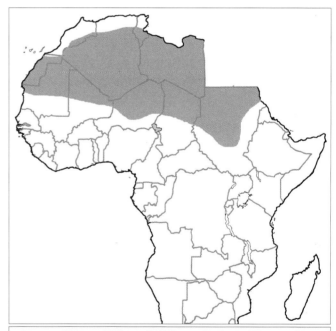

Map 188. Range of the Sahara Horned Viper, *Cerastes cerastes* in the USAFRICOM region.

Venom and Bite: Deaths are known from the bite of Sahara Horned Vipers, but Tony Phelps in his book *Old World Vipers* states that "there are no recent reports" (of deaths). Clinical Toxinology Resources website (viewed 2012), lists only procoagulants and possibly haemorragins. However, Spawls & Branch in their book *The Dangerous Snakes of Africa* (1995), make the following statement in regards to the venom of the Sahara Horned

Viper. "in experimental studies in rats caused cardiotoxicity, myotoxicity, and oedma. It acts as an anticouagulant and may cause pre-synaptic neurotoxicity."

A number of antivenoms are listed by the World Health Organization and Toxinology Resources websites. Including: Anti-viperin (Bi-valent) by Institute Pastuerd'Algerie Polyvalent Snake Antivenom by National Antivenom and Vaccine Production Center in Saudi Arabia; Polyvalent Anti-viper Venom made by VACSERA in Egypt; and Antiviperin Sera from Institut Pastuer de Tunis in Tunisia.

Sahara Sand Viper

Cerastes vipera

Description and Identification: Another short, very stout bodied desert adapted viper. This species lacks horns. The head is quite broad, very distinct from the neck and the snout is rounded and lacks a distinct canthus. The eyes are situated on the top of the head. Maximum length is just under 2 feet but most are even smaller. Its coloration a light, sandy brown, varying from yellowish to grayish. There is a row of indistinct darker blotches down the center of the back. Overall color matches the color of the sands in the snake's environment.

Distribution, Habitat, and Biology: This desert adapted snake has eyes situated high on the head to facilitate ambush hunting from a position with the body buried beneath the sand. They will wriggle the tip of the

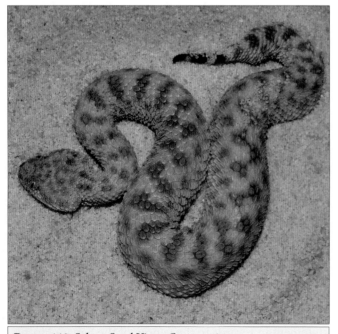

Photo 162. Sahara Sand Viper, *Cerastes vipera*

tail on the surface of the sand to lure in lizards and other small prey. Different populations reproduce by both egg-laying and live-bearing. Sahara Sand Vipers range across the Sahara Desert region of North Africa from Western Sahara to the Arabian Peninsula. It thus is also found in the USCENTCOM region (northern Egypt, Sinai, and western Yemen.).

Venom and Bite: The venom is presumed to be similar to that of the preceding species, but there is little information available and the author could find no references of antivenom availability for this species. It is likely that antivenoms listed for the preceding species (Desert Horned Viper) would be effective in treating bites by this snake.

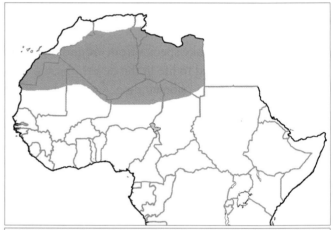

Map 189. Range of the Sahara Sand Viper, *Cerastes vipera*, in the USAFRICOM region.

Additional Species: Recently, a new species of this genus (*Cerastes boemei*, no common name) was discovered in Tunisia. Very little is known about this new species.

Family - Viperidae

Subfamily - Viperinae - True Vipers

Genus- Adenorhinos

Uzungwe Viper

This unusual genus consists of a single species of terrestrial viper that is possibly related to the Bush Vipers (*Atheris*). They are rare snakes found only in a tiny region of western Tanzania.

Definition: Head small and short, only slightly distinct from neck, snout short and rounded; canthus rostralis obtuse. Body moderately slender; tail moderate in length.

Eyes very large. Pupils vertically elliptical.

Head scales: No enlarged scutes on the crown, covered with small imbricate keeled scales. Laterally, nostril in anterior part of single nasal, which has a posterior row of suboculars separating eye from upper labials; anterior and posterior temporals single.

Body scales: Heavily keeled and somewhat imbricate anteriorly and along the vertebral line. Scale rows 19-23 at midbody. Ventrals 116-122, subcaudals 19-23, anal scute entire.

In the 1965 edition of the U.S. Navy Manual, *Poisonous Snakes of the World,* this species was known as the Worm-eating Viper.

Uzungwe Viper,
Adenorhinos barbouri

Description and Identification: These are small snakes that are less than 18 inches in length when fully grown. Ground color is brownish. A reticulated pattern of light brown markings down the dorsum.

The top of the head is covered with small, heavily keeled scales.

Distribution, Habitat and Biology: This is a very rare species that is found only in the Uzungwe and Ukinga Mountains of Tanzania.

Venom and Bite: Nothing is known about the venom of this species, but given its rarity it does not pose a significant threat of snakebite. There is no antivenom.

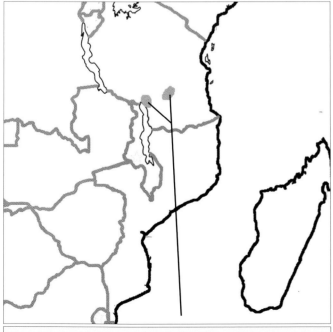

MAP 190. Range of the Uzungwe Viper, *Adenorhinos barbouri.*

Family - Viperidae

Subfamily - Viperinae - True Vipers

Genus- Causus

Night Adders

There are 7 species and all are native to the African continent. This is the most unusual genus in the viper family. In appearance they are quite un-viper-like. The head is small and not distinct from the neck, the pupils are round, and the body shape is only moderately stout. The scales are smooth or weakly keeled. They are all egg layers, an unusual trait for a viper (although a few other vipers are also egg-layers). These are small snakes that reach a maximum length of just over 3 feet.

The fangs are small and the venom is not highly toxic. No deaths are known but the bite of some species can produce significant local symptoms (swelling, intense pain).

Definition: Head not noticeably distinct from neck. Pupils round. Body moderately stout to slender. Top of head covered with large plates.

Body scales: Dorsals smooth or weakly keeled in 15-23 oblique rows at mdibody. Ventrals 108-166. Caudals 14-36, anal divided or entire.

West African Night Adder,
Causus maculatus

Description and Identification: Dorsal coloration brown or olive green. Darker vertebral blotches are indistinct.

Distribution, Habitat, and Biology: Found in virtually all habitats within its range except aquatic situations. Diet and activity similar to the previous species.

Venom and Bite: The bite is not life threatening and thus no antivenom is produced.

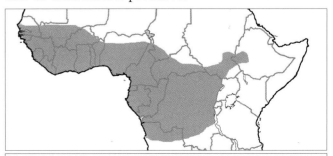

MAP 191. Range of the West African Night Adder, *Causus maculatus.*

Common Night Adder,
Causus rhombeatus

Description and Identification: There is a distinct dark chevron marking on the top of the head. The ground color is brown or grayish brown and the top of the back has a series of dark brown to black blotches that are more or less rhomboid in shape and are edged in white. Smaller dark blotches edged in white occur laterally. Average size about 2.5 feet. Maximum 39 inches (Phelps 2010).

Distribution, Habitat, and Biology: A common species throughout its range including urban areas. Occupies a wide variety of habitats. Feeds on frogs and toads. Both diurnal and nocturnal in habits.

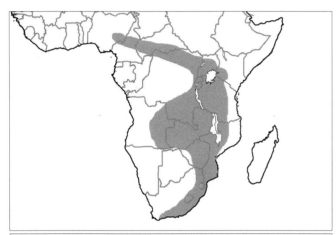

Map 192. Range of the Common Night Adder, *Causus rhombeatus.*

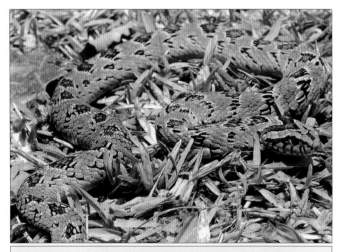

Photo 163. Common Night Adder, *Causus rhombeatus*

Venom and Bite: Bites by this species are fairly common but not life threatening. Swelling and pain can sometimes be severe and may last up to several days. No antivenom is produced for this species.

Snouted Night Adder,
Causus defilippii

Description and Identification: A typical Night Adder with an upturned rostral which gives it a distinct "hognosed" appearance.

Distribution, Habitat, and Biology: Another common Night Adder that occurs in a wide variety of habitats. Habits similar to others of its genus.

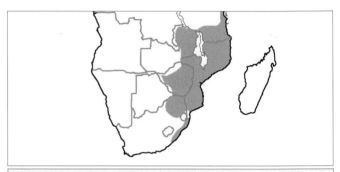

Map 193. Range of the Snouted Night Adder, *Causus defilippii*

Venom and Bite: The bite is not life threatening and thus no antivenom is produced.

Additional Species: Three other Night Adder species are found in the USAFRICOM region (see map 194.) All are similar in habits and biology. None are considered to be deadly to man.

The three additional species are:
Velvety Green Night Adder- *Causus resimus*
Forest Night Adder - *Causus lichensteinii*
Two-striped Night Adder - *Causus bilineatus*

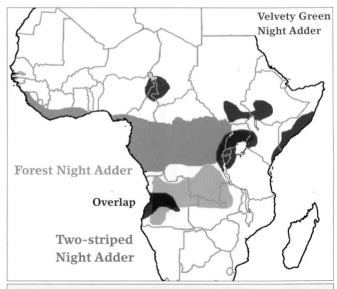

Map 194. Ranges of 3 Night Adder species. *C. resimus*, (Green) *C. lichensteinii*, (Forest) & *C. bilineatus* (Two-striped). Purple areas are range overlaps by *C. resimus*.

Family - Elapidae: Genus -Paranaja

Burrowing Cobras

There is a single species with 3 recognized subspecies. These are small snakes that never exceed 3 feet in length. They are shy and secretive, thus they probably do not pose much of a threat to humans. They do possess large front fangs, but little is known of their venom.

Most experts now assign the Burrowing Cobra (also known as the Many-banded Snake) to the genus *Naja* (the true cobras).

Definition: Head short, flattened slightly distinct from body. Body moderately slender, cylindrical, apparently without hood; tail short.

Eyes of moderate size, pupil round.

Head scales: The usual 9 scales on the crown; rostral broad, rounded, internasals short. Laterally nasal in broad contact with single preocular.

Body scales: Dorsals smooth in 15-17 oblique rows at midbody, more (17-19) on neck, fewer (13) posteriorly. Ventrals 150-175; anal plate entire; subcaudals 30-39, all or mostly paired.

Many-banded Snake,

Paranaja multifasciata

Description and Identification: Small, never exceeding 3 feet. A black snake with a yellow or greenish yellow spot on each scale. There is a yellow band around the nape, and the side of the head are yellow with black lines below the eye and on the posterior upper labials.

Distribution, Habitat, and Biology: In spite of the fact that this species does not spread the neck into a hood, it is today regarded by most experts as belonging to the genus *Naja* (true cobras that have the ability to spread the neck into a hood). These snakes are apparently burrowers that inhabit forested areas of west-central Africa.

Venom and Bite: There seems to be very little information available on the venom of this snake. Stephen Spawls and Bill Branch in their 1995 book *Dangerous Snakes of Africa* write that the venom is "probably a weak neurotoxin." There is no antivenom produced for this species.

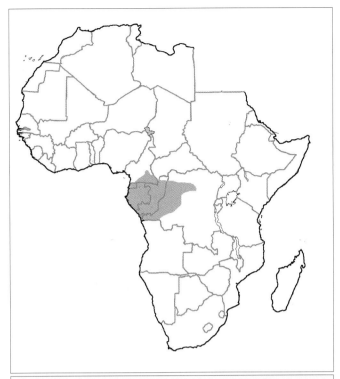

MAP 195. Range of the Many-banded Snake, *Paranaja multifasciata*

Family - Elapidae: Genus - Naja

True Cobras

As many as 28 species are recognized. These snakes are mostly African or Asian but there are some species in the Pacific region of Indonesia and the Philippines. Fifteen species are found in the USAFRICOM region. This genus has seen much revision since the classic work *Poisonous Snakes of the World* was first published in 1965. For example, the next 3 species described were all once considered to be a varieties of the Egyptian Cobra. Additional taxonomic changes are possible in the future. *Naja* cobras are moderate to large in size (4 to 8 feet as adults). They have large fangs and toxic venom. Some species are capable of "spitting" venom into the eyes of an aggressor and all members of this genus will react to threats by raising the anterior portion of the body and spreading the neck into a hood.

Identification of *Naja* species in the USAFRICOM region is complicated by the fact that many species exhibit as young snakes a different color and pattern from the adults. All *Naja* species in the USAFRICOM region are potentially deadly snakes, and several are extremely dangerous.

Definition: Head rather broad, flattened, only slightly distinct from the neck. Snout rounded, a distinct canthus. Body moderately slender, slightly depressed, tapered, neck capable of expansion into a hood. Tail of moderate length.

Eyes moderate in size; pupils round.

Head Scales: The usual 9 on the crown; frontal short; rostral rounded. Laterally, nasal in contact with the one or two preoculars.

Body scales: Dorsals smooth in 17-25 oblique rows at midbody, usually more on the neck, fewer posteriorly. Ventrals 159-232, subcaudals 42-88, mostly paired.

Maxillary teeth: Two rather large tubular fangs.

Non-Spitting Cobras

The difference between cobras that are capable of "spitting" their venom and those that are not is a nontaxonomic distinction. Thus, both are considered to be members of the *Naja* genus. Of the 15 species of *Naja* cobras in the USAFRICOM region, 8 are "non-spitters." The venom of these snakes tends to be more neurotoxic than that of the "spitters" whose venom is more cytotoxic.

Egyptian Cobra,
Naja haje

Description and Identification: This snake also often goes by the name Brown Cobra, a good description of its overall appearance. Many specimens are indeed tan, brown, or gray brown. However, this species does show extensive variation and there is a very dark, sometimes solid black phase that occurs in northwestern Africa. These are large snakes that can reach 8.5 feet in length (average about 5 feet).

Distribution, Habitat, and Biology: In spite of its common name this species is only found in a small area of Egypt (northern). It is, however, widespread across much of the rest of northern Africa. It inhabits most habitats within its range except rainforest and extreme desert. Feeding mostly on small mammals it is most active at dusk and into the night.

Venom and Bite: Post-synaptic neurotoxins, possibly myotoxins. These very large cobras produce huge quantities of mainly neurotoxic venom and their bite has killed many humans. Death can occur within a few

hours in severe envenomations. Egyptian Cobras are non-spitters.

The World Health Organization (www.who.int/blood-products/snakeantivenoms), viewed 2012, lists the following antivenoms for this snake:

Product: Polyvalent Snake Antivenom
Manufacturer: National Antivenom and Vaccine Production Center
Country of Origin: Saudi Arabia
Product: Bivalent Naja/Walterinnesia Snake AV
Manufacturer: National Antivenom and Vaccine Production Center
Country of Origin: Saudi Arabia
Product: FAV-Afrique
Manufacturer: Sanofi-Pastuer
Country of Origin: France

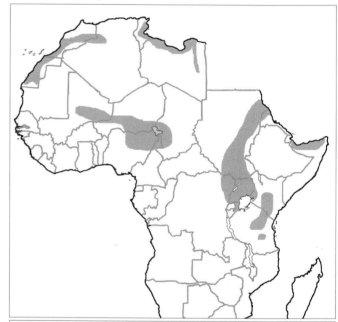

MAP 196. Range of the Egyptian Cobra, *Naja haje* in the USAFRICOM region.

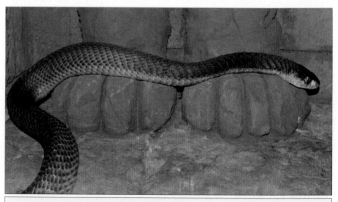

PHOTO 164. Egyptian Cobra, *Naja haje*

Snouted Cobra,
Naja annulifera

Description and Identification: Very similar to the preceding species and once considered a subspecies of *N. haje.* Typical adult is brown or olive dorsally. Young snakes are yellowish, usually with dark transverse bands. A banded phase also occurs among adults in which there are a series of broad yellowish bands on a dark brown ground color. The snout is pointed when viewed from above and the head is slightly larger than the neck. When hooded it may show a dark brown neck band on the lower neck.

Distribution, Habitat ,and Biology: Found in savanna and grassland habitats. Avoids deep forest.

Mainly nocturnal and crepuscular in habits, but may be seen basking during the day. Primary prey is rodents which it often hunts near human habitations.

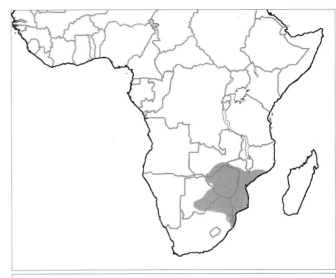

MAP 197. Range of the Snouted Cobra, *Naja annulifera.*

Venom and Bite: With a maximum length of up to 8 feet this large cobra with subsequently large amounts of venom is quite capable of killing. Numerous deaths are known to have occurred from its bite. Does not spit.

The World Health Organization (www.who.int/blood-products/snakeantivenoms), viewed 2012, lists the following antivenom for this snake:

> Product: SAIMR Polyvalent Snake Antivenom
> Manufacturer: South African Vaccine Producers (SAVP)
> Country of Origin: South Africa

Similar Species: Anchieta's Cobra, *N. anchietae* is similar to the Snouted Cobra in its morphology and biology. It is a dangerous species. Antivenom is the same as for the Snouted Cobra. Range map below.

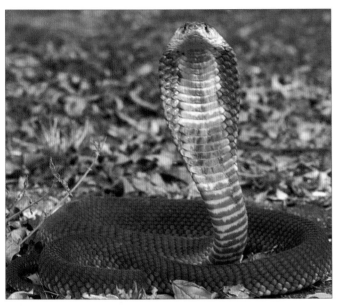

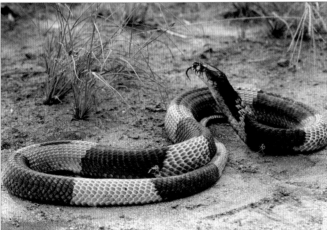

PHOTOS 165 & 166. Snouted Cobra, *Naja annulifera*, Typical (top) and banded phase (bottom).

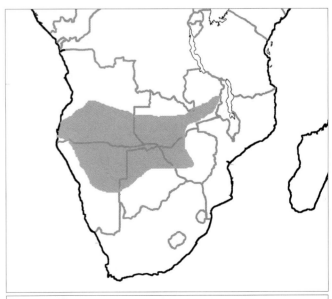

MAP 198. Range of the Anchieta's Cobra, *Naja anchietae.*

Cape Cobra,
Naja nivea

Description and Identification: This is a variable species that may be brown, yellow, chocolate, or reddish brown with yellow speckling, yellow with brown speckling, or a mottling of yellow and brown. Solid chocolate brown or nearly black specimens are also known occasionally. It is a medium to large cobra that averages about 4 feet but may reach a length of 6 feet. The head is only slightly distinct from the neck. When hooded it may or may not show a dark band on the throat. The snout is rounded and there is a distinct canthus. Dorsal scales are smooth and in 19-21 rows at midbody. Ventrals 195-227. Subcaudals 50-68.

Distribution, Habitat and Biology: Arid and semi-arid habitats often in the vicinity of water. These snakes can be common around farms where they hunt rodents. They may also be found in small villages and even suburbs. In addition to small mammals they also feed on anurans, lizards, and other snakes. Although mainly a terrestrial species they will climb trees to raid bird nests. Mainly crepuscular but also diurnal in activity.

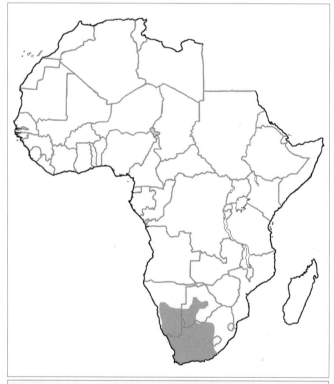

MAP 199. Range of the Cape Cobra, *Naja nivea.*

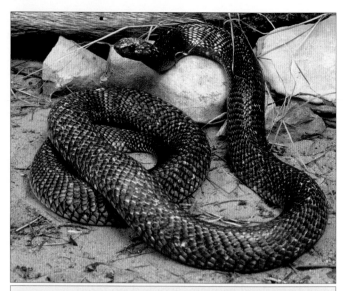

PHOTO 167. Cape Cobra, *Naja nivea*, brown phase

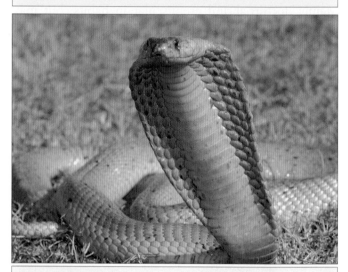

PHOTO 168. Cape Cobra, *Naja nivea,* yellow phase

Venom and Bite: Post-synaptic neurotoxins and possibly cardiotoxins. These are alert and active snakes that can be found in proximity to human habitations. While they usually flee from people, they will defend themselves vigorously when threatened and may advance if cornered and there is no avenue of escape. It would be hard to overstate the gravity of a bite by this snake. Its venom (post-synaptic neurotoxin) is extremely potent and it is regarded as the most dangerous cobra in Africa. Bites by this snake are fairly common and have resulted in many deaths.

Recommended antivenom is:

    Product: SAIMR Polyvalent Antivenom

    Manufacturer: South African Vaccine Producers (SAVP)

    Country of Origin: South Africa

Forest Cobra,

Naja melanoleuca

Description and Identification: This is Africa's largest cobra species and the biggest individuals can be 10 feet in length. Most adults are uniformly glossy black above, but they can also be gray or brownish. When hooded there is a broad black ring that shows on the ventral surface of the neck and often there are additional black rings below that. The ventral surface of the hood is frequently marked with dark spots. The face is distinctly marked with black and white.

Dorsals 17-21 at midbody (23-29 on neck), Ventrals 197-226; subcaudals 57-74.

Distribution, Habitat, and Biology: Inhabits the tropical forests and brush-grass savanna regions of eastern and central Africa. Often found near water and near human habitations. Fast moving and alert, these large snakes will raise the body several feet off the ground when hooding.

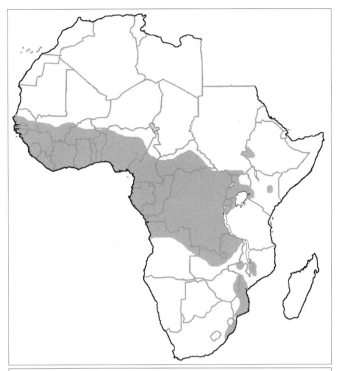

Map 200. Range of the Forest Cobra, *Naja melanoleuca*.

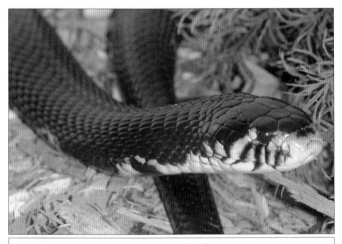

Photo 169. Forest Cobra, *Naja melanoleuca*

Venom and Bite: A non-spitter that is quick to bite if provoked. Though bites by this species are not common, it is a large and very deadly snake possessing significant quantities of potent neurotoxic venom (post-synaptic).

The World Health Organization (www.who.int/blood-products/snakeantivenoms), viewed 2012, lists the following antivenoms for this snake:

    Product: SAIMR Polyvalent Snake Antivenom
    Manufacturer: South African Vaccine Producers (SAVP)
    Country of Origin: South Africa
    Product: FAV-Afrique
    Manufacturer: Sanofi-Pastuer
    Country of Origin: France

Banded Water Cobra,

Naja annulata

Description and Identification: A very distinctly banded cobra. The ground color is usually yellowish brown but can be orange or gray. There is a variable number of narrow black bands that cross the entire body both dorsally and ventrally. Individuals from the eastern part of its range have the bands greatly reduced or even absent, especially posteriorly. This is a large, robust cobra with a relatively thick body that can reach 9 feet in length.

Distribution, Habitat, and Biology: A thoroughly aquatic cobra species that inhabits rivers and lakes throughout the forest regions of central Africa. Also found in woodland savanna in aquatic situations. Feeds on fish.

Until recently this snake was considered to be distinct from other African cobras and was assigned to its own genus (*Boulengerina*). It is now regarded by some taxonomists as a member of the *Naja* genus. It is also apparently closely related to the Forest Cobra, Van Wallach, et al. (2009).

Venom and Bite: There is little information available on the venom of this species or its effect on humans. Given its large size, it is quite likely a dangerous species. No antivenom is produced.

Similar Species: The Congo Water Cobra *Naja christyi* is a rare and poorly known species that occurs around the mouth of the Zaire River in Congo and adjacent Angola.

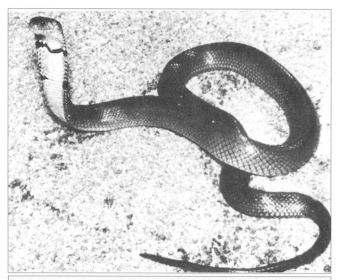

Photo 170. Banded Water Cobra, *Naja annulata*

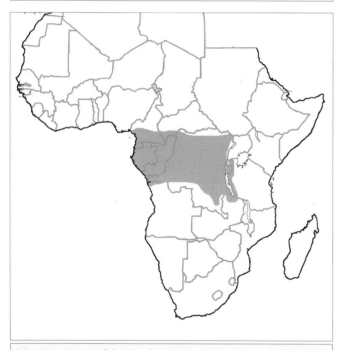

Map 201. Range of the Banded Water Cobra, *Naja annulata*.

Additional Species: In addition to those species already discussed, there is one other species of non-spitting cobra in the USAFRICOM region. The Senegal Cobra, *Naja senegalensis,* is a non-spitter once included in the *N. haje* species complex. Many specimens show a light marking on the hood, similar to Asian *Naja*. It is found in the west African Savannah region from Senegal to southern Niger and northern Nigeria. The World Health Organization lists FAV-Afrique antivenom for treating bites by *N. senegalensis.*

Spitting Cobras

This group of cobras, though not taxonomically distinct from the rest of the *Naja* genus, are different in that they have fangs that possess a modified orifice for discharging venom which allows these snakes to "spit," or more descriptively, "spray" their venom. This defensive technique is directed at the eyes of a protagonist and most "spitters" can accurately eject a stream of venom up to 10 feet. Of course, they also bite and they are known for producing large quantities of venom. There are currently 7 species of *Naja* in the USAFRICOM region that are spitters.

Red Spitting Cobra,
Naja pallida

Description and Identification: The aptly named Red Spitting Cobra is uniformly red or reddish brown with an orange to red belly. In some regions they may be brown or even grayish, but orange, red, or reddish brown is typical. There is a broad black neck band on the throat that is easily visible when the snake hoods. These are smallish cobras that average about 3 to 4 feet, with a maximum length of about 5 feet.

Distribution, Habitat, and Biology: Distributed across "the horn" of Africa, these snakes are found in semi-arid savannas and grasslands, but avoid true desert. Primarily nocturnal and terrestrial in habits.

Venom and Bite: While this snake will spit readily, it is less inclined to bite. There does not seem to be much information available on the venom of this snake or the dangerousness of its bite (post-synaptic neurotoxins and necrotoxins listed by Clinical Toxinology Resources website). Like most spitters it can reportedly yield large amounts of venom and it should be considered a dangerous snake. There is no specific antivenom produced and neither the WHO antivenom index or the Munich Antivenom Index (MAVIN) lists a cross reactive antivenom for *N. pallida.* However, both list a number of antivenoms for the Black-necked Spitting Cobra, *N. nigricollis,* that may be effective against *N. pallida.*

Finally, the Clinical Toxinology Resources website (www.toxinology.com) viewed 2012 does list the following antivenom for this species: Bivalent *Naja* / Walternnesia Snake Antivenom manufactured by National Antivenom and Vaccine Production Centre in Saudi Arabia.

Similar Species: The Nubian Spitting Cobra, *Naja nubia*, is another type of spitting cobra that is found in widely disparate populations across north Africa. It is a small, relatively rare snake that does not pose much threat of snakebite and its venom is less potent than many other cobras in Africa. Until recently it was considered to be a subspecies of the Red Spitting Cobra. The venom of the spitting cobras tend to be more cytotoxic than neurotoxic.

Black-necked Spitting Cobra,
Naja nigricollis

Description and Identification: Maximum length up to 6.5 feet (average about 4 feet.). Like many African cobras this is a variable species that can be brown, gray, or solid black. The name is derived from the fact that most lighter colored specimens reveal a black throat when hooded.

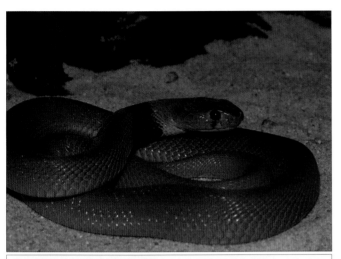

Photo 171. Red Spitting Cobra, *Naja pallida*

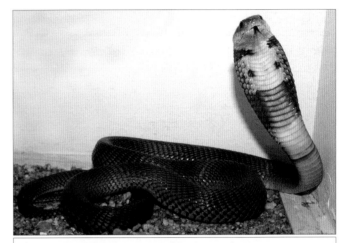

Photo 172. Nubian Spitting Cobra, *Naja nubia*

Distribution, Habitat, and Biology: This is a wide-ranging species that is found across a broad swath of tropical Africa below the Sahara Desert. Natural regions within its range are the deciduous forests-woodland savannas and brush grass savannas of western and central Africa and those same habitats plus grassland and semi-desert in eastern Africa.

Venom and Bite: Post-synaptic neurotoxins, necrotoxins, and possibly cardiotoxins.

This snake is quick to spit and also bites readily when cornered. As with most spitting cobras, it has a lot of venom and human fatalities from its bite are known to occur. Three antivenoms are listed by the World Health Organization's snake antivenom database (viewed 2012), they are:

Product: FAV-Afrique
Manufacturer: Sanofi-Pasteur
Country of Origin: France
Product: Favirep
Manufacturer: Sanofi-Pasteur
Country of Origin: France
Product: Polyvalent Snake Antivenom
Manufacturer: VACSERA
Country of Origin: Egypt

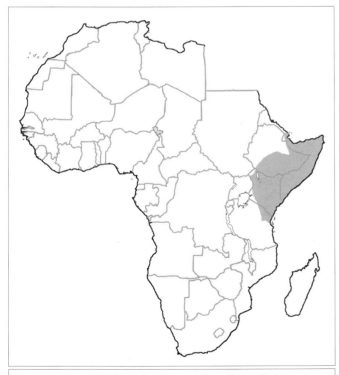

Map 202. Range of the Red Spitting Cobra, *Naja pallida.*

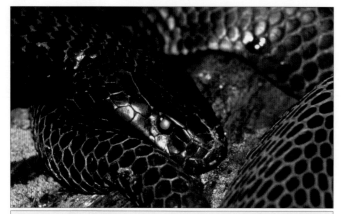

PHOTO 173. Black-necked Spitting Cobra, *Naja nigricollis*

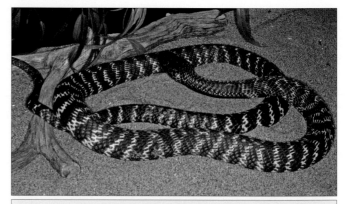

PHOTO 174. Western Barred Spitting Cobra, *Naja nigricincta* (barred phase)

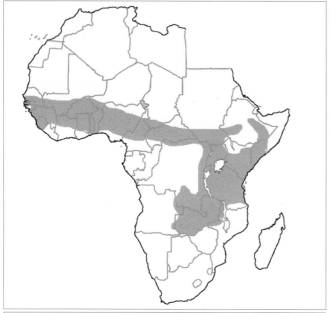

MAP 203. Range of the Black-necked Spitting Cobra, *Naja nigricollis.*

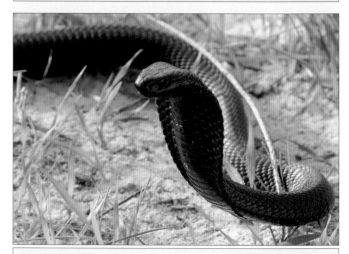

PHOTO 175. Western Barred Spitting Cobra, *Naja nigricincta* (black phase)

Western Barred Spitting Cobra,

Naja nigricincta

Description and Identification: Typical specimens are distinctively marked with black and white "zebra" barring around the body. Snakes from the southern portion of the range in southern Namibia and South Africa are solid black and are regarded as a distinct subspecies.

Distribution, Habitat, and Biology: Found in the Namib Desert and in semi-desert and brush grass savanna regions of Namibia and South Africa. Formerly regarded as a subspecies of the preceding snake, *N. nigricollis.*

Venom and Bite: Post-synaptic neurotoxins, necrotoxins and possibly cardiotoxins.

Antivenoms are the same as listed for the *N. nigricollis.*

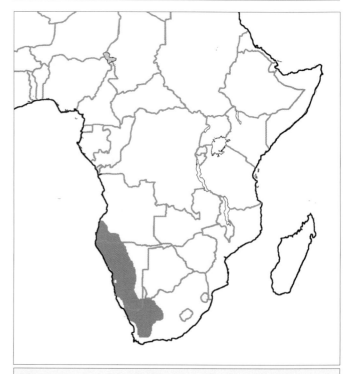

MAP 204. Range of the Western Barred Spitting Cobra, *Naja nigricincta.*

Mossambique Spitting Cobra,

Naja mossambica

Description and Identification: A fairly nondescript, brown cobra that can reach a length of 5 feet. When hooded shows a cream to yellowish throat with one broad and one narrow black band. Sometimes only the broad dark band is present, but above it the cream/yellow throat is heavily marked with dark square edged blotches. Scale rows at midbody 23-25.

Distribution, Habitat, and Biology: This species is quick to "spit" if threatened or cornered, but like many other spitting cobras it rarely bites. This is a terrestrial snake that lives mainly in open areas of brush-grass savanna or woodland savanna. Adults are primarily nocturnal in habits but young snakes may be abroad during the day.

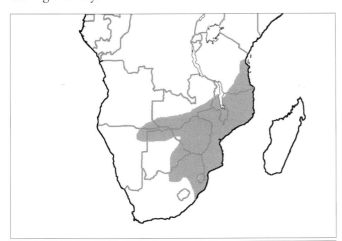

MAP 205. Range of the Mossambique Spitting Cobra, *Naja mossambica.*

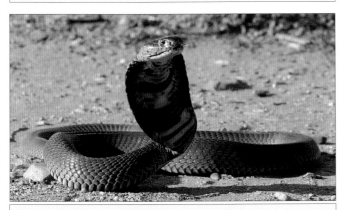

PHOTO 176. Mossambique Spitting Cobra, *Naja mossambica.*

Venom and Bite: Post-synaptic neurotoxins, necrotoxins, and possible cardiotoxins. The venom of this species is known to cause significant necrosis and tissue damage. Human deaths are known.

Recommended antivenom:

Product: SAIMR Polyvalent Antivenom

Manufacturer: South African Vaccine Producers (SAVP)

Country of Origin: South Africa

Additional Species: In addition to the previously described species there are two other spitting cobra species found in the USAFRICOM region.

Ashe's Sptting Cobra, Naja ashei: A nondescript usually uniformly olive brown cobra found in portions of Kenya, Somalia, Ethiopia, and in northeastern Uganda. These are large cobras that can reach a length of 7 feet. They also produce large quantities of venom, perhaps more than any other African cobra, and thus must be regarded as very dangerous snakes. These cobras are closely related to the Black-necked Spitting Cobra.

Brown Spitting Cobra, Naja katiensis: Found in a broad swath across west Africa from Senegal and Guinea-Bissau east to Cameroon. Major habitat types found within its range are deciduous forest-woodland savanna and brush-grass savanna. This species has caused human fatalities. Once thought to be a subspecies of the Black-necked Spitting Cobra, *N. nigricollis.*

Toxinology Resources website viewed 2012 lists Bivalent *Naja*/Walternnesia Snake Antivenom for treating bites by *N. katiensis*. Meanwhile the World Health Organization website (viewed 2012) showed no antivenoms listed for either species.

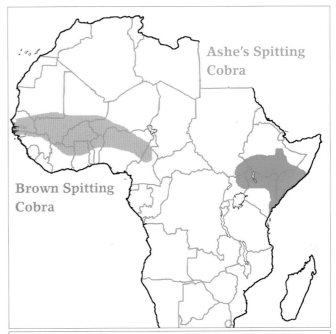

MAP 206. Range of the Brown Spitting Cobra *Naja katiensis,* and the presumed range of the Ashe's Spitting Cobra, *Naja ashei.*

Family - Elapidae: Genus - Hemachatus

Rinkhals

A single species is recognized. It is confined to southern Africa. It is a highly developed "spitting" cobra and is a dangerous species.

Definition: Head rather broad, flattened, not distinct from neck; distinct canthus; snout obtusely pointed. Body moderately slender, slightly depressed, tapering; neck region capable of expanding into hood; tail moderately long.

Eyes moderate in size, pupils round.

Head scales: The usual 9 on the crown; rostral large and obtusely pointed. Laterally, nasal in contact with single preocular.

Body scales: Dorsals distinctly keeled, in 19 oblique rows at midbody, fewer (15) posteriorly. Ventrals 116-150; anal plate entire; subcaudals 33-47, the first 3-4 frequently single, the remainder paired.

Rinkhals,
Hemachatus hemachatus

Description and Identification: This unique spitting elapid is easily told from all *Naja* cobras by its keeled scales. The Rinkhals is a modest sized snake that may reach 5 feet but averages 3 to 4 feet.

Many specimens are barred black and white or black and yellow in a "zebra striped" pattern. Others may be uniformly dark brown or black with light, irregular spotting. The belly is uniformly black except for two white bars across the throat that are visible when the snake is hooded. Melanistic specimens may lack the white throat bars.

Distribution, Habitat, and Biology: Endemic to southernmost Africa where it lives from sea level to over 7,000 feet. It is common in the habitat known as veldt which is a grassland region occupying a large swath of South Africa. Mainly nocturnal in activity but basks frequently during the day. Feeds on small vertebrates of all kinds including anuran amphibians, birds, and small mammals. This is the only elapid snake in Africa that is viviparous (live bearing). In another unusual characteristic, these snakes are known to play dead at times when cornered.

Venom and Bite: Well known for its highly developed spitting abilities, the Rinkhals can direct a stream of ven-

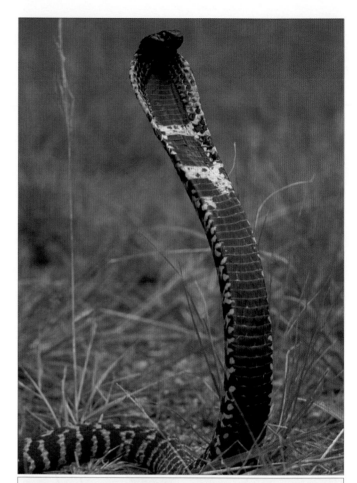

Photo 177. Rinkhals, *Hemachatus hemachatus*

om into the eyes of an adversary for a distance of at least 10 feet. The estimated lethal dose for a human is 50-60 mg. and this snake can yield 80-120 mg. (Spawls and Branch, 1995). Thus, it would appear that this species is more than capable of inflicting a fatal bite.

The MAVIN Antivenom Index (viewed 2012) lists:

Product: SAIMR Polyvalent Antivenom
Manufacturer: South African Vaccine Producers (SAVP)
Country of Origin: South Africa

Venom spit into the eye should be treated by washing the eye repeatedly and thoroughly. In severe cases the eye should be rinsed with diluted antivenom. Venom toxins include neurotoxins, cardiotoxins, and possibly haemorragins.

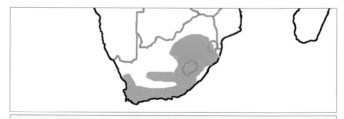

Map 207. Range of the Rinkhals, *Hemachatus hemachatus*.

Family - Elapidae: Genus - Pseudohaje

Tree Cobras

Two species are recognized; both inhabit the tropical rain forest region of central and western Africa. They have average adult lengths of about 6 feet and individuals occasionally approach 8 feet. Both species are considered dangerous.

Definition: Head short and narrow, slightly distinct from neck; snout broad, rounded, canthus distinct.

Body slender, tapering; neck region with very slight suggestion of a hood; tail long.

Eyes very large; pupils round.

Head scales: The usual 9 on the crown; rostral broad. Laterally, nasal in contact with preocular or separated from it by a loreal scale that is occasionally formed by a vertical suture across the unusually elongate preocular.

Body scales: Dorsals smooth and glossy, in 13-15 oblique rows at midbody, the same number or more (15) on the neck, fewer (9-11) posteriorly. Ventrals 180-205; anal plate entire; subcaudals 74-94, paired.

The two Tree Cobras are so similar in appearance and biology that the author has elected to treat them here in a single account. They are best distinguished based on range.

Gold's Tree Cobra &
Black Tree Cobra,
Pseudohaje goldii & Pseudohaje nigra

Description and Identification: These are large snakes that can reach 9 feet. They are slim bodied with a rather short head. The most diagnostic feature is the huge, dark eye. Dorsally they are quite dark, being either black or very dark brown and the skin is smooth and glossy. The top of the head is dark, but the scales of the face and throat are yellow or greenish yellow and each yellow scale is edged in black.

These snakes are very similar in appearance and habits to the Blandings Tree Snake, but that species has an elliptical pupil. Their ability to hood is reduced to a narrow flattening of the neck

Distribution, Habitat, and Biology: These are alert, agile, and fast moving snakes. They are decidedly arboreal in habits and with their lithe bodies move easily through the branches. When travelling on the ground they often raise the fore body and hold the head well off ground. They are often described as being intermediate in appearance and habits between the true cobras (*Naja*) and the Mambas (*Dendroaspis*). Little is known of their habits, but the large eye suggests a snake that sees well and may be well suited for nocturnal activity. The Tree Cobras are snakes of the tropical forests of western and central Africa.

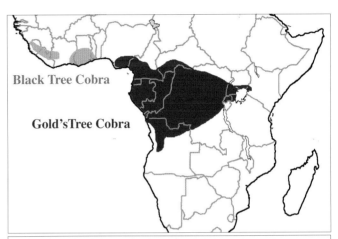

MAP 208. Range of the Tree Cobras, *Pseudohaje goldii* and *Psuedohaje nigra.*

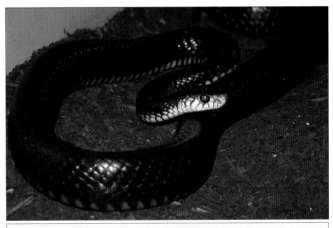

PHOTO 178. Gold's Tree Cobra, *Pseudohaje goldii*

Venom and Bite: There is not much information available on the venom or bite of this species. The venom yield is reported to be low, however there is evidence that the venom may be extremely potent. Both species should be regarded as potentially deadly to man.

Neither the MAVIN Antivenom Index, the Clinical Toxinology Resources website, or the WHO snake antivenom database lists an antivenom for this species. The book *Dangerous Snakes of Africa* (1995) by Stephen Spawls and Bill Branch states that "SAIMR Polyvalent Antivenom, although not specific against the bite of this snake, is reported successfully to neutralize its venom."

Family - Elapidae: Genus - Dendroaspis

Mambas

Four species are recognized. They range over most of central and southern Africa. Due to their size, speed, and highly toxic venom, they are considered among the most dangerous of all snakes. All are large snakes averaging between 6 and 10 feet as adults and one species, the Black Mamba (*D. polylepis*) may reach 14 feet.

Definition: Head narrow and elongate, slightly distinct from neck; a distinct canthus. Body slender and tapering, slightly compressed; neck may be flattened when snake is aroused, but there is no real hood; tail long and tapering.

Eyes moderate in size; pupils round.

Head scales: The usual 9 on the crown; frontal broad anteriorly, narrow posteriorly. Laterally nasal widely separated from preoculars by prefrontal.

Body scales: Dorsals smooth and narrow, in 13-25 distinctly oblique rows at midbody, the same or more rows anteriorly, fewer posteriorly. Ventrals 201-282; anal plate divided; subcaudals paired, 99-131.

Maxillary teeth: Two large tubular fangs without external grooves; no other teeth on bone.

Black Mamba,
Dendroaspis polylepis

Description and Identification: A long, slender, lithe-bodied serpent with a long, narrow head that is only very slightly wider than the neck. There is a very distinct canthus. The overall appearance of the head is that of a box-like, flat sided rectangle. The body color is typically a uniform slaty gray, but may sometimes tend towards an olive or brownish gray. There is often no dorsal pattern at all, but some may show a very indistinct tendency towards light lateral stripes posteriorly. The belly is light gray or whitish. This is the largest venomous snake in Africa and adults will average 9-10 feet in length. The record length is at least 11.5 feet and some authors claim they can reach a length of just over 14 feet! The membrane of the inside of the mouth is black and this trait is responsible for the snake's name.

Distribution, Habitat, and Biology: The Black Mamba is widespread across sub-saharan Africa. It is found throughout eastern and southern Africa (except much of the Cape) and occurs in disjunct locales in west Africa. It is primarily a savanna species and it avoids the dense tropical forests of central Africa.

These snakes are diurnal in habits and have a strong arboreal tendency. They can glide quickly and effortlessly through trees and bushes, but they are also quite at home on the ground, where they are also capable of astonishing speed. They are alert and seemingly intelligent snakes. If threatened, they may raise the front half of the body, hiss menacingly, and gape open the mouth revealing the black membrane inside the mouth. This gaping behavior is so instinctive that captive snakes startled by the flash of a photographer's camera will invariably throw open the mouth with each flash of the camera.

These snakes are often reported to be aggressive animals that will attack unprovoked. Though this is an exaggeration, the Black Mamba when cornered or hard pressed will not hesitate to resort to offensive action and they are quick to bite when threatened.

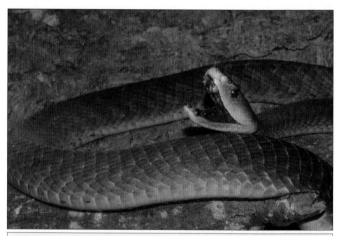

PHOTO 179. Black Mamba, *Dendroaspis polylepis*

Venom and Bite: Many experts regard this as the world's most dangerous snake. The combination of speed, agility, and a tendency to resort to biting at little provocation, coupled with large quantities of a highly potent venom, equals a very deadly serpent. The venom contains virulent neurotoxins and a large specimen may have enough venom to kill 10-15 humans. The fangs are situated near the tip of the snout, and unlike most elapid snakes they are capable of some forward movement. The strike of the Black Mamba is so quick and envenomation is achieved with often such a light touch that victims lucky enough to survive the bite sometimes report that at first they did not realize the snake had succeeded in biting them.

Before the advent of antivenom, bites from this snake were nearly 100 percent fatal. Even today a significant percentage of its victims die from its bite, especially in rural areas that may be hours from medical treatment.

World Health Organization and Munich Antivenom Index listings of recommended antivenoms (viewed 2012):

Product: SAIMR Polyvalent Antivenom

Manufacturer: South African Vaccine Producers (SAVP)

Country of Origin: South Africa

Product: FAV-AFRIQUE

Manufacturer: Sanofi-Pastuer

Country of Origin: France

Product: ISPER AFRIQUE-PASTEUR

Manufacturer: Sanofi-Pastuer

Country of Origin: France

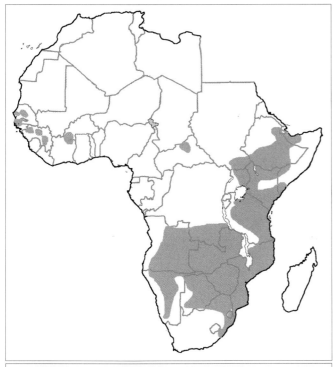

MAP 209. Range of the Black Mamba, *Dendroaspis polylepsis.*

East African Green Mamba,
Dendroaspis angusticeps

Description and Identification: Appropriately named, the East African Green Mamba is uniformly bright green in color. Like the Black Mamba the head is elongate and box shaped and about the same diameter as the neck. These are large snakes that can reach a length of at least 6.5 feet. However, they are a much slimmer snake than a comparable size cobra.

Distribution, Habitat, and Biology: Restricted to forests and thick brush in eastern Africa. These are arboreal snakes that are quite at home in the trees and will ascend to the very top of large trees. They move with equal agility through tree tops or low bushes nearer the ground. They are diurnal snakes that usually spend the night coiled high in a tree rather than seeking refuge below ground in the manner of most snakes, Spawls & Branch (1995). Does not "gape" in the manner of the Black Mamba and is usually inoffensive in behavior. Although the two species share much of this snake's range, they are partitioned by habitat preferences. The Black Mamba occupies more open areas, with the East African Green sticking to dense woodland and thickets.

Venom and Bite: Though not as dangerous as the preceding species, this snake is more than capable of killing a human. Antivenoms are the same as for the Black Mamba.

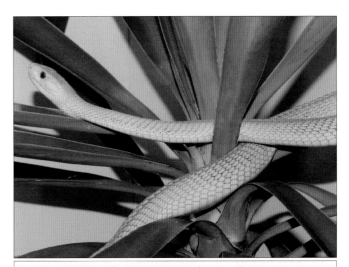

PHOTO 180. East African Green Mamba, *Dendroaspis angusticeps*

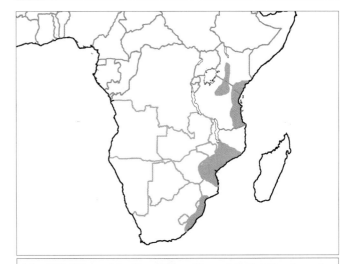

MAP 210. Range of the East African Green Mamba, *Dendroaspis angusticeps.*

West African Green Mamba,

Dendroaspis viridis

Description and Identification: This is another arboreal mamba. Like many forest snakes it has an overall green or yellowish color, but each of the dorsal scales, as well as the head scales, is edged with black. The dorsal scales are extremely large and narrow; each dorsal except the one bordering the ventral row is equal to two ventrals in length. This snake has few dorsal rows than any of the other snakes with which it might be confused and also lacks the loreal scale typical of harmless colubrid snakes. No other mamba occurs within its range. Adults average 6-7 feet in length. Large individuals may approach 8 feet in length.

Dorsal in 13 rows at midbody, more (15) on the neck, fewer (9) posteriorly. Ventrals 211-225; subcaudals 105-119.

Distribution, Habitat, and Biology: The West African Green Mamba is a tree dwelling species that ranges throughout the equatorial forests of western Africa. It is active by day but is normally non-aggressive. It will usually flee up into the trees or bushes if encountered.

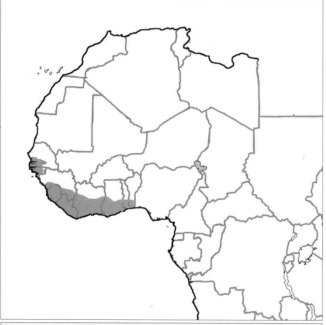

MAP 211. Range of the West African Green Mamba, *Dendroaspis viridis.*

Venom and Bite: The venom is suspected to be a potent neurotoxin similar to that of the Black Mamba. Venom yields approach that of the Black Mamba, and this species is a highly dangerous snake.

World Health Organization and Munich Antivenom Index recommended antivenoms are:

Product: FAV-AFRIQUE

Manufacturer: Sanofi-Pastuer

Country of Origin: France

Product: ISPER AFRIQUE-PASTEUR

Manufacturer: Sanofi-Pastuer

Country of Origin: France

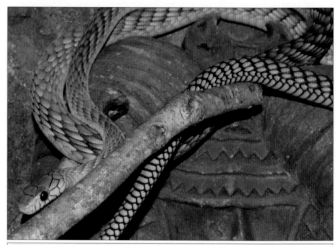

PHOTO 181. West African Green Mamba, *Dendroaspis viridis*

Jameson's Mamba,

Dendroaspis jamesoni

Description and Identification: A mainly green tree snake with scales usually edged in black, the overall coloration becoming darker posteriorly, with the tail entirely black in some individuals. This snake may be confused with the preceding species and range is the easiest way to differentiate between the two.

Distribution, Habitat, and Biology: Like the preceding species this is an arboreal snake of the equatorial forest. The range of the Jameson's Mamba is much larger, including most of central Africa, although it does overlap that of the East African Green Mamba in southern Ghana and Togo.

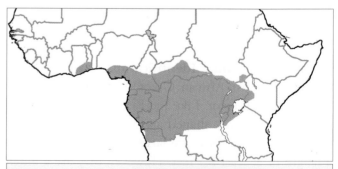

MAP 212. Range of the Jameson's Mamba, *Dendroaspis jamesoni.*

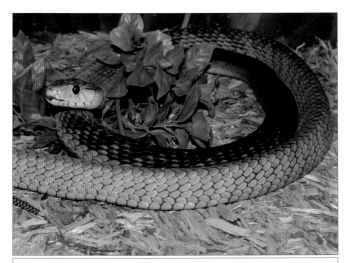

PHOTO 182. Jameson's Mamba *Dendroaspis jamesoni*

Family - Elapidae: Genus - Aspidelaps

African Coral Snakes

There are two species of African Coral Snakes.They are also known as Shield-nosed Snakes on account of the specialized rostral scale which forms a large "shield" on the front of the snout and is an adaptation for a burrowing lifestyle. In the U.S. Navy's 1965 manual for the military entitled *Poisonous Snakes of the World,* these small elapids were not regarded as dangerous to man. It is now known that both species are capable of killing a human.

Definition: Head short and only slightly distinct from neck; a broad snout modified for burrowing; canthus indistinct. Body cylindrical or somewhat depressed, stout; tail short, obtusely pointed.

Eyes moderate in size; pupils round or vertically elliptical.

Head scales: The usual 9 on the crown; rostral very large, concave below, curved backward over snout. Separated from other scales on sides; prefrontals very short. Laterally, nasal in broad contact with single preocular.

Body scales: Dorsals smooth or faintly keeled (in A. scutatus) in 19-23 oblique rows anteriorly and at midbody, fewer (15) posteriorly. Ventrals 115-172,

Anal plate entire; subcaudals paired, 20-38.

Shield-nosed Snake,
Aspidelaps scutatus

Description and Identification: A short, very heavy bodied snake that reaches a maximum length of about 30 inches (most are smaller). The most diagnostic feature is the greatly enlarged rostral scale.

The head is short and wide and the neck has one or more dark bands that usually encircle the entire neck region (except for the throat which is white). Another unusual character is the fact that the body scales are nearly smooth anteriorly, but become heavily keeled posteriorly. The ground color is brown or reddish brown and the anterior portion of most of the dorsal scales have a black spot.

Distribution, Habitat, and Biology: The Shield-nosed Snake ranges across a broad swath of the northern portions of southern Africa just north of the Cape region. Its habitat is savanna and dry grassland regions, especially areas with sandy soil which facilitates easy burrowing. Mainly nocturnal when above ground.

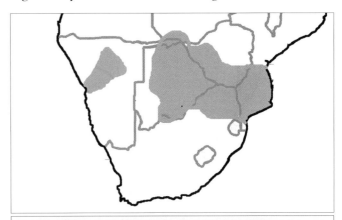

MAP 213. Range of the Shield-nosed Snake, *Aspidelaps scutatus.*

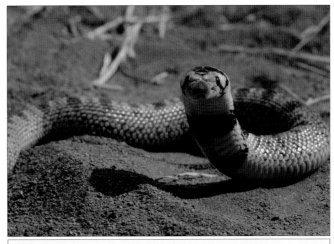

PHOTO 183. Shield-nosed Snake, *Aspidelaps scutatus*

Venom and Bite: Though once regarded as not deadly to man, it is now known that this species is capable of killing a human (although deaths are quite rare). There is no specific antivenom produced and none of the antivenoms available for other deadly African species are known to work on the bite of this snake.

Western Coral Snake,
Aspidelaps lubricus

Description and Identification: In size this snake is similar to the preceding species, but can get a just a bit longer (32 inches). The color is variable, but usually is reddish or orange with distinct black bands around the dorsum. As with the Shield-nosed Snake, the most diagnostic feature on this snake is the enormous rostral scale.

Distribution, Habitat, and Biology: Lives in semi-arid regions of the western side of southern Africa. When threatened this snake will rear the fore part of the body and spread its neck in a narrow hood similar to the cobras.

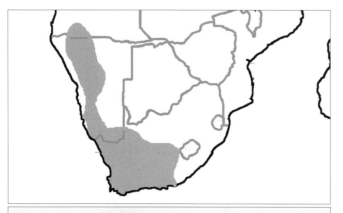

MAP 214. Range of the Western Coral Snake, *Aspidelaps lubricus.*

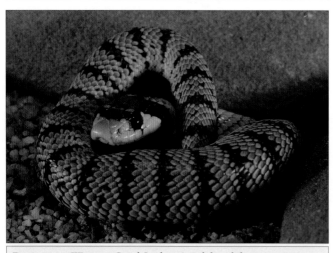

PHOTO 184. Western Coral Snake, *Aspidelaps lubricus*

Venom and Bite: As with the previous species, these snakes were once regarded as not being deadly to man. But at least two deaths have now been attributed to this snake (Spawls & Branch, 2012). The venom is probably neurotoxic and there is no specific antivenom produced. More importantly, none of the other antivenoms available are known to have any effect on neutralizing the effects of its bite.

Family - Colubridae: Genus - Dispholidus
Boomslang

A single species, D. typhus. This snake, found only in tropical and southern Africa is the most dangerous member of the family Colubridae.

Definition: Head oval, but distinct from slender neck; crown of head convex. Snout short with a distinct canthus. Body slender and elongate, moderately compressed; tail long and slender.

Eyes very large; pupils round.

Head scales: The usual 9 on the crown. Laterally, a single loreal scale separates the nasal from the one or two preoculars.

Body scales: Dorsals narrow, distinctly keeled and with apical pits; in 17-21 rows at midbody, more (21-25) anteriorly, fewer (13) posteriorly. Ventrals of normal size, obtusely angulate laterally, 164-201; anal plate divided (like most scale characteristics this is not true 100 percent of the time); and the anal plate is rarely entire.

Boomslang,
Dispholidus typus

Distribution, Habitat, and Biology: These are highly variable snakes in coloration and they also exhibit sexual dimorphism (a trait in which the sexes are different in color or pattern). To further complicate things, they, like many snake species, also are subject to ontogenic changes in color and pattern (difference in color or pattern between the young and the adult). Typical adult males can be beautiful snakes with greenish yellow scales highlighted by black between each scale, giving the appearance of a black snake speckled with yellow or green. Other males may be uniformly dark brown or black above with a pale belly. The labial scales are also often a pale color (yellowish to orange) and in sharp contrast to the normally dark dorsal surface of the head. Females tend to be uniformly olive, brown, or rust above. The most obvious feature of these snakes is the short head with an enormous eye and a long, slender body and long tail.

Distribution, Habitat, and Biology: Boomslangs are one of the most wide-ranging venomous snakes in the USAFRICOM region and are found throughout most of sub-saharan Africa except the rainforest region of central Africa. Active by day and non-aggressive unless captured or cornered. They are highly arboreal and are usually seen in trees or shrubs. When threatened they will flatten the neck laterally into a flat oval shape. These snakes are easily confused with a number of other harmless tree snakes in the region which may also flatten the neck laterally when disturbed.

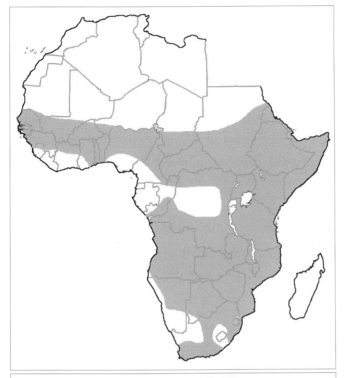

MAP 215. Range of the Boomslang, *Dispholidus typus*

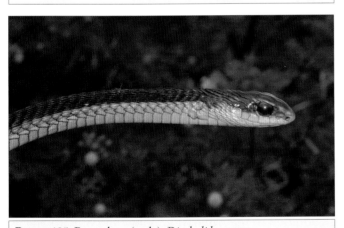

PHOTO 185. Boomslang (male), *Dispholidus typus*

Venom and Bite: The venom of the Boomslang is a powerful haemotoxin. Despite the fact that the venom-conducting fangs are in the back of the upper jaw, these snakes are capable of injecting venom without chewing, although most such bites would result in minimal envenomations. When the snake does achieve a significant envenomation it is a life threatening situation. Most fatalities have been to snake enthusiasts including a well known American herpetologist who was killed by a captive specimen in 1957.

Fortunately, a highly effective specific antivenom is available for this species.

Product: SAIMR Boomslang Antivenom

Manufacturer: South African Vaccine Producers (SAVP)

Country of Origin: South Africa

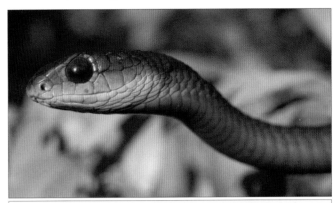

PHOTO 186. Boomslang (female), *Dispholidus typus*

Family - Colubridae: Genus - Thelotornis

African Vine Snakes

There are two species known. Like the Boomslang these snakes are members of the Colubridae family which contains most of the world's snake species, all but a handful of which are harmless to man.

Definition: Head elongate, flattened, and distinct from the neck. A distinct and projecting canthus which forms a shallow groove below it on the side of the snout. Body slender and elongated. Tail long.

Eyes large; pupils horizontally elliptical (keyhole shaped).

Head scales: The usual 9 on the crown. Internasals large; parietals bordered posteriorly by 3 large scales. Laterally, 1-3 loreal scales separate the nasal from the preocular.

Body scales: Dorsals narrow, feebly keeled, with apical pits, in 19 oblique rows at midbody. Fewer (11-13) posteriorly. Ventrals rounded, 147-189; anal plate divided; subcaudals paired, 131-175.

Savanna Vine Snake,
Thelotornis capensis

Description and Identification: An extremely slender bodied snake with a very long, tapering tail.

These are not large snakes and average just under 3 feet in length (maximum of about 3.5 feet). The ground color is light gray or light brownish with a dorsal pattern of diagonal bars that may alternate between dark and light. The head is very slender and lance-shaped.

Distribution, Habitat, and Biology: Another decidedly arboreal species. It rarely leaves the sanctuary of trees and shrubs where it is very cryptic and difficult to detect. Quick moving and agile it glides effortlessly through the branches. Strictly diurnal. Like the Boomslang and several other tree snake species, the Savanna Vine Snake will inflate the throat in a threat display when molested.

Venom and Bite: Though not prone to bite unless severely molested or restrained, this snake's venom is quite potent and a number of human deaths have been recorded. One of them was a herpetologist killed by this snake in 1975.

Similar species: The Forest Vine Snake *Thelotornis kirtlandi,* is a very similar species and in fact the two snakes were once regarded as the same animal. The Forest Vine Snake as its name implies inhabits the continuous rainforest region of central and western Africa.

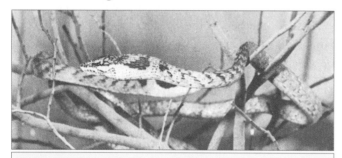

Photo 187. Forest Vine Snake, *Thelotornis capensis*

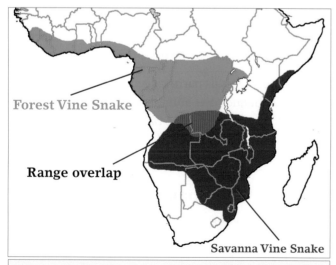

Forest Vine Snake

Range overlap

Savanna Vine Snake

Map 216. Range of the African Vine Snakes, *Thelotornis capensis & Thelotornis kirtlandi*

Family - Lamprophiidae:

Genus - Atractaspis

Mole Vipers (Burrowing Asp)

Twenty-one species are known, all but 2 are endemic to Africa. The other two species occur in the USCENTCOM region on the Arabian peninsula. These are all small snakes, less than 3 feet in length. However, they have large fangs (which look enormous in the small mouth) and are capable of inflicting serious bites on those who attempt to pick them up or who step on them with bare feet.

Defiinition: Head short and conical, not distinct from neck, no canthus; snout broad, flattened, often pointed. Body cylindrical, slender in small individuals, stout in larger ones; tail short, ending in distinct spine.

Eyes very small, pupils round.

Head scales: The usual 9 crown scales, rostral enlarged, extending between internals to some degree, often pointed; frontal large and broad, supraoculars small. Laterally, nasal in contact with single preocular (no loreal), usually one postocular.

Body scales: Dorsals smooth without apical pits, in 19-37 nonoblique rows at midbody. Ventrals 178-370; anal plate entire or divided; subcaudals single or paired.

These snakes also frequently go by the name "stiletto snakes" in reference to the their extremely long fangs. They are well known among reptile keepers and venom lab personnel as being nearly impossible to handle without being bitten. If grasped behind the head in the manner used in typical venom extraction techniques, these snakes may slip their long fangs outside their still closed mouth where they wield them with uncanny ability. The result is often an envenomed thumb or finger of the unfortunate handler.

In addition to the name Mole Viper and Stiletto Snake, they are also frequently referred to as Burrowing Asps.

Although this a rather large genus, they are all remarkable similar and are thus treated here in a single account.

Mole Vipers,
Atractaspis species

Description and Identification: To the North American herpetologist, these snakes could easily be mistaken for a harmless colubrid. Their small head, round pupils, smooth scales and monotonously colored bodies, coupled with their burrowing habits, gives an impression easily associated with a non-venomous worm snake (although they are much larger).

In color they are uniformly dark brown or black and devoid of any dorsal pattern (a few species may have light markings on the head). In size they range from barely a foot to over 3 feet in length.

Distribution, Habitat, and Biology: As the name implies, these are fossorial snakes that spend much time in underground burrows or moving through loose soil or vegetative litter. They do sometimes emerge to prowl above ground at night.

They occur in most habitats except for true desert.

Venom and Bite: Smaller species may not be capable of killing, but deaths have been recorded from larger species. There is no antivenom available for bites by *Atractaspis* species. Indirect cardiotoxicity is reported from one of the larger and more dangerous species (*A. microlepidota*). This is one of the few species that have been known to kill humans.

In addition to the Small-scaled Mole Viper shown in photo 188. There are 19 other *Atractaspis* species found within the USAFRICOM region. Those species are:

Slender Mole Viper - *A. aterrima*

Battersby's Burrowing Asp - *A. battersbyi*

Southern Mole Viper - *A. bibroni*

Central African Mole Viper - *A. boulengeri*

Congo Burrowing Asp - *A. congica*

Black Mole Viper - *A. coalescens*

Fat Mole Viper - *A. corpulenta*

Dahomey Mole Viper - *A. dahomeyensis*

Beaked Burrowing Asp - *A. duerdeni*

Engdahl's Burrowing Asp - *A. engdahli*

Variable Burrowing Asp - *A. irregularis*

Reticulated Mole Viper - *A. reticulata*

Peter's Mole Viper - *A. fallax*

Ogaden Mole Viper - *A. leucomelas*

Magretti's Burrowing Asp - *A. magrettii*

Sahelian Burrowing Asp - *A. miropholis*

Phillips' Burrowing Asp - *A. phillipsi*

Somalia Burrowing Asp - *A. scortecci*

Watson's Burrowing Asp - *A. watsoni*

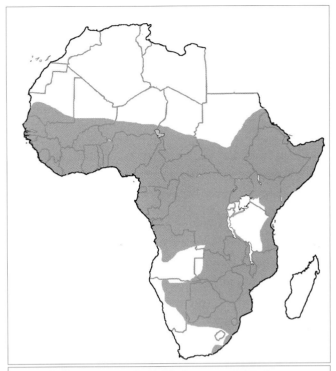

MAP 217. Combined range of all Mole Vipers, species (genus *Atractaspis*) found in the USAFRICOM region.

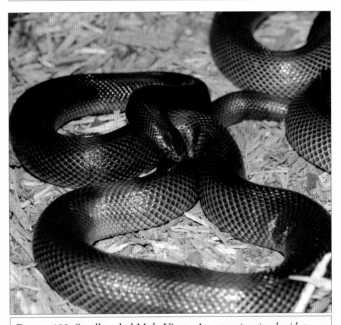

PHOTO 188. Small-scaled Mole Viper, *Atractaspis mircolepidota*

Current References

Books & Publications

Dobiey, Maik & Gernot Vogel. 2007. *Venomous Snakes of Africa.* TERRALOG Vol. 15. Edition Chimaira, Frankfort, Germany.

Dowling, Herndon G., Sherman A. Minton, and Findlay E. Russell. 1965. *Poisonous Snakes of the World.* Department of the Navy Bureau of Medicine and Surgery. Washington, DC.

Phelps, Tony. 2010. *Old World Vipers, A Natural History of the Azemoipinae and Viperinae.* Edition Chimaira. Frankfurt, Germany.

Spawls, Stephen & Bill Branch. 1995. *The Dangerous Snakes of Africa.* Blandford, England.

Guidelines for the Prevention and Clinical Management of Snakebite in Africa. 2010. World Health Organization Regional Office for Africa. Republic of Congo.

Journals

Trape, J.F; Chiro,L.; Broadley, D.J. & Wuster, W. 2009. "Phylogeography and systematic revision of the Egyptian Cobra (Serpentes: Elapidae: *Naja haje*) species complex, with the description of a new species from west Africa". Zootaxa 2236: 1-25.

Wallach, V., Wuster, W., & D.G.Broadley (2009). "In Praise of Subgenera: Taxonomic Status of Cobras in the the Genus *Naja* Laurenti (Serpentes: Elapidae)". Zootaxa 2236: 26-36.

Wuster, W. & Broadley, D.G. (2007). "Get an eyeful of this: a new species of giant spitting cobra from eastern and northeastern Africa (Squamata: Serpentes: Elapidae: *Naja*)". Zootaxa 1532: 51-68.

---, (2003). "A New Species of Spitting Cobra (*Naja*) from north-eastern Africa (Serpenties: Elapidae)". J. Zoo., Lond. 259, 345-359.

Wuster, Wolfgang; Steven Crookes, Ivan Ineich, Youssouph, Mane, Catharine E. Pook, Jean-Francois Trap 2007. "The phylogeny of cobras inferred from mitochondrial DNA sequences: Evolution of venom spitting and phylogeography of African spitting cobras (Serpentes; Elapidae: *Naja nigricollis* complex)". Molecular Phylogenetics and Evolution 45: 437-453.

Websites

Munich Antivenom Index (MAVIN) - www.toxinfo.org/antivenoms

University of Adelaide, Clinical Toxinology Resources Wesbsite (2012) - www.toxinology.com

World Health Organization - www.who.int/bloodproducts/snakeantivenoms/database

The Reptile Database - http//www.reptiledata-base.org, moroccoherps.com

Catalogue of Life - www.catalogueoflife.org

Armed Forces Pest Managment Board - www.afpmb.org/content/living-hazards-database

Original References

BONS, J. and B. GIROT. 1962. Cle Illustree des Reptiles du Maroc. Trav. Inst. Sci. Cherifien Ser. Zool. No. 26, p. 1–62, figs. 1–15.

KRAMER, Eugen and H. SCHNURRENBERGER. 1963. Systematik, Verbreitung und Okologie der Libyschen Schlangen. Rev. Suisse de Zool., vol. 70, pp. 453–568, pls. 1–4, figs. 1–13.

MARX, Hymen. 1956. Keys to the Lizards and Snakes of Egypt. Research Rpt. NM 005 050.39.45, NAMRU-3, Cairo pp. 1–8.

SAINT-GIRONS, H. 1956. Les Serpents du Maroc. Var. Scient. Soc. Sci. Nat. Psyc. Maroc, vol. 8, pp. 1–29, pls. 1–3, figs. 1–9.

VILLIERS, Andre. 1950. Contribution a l'etude du peuplement de la Mauritanie. Ophidiens. Bull. Inst. Francais d'Afrique Noire, vol. 12, pp. 984–998, figs. 1–2, tables.

ANGEL, F. 1933. Les serpents de l'Afrique occidentale Francaise. Larose Ed., Paris. 246 p., 83 figs.

BOGERT, Charles M. 1940. Herpetological Results of the Vernay Angola Expedition, with Notes on African Reptiles in Other Collections. Part I. Snakes, Including an Arrangement of African Colubridae. Bull. Amer. Mus. Nat. Hist., 77 (Art 1) : 1–107, figs. 1–18, pl. 1.

BOGERT, Charles M. 1942. *Pseudohaje* Gunther, A Valid Genus for Two West African Arboreal Cobras. Amer. Mus. Novitates (1174) : 1–9, figs. 1–8.

BROADLEY, Donald G. 1959. The Herpetology of Southern Rhodesia. Part 1. Snakes. Bull. Mus. Comp. Zool., 120 (1) : 1–100, figs. 1–10, pls. 1–6.

Original References (cont.)

CANSDALE, George S. 1961. West African Snakes. Longmans Green & Co., Ltd. London. 74 p., 34 figs. (most in color).

CORKILL, N. L. 1935. Notes on Sudan Snakes. Publ. Sudan Govt. Mus. (Nat. Hist.), (3) : (*not seen*).

CORKILL, Norman L. 1956. Snake Poisoning in the Sudan, p. 331–339, figs. 1–5. *In* E. E. Buckley and N. Porges, Venoms, Pub. Am. Assoc. Advanc. Sci. (44). 467 p.

DOUCET, Jean. 1963. Les serpents de la Republique de Cote d'Ivoire. Acta Tropica, 20 (3 & 4) : 201–340, figs. 1–57, pls. 1–10.

FITZSIMONS, Vivian F. M. 1962. Snakes of Southern Africa. Macdonald & Co., Ltd., London. 423 p., 74 color pls., 106 figs., 78 maps.

KNOEPFFLER, Louis-Philippe. 1965. Auto-observation par morsure d'*Atheris* sp. Toxicon, 2 : 275–276.

KRAMER, Eugen. 1961. Uber zwei afrikanische Zwergpuffottern, *Bitis hindii* (Boulenger, 1910) und *Bitis superciliaris* Peters, 1854). Vierteljahrsschrift naturf. Ges. Zurich, 106 : 419–423, fig. 1.

LAURENT, Raymond F. 1956. Contribution a l'Herpetologie de la region des Grands Lacs de l'Afrique central. Parts 1–3. Ann. Mus. Royal Congo Belgie, ser. 8 (sci. zool.), 48 : 1–390, figs. 1–50, pls. 1–31.

LAURENT, Raymond F. 1956. Esquisse d'une faune herpetologique du Ruanda-Urundi. Bull. Nat. Belges, nov-dec. 1956 : 280–287.

LAURENT, Raymond F. 1964. Reptiles et Amphibiens de l'Angola. Pub. Culturais Mus. Dundo (67) : 1–165, figs. 1–40.

LEESON, Frank. 1950. Identification of Snakes of the Gold Coast. Crown Agents for the Colonies, London. 142 p., 65 figs., 33 pls. (13 color).

LOVERIDGE, Arthur. 1953. Zoological Results of a Fifth Expedition to East Africa. III. Reptiles from Nyasaland and Tete. Bull. Mus. Comp. Zool., 110 (3) : 143–322, figs. 1–4, pls. 1–5.

LOVERIDGE, Arthur. 1957. Check List of the Reptiles and Amphibians of East Africa (Uganda; Kenya; Tanganyika; Zanzibar). Bull. Mus. Comp. Zool., 117 (2) : 153–362.

MANACAS, Sara. 1956. Ofidios de Mocambique. Mem. Junta Invest. Ultram., 8 : 135–160.

MERTENS, Robert. 1938. Herpetologische Ergebnisse einer Reise nach Kamerun. Abh. senckenbergischen naturf. Ges., 442 : 1–52, pls. 1–10.

MERTENS, Robert. 1955. Die Amphibien und Reptilien Sudwestafrikas. Aus den Ergebmissen einer im Jahre 1952 ausgefuhrten Reise. Abhandl. senckenbergischen naturf. Ges., 490 : 1–172, 24 pls. (1 color).

PARKER, H. W. 1949. The Snakes of Somaliland and the Sokotra Islands. Zool. Verh. Rijksmus. Nat. Hist. Leiden (6) : 1–115, figs. 1–11, map.

PERRET, J. L. 1960. Une nouvelle et remarquable espece d'Atractaspis (Viperidae) et quelques autres Serpents d'Afrique. Rev. Suisse Zool., 67 (5) : 129–139, figs. 1-4.

PITMAN, Charles R. S. 1938. A Guide to the Snakes of Uganda. Pub. Uganda Soc., Kampala, Uganda. 362 p., 2 figs., 23 color pls.

POPE, Clifford H. 1958. Fatal Bite of Captive African Rear-fanged Snake (*Dispholidus*). Copeia, 1958 (4) : 280–282.

SCHMIDT, Karl P. 1923. Contributions to the Herpetology of the Belgian Congo Based on the Collection of the American Museum Congo Expedition, 1909–1915. Part II. Snakes. Bull. Amer. Mus. Nat. Hist., 49 (art. 1) : 1–146, figs. 1–15, pls. 1–22, maps 1–19.

SWEENEY, R. C. H. 1961. Snakes of Nyasaland. Nyasaland Soc. & Nyasaland Govt. Zomba, Nyasaland. 200 p., 43 figs., map.

VISSER, John. 1966. Poisonous Snakes of Southern Africa and the Treatment of Snakebite. Howard Timmins: Capetown, 60 pp., 65 figs. (60 col.).

WITTE, Gaston-Francois de. 1941. Batraciens et reptiles. *In* Exploration du Parc National Albert, Mission G. F. de Witte (1933–1935). Pub. Inst. Parc Nationaux Congo Belge, fasc. 33 : 1–261, figs. 1–54, pls. 1–76.

WITTE, Gaston-Francois de. 1962. Genera des serpents du Congo et du Ruanda-Urundi. Ann. Mus. Royal Afrique Central, ser. 8 (104) : 1–203, figs. 1–94, pls. 1–15.

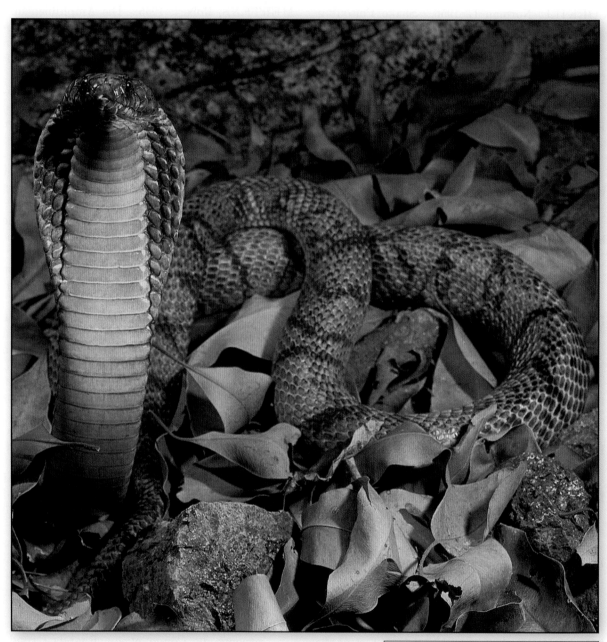

Andaman Cobra, *Naja sagittfera*

CHAPTER **13**

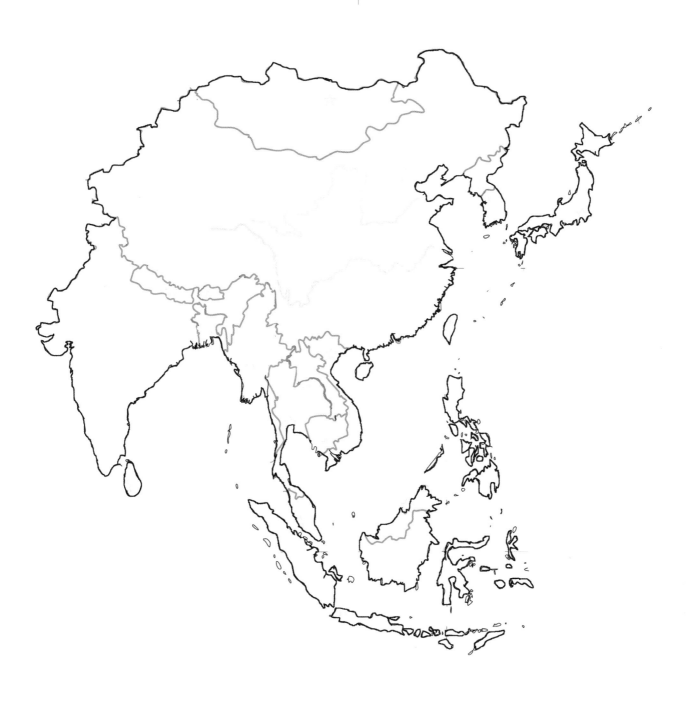

MAP 218. Region 6, Part One - United States Pacific Command. Southeast Asia, the Indo Pacific.

Introduction

The USPACOM region leads every other region in this volume for the total number of dangerously venomous snake species. There are at least 130 Elapids (cobra-like snakes) and as many as 91 vipers and pit vipers for a minimum of 231 venomous snakes within the region which may pose a significant threat to man.

The Colubridae family also has in the region some rear-fanged, mildly venomous genera including the *Boiga* and *Rhabdophis.* The latter is a genus that has at least one species that has killed a few people. None of the above mentioned species are included in this volume because these snakes are not usually considered a significant threat to man.

Snakebite in this region is a serious health problem and as many as 35,000 people per year may die as a result of snake envenomation. As high as this current number is, it is most certainly but a fraction of the number of deaths that must have occurred just a few decades ago before the advent of antivenoms and advanced trauma therapy.

In the original version of *Poisonous Snakes of the World* (1965), the current region of command known as US-PACOM was divided into three regions. In keeping with the intent of this volume to utilize the U.S. military's current regions of command, those three regions have been consolidated into the region now known as the United States Pacific Command (USPACOM). Although this regional designation fits well into the format of this book, it does present some problems for both the writer and the reader, as the USPACOM region encompasses such a huge geographical area. Moreover, there are more species of venomous snakes to be described in this region than any other in this book.

In an attempt to simplify the complex task of dealing with so many species throughout such an enormous area, the author has deemed it useful to divide the US-PACOM region into two parts. Part one will include all of the Asian continent not included in other chapters, as well as the Indo-Pacific islands. Part two shall deal with Australia and the Papuan archipelago.

In part one of the USPACOM region the most well represented venomous snakes are the Pit Vipers (family Crotalidae) with approximately 91 species endemic to the region. In fact, southeast Asia is considered by most experts to be the cradle of evolution for this family of snakes.

The Elapidae (cobra family) is also well represented here, but it is in part 2 of the USPACOM that these snakes really dominate. In fact, in USPACOM part two all dangerously venomous snakes are members of the cobra family.

The absence of viperids and pit vipers throughout the Australia / New Guinea region has resulted in several elapid species evolving to occupy ecological niches normally filled by viperids throughout the rest of the world. Some species even resemble the vipers and pit vipers in morphology and biology; that is, triangular head distinct from neck, elliptical pupils, stout bodies, live bearing, etc.

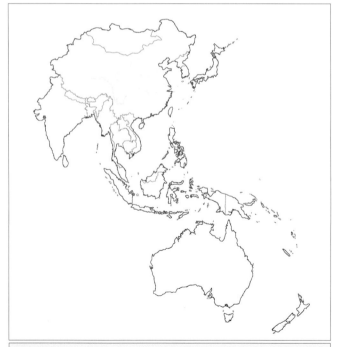

MAP 219. Region 6, United States Pacific Command. Southeast Asia, the Indo Pacific, and Australia.

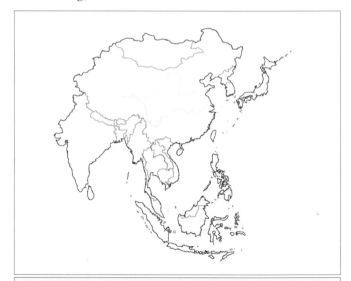

MAP 220. Region 6, Part One - United States Pacific Command. Southeast Asia, the Indo Pacific.

Generic And Species Descriptions

Family - Elapidae: Genus - Naja

True Cobras

As many as 28 species are recognized. These snakes are also found in the USAFRICOM and USCENTCOM regions. In the USPACOM region they range from India eastward across southeast Asia as far as Taiwan, and southward into the Indo-Pacific. At least 11 species are found in the USPACOM region (at one time all were considered to be subspecies of *Naja naja*). *Naja* cobras are moderate to large in size (4 to 8 feet as adults). They have large fangs and toxic venom. Some species are capable of "spitting" venom into the eyes of an aggressor and all members of this genus will react to threats by raising the anterior portion of the body and spreading the neck into a hood.

All *Naja* species in the USPACOM region are potentially deadly snakes, and several are extremely dangerous.

Definition: Head rather broad, flattened, only slightly distinct from the neck. Snout rounded, a distinct canthus. Body moderately slender, slightly depressed, tapered, neck capable of expansion into a hood. Tail of moderate length.

Eyes moderate in size; pupils round.

Head Scales: The usual 9 on the crown; frontal short; rostral rounded. Laterally, nasal in contact with the one or two preoculars.

Body scales: Dorsals smooth in 17-25 oblique rows at midbody, usually more on the neck, fewer posteriorly. Ventrals 159-232, subcaudals 42-88, mostly paired.

Maxillary teeth: Two rather large tubular fangs.

Common Cobra,

Naja naja

Description and Identification: The most readily recognizable feature of the Common Cobra is the classic "spectacled" markings on the hood. In fact, the name "Spectacled Cobra" is often used along with the name "Indian Cobra." Both these common names are appropriate since the hood markings of this species resemble a pair of spectacles and its range coincides closely to the Indian subcontinent.

A few individuals may have the spectacled hood markings reduced or occasionally even absent. The overall color is drab gray or brown. There is often no dorsal pattern at all and uniformly brown or grayish specimens are common. Some are more interestingly marked with narrow, irregular light bands across the body or alternating light and dark bands. Light color on the skin between the scales is also seen and when present produces a mottled effect. An all black population occurs in Pakistan. When spectacles are present they are sometimes seen on the ventral surface of the hood as a light circle containing two dark spots, one on each side of the hood. Average size is 3.5 to 4 feet, but can reach a maximum of just over 6 feet.

Distribution, Habitat, and Biology: At one time all the cobras of Asia were attributed to this species which was divided into numerous subspecies. It is now known that those subspecies are in fact full species. *Naja naja* ranges throughout India and the island of Sri Lanka as well as into portions of Pakistan and Nepal and Bangladesh. Common Cobras are indeed common animals throughout much of their range and they inhabit a wide variety of environments. Their food is almost anything that can be swallowed, from rodents to frogs and other snakes.

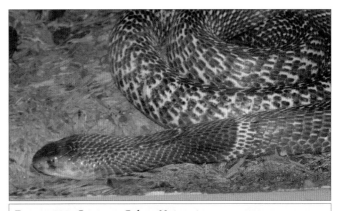

Photo 189. Common Cobra, *Naja naja*

Venom and Bite: These cobras are non-spitters and their venom is mainly neurotoxic, but it does contain some cytotoxic properties. The venom is potent and many human deaths are recorded each year. The Common Cobra, along with the similar Monocle Cobra (page 212) together range throughout some of the most densely populated regions of the world. A big portion of the ranges of these two snakes includes agricultural areas and rural communities where the human population comes into frequent contact with snakes. As a result, the Common Cobra along with the Monocle Cobra are responsible for more human fatalities than any other cobra species.

The World Health Organization (www.who.int/blood-products/snakeantivenoms), viewed 2012, lists the following antivenoms for this snake:

Product: Polyvalent Snake Antivenin
Manufacturer: Biological Limited
Country of Origin: India
Product: Polyvalent Snake Antivenom (Asia)
Manufacturer: Bharat Serums and Vaccines
Country of Origin: India
Product: Snake antivenin I.P. (Asia)
Manufacturer: Haffkine Biopharmaceutical Corp. Ltd.
Country of Origin: India
Product: Snake Venom Antiserum I.P. (Asia)
Manufacturer: VINS Bioproducts Ltd.
Country of Origin: India

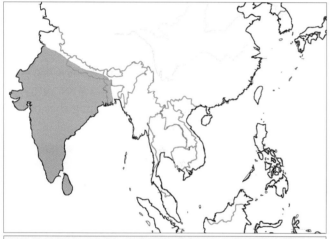

MAP 221. Range of the Common Cobra, *Naja naja*, in the USPACOM region.

Similar Species: The Central Asian Cobra (*N. oxiana*) is a very similar species found mostly in the USCENTCOM region but also ranging into the USPACOM region in extreme northwest India. For photo and information see chapter 11 (USCENTCOM), page 157.

Monocle Cobra,
Naja kouthia

Description and Identification: Similar in many respects to the Common Cobra, but has a single rounded hood marking reminiscent of the old time "monocle" eyepiece that was commonly used in colonial times. In color they are also similar to the Common Cobra, ranging from light brown to gray to nearly black. Most are uniformly colored dorsally, but some specimens have light, irregular crossbars or light blotches on the back.

These are rather stout bodied cobras that can reach a length of up to 6 feet.

Distribution, Habitat, and Biology: Found from northern India and southern Nepal eastward through Bangladesh, Bhutan, and Myanmar; then southeastward all the way to southern Vietnam. It ranges well onto the Malay Peninsula as far south as northern Malaysia. These are common snakes in most of their range and they can be found in both forests and agricultural areas. Rodents, anurans, and other snakes are listed as prey.

Venom and Bite: A non spitter whose venom is mainly postsynaptic neurotoxins. Cardiotoxins may also be present. There is evidence that specimens from different regions have different venom properties, with some possessing more neurotoxins and being more potent. These snakes kill many people each year throughout their range. In fact, the Monocle Cobra and the Common Cobra are together responsible for more human fatalities than any other members of the *Naja* genus.

The World Health Organization (www.who.int/blood-products/snakeantivenoms), viewed 2012, lists the following antivenoms for this snake:

Product: Cobra Antivenin
Manufacturer: Myanmar Pharmaceutical Factory
Country of Origin: Myanmar
Product: Cobra Antivenin (QSMI)
Manufacturer: Queen Saovabha Memorial Institute
Country of Origin: Thailand
Product: Neuro-polyvalent snake antivenom
Manufacturer: Queen Saovabha Memorial Institute
Country of Origin: Thailand
Product: SAV-Naja
Manufacturer: Institute of Vaccines and Biological Substances
Country of Origin: Vietnam

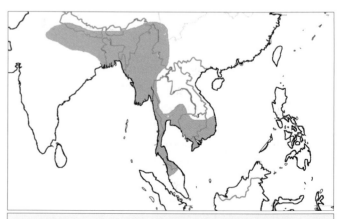

MAP 222. Range of the Monocle Cobra, *Naja kouthia*.

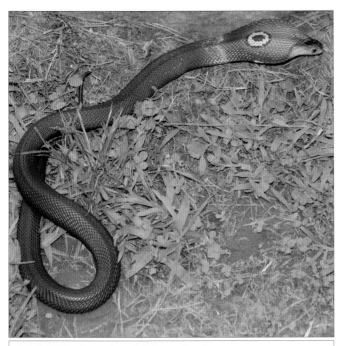

Photo 190. Monocle Cobra, *Naja kouthia*

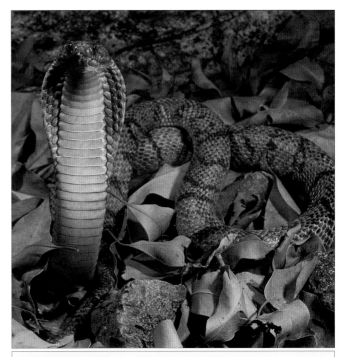

Photo 191. Andaman Cobra, *Naja sagittfera*

Andaman Cobra,
Naja sagittfera

Description and Identification: In color they vary from brown or gray to black. Many show faint dark bands across the back, and juvenile specimens can be black with light bands. A well defined monocle marking on the hood is common.

Distribution, Habitat, and Biology: The Andaman Cobra is an insular species found on the Andaman Islands west of the Malay Peninsula in the Andaman Sea.

Venom and Bite: No specific antivenom is listed for this species by the World Health Organization. Antivenoms for the Monocle Cobra may have some effectiveness against the Andaman Cobra, but this is unknown.

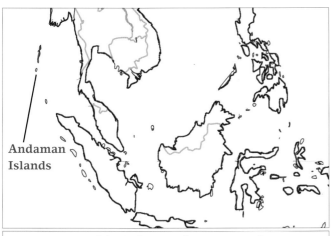

Map 223. Range of the Andaman Cobra, *Naja sagittfera*.

Chinese Cobra,
Naja atra

Description and Identification: Chinese Cobras are typically dark in color. They may be dark brown, charcoal gray, or nearly black. Many show a series of thin light crossbands that are widely spaced down the back. The hood is marked with a well defined marking which may extend laterally across the entire dorsal surface of the hood. These snakes can reach a maximum of 6.5 feet in length. There are 19-21 mid-body scale rows with 23-27 at the neck.

Distribution, Habitat, and Biology: Most of this snake's range is contained in southeastern China. It also occurs in northern Vietnam and northern Laos as well as the islands of Taiwan and Hainan. These snakes inhabit most habitats within their range except for dense, closed canopy forests and they are most common around areas of human habitat alterations (edges of clearings, second growth, rice paddies, etc.) (Orlov et al., 2003). They are most active during the day and early evening hours. Like most cobras they are very catholic in their diet and eat most any type of terrestrial vertebrate they can swallow.

Venom and Bite: Mainly a non spitter, but some specimens may be capable of spitting. The venom is quite toxic and consists of both neurotoxins and cytotoxins. The cytotoxins can cause necrosis and more significantly can act as a cardiotoxin.

The World Health Organization (www.who.int/blood-products/snakeantivenoms), viewed 2012, lists the following antivenoms for this snake:

Product: Naja naja (atra) antivenom

Manufacturer: Shanghai Institute Biological Technology Co. Ltd.

Country of Origin: China

Product: Antivenom B. multicinctus/N.n.naja

Manufacturer: National Institute of Preventative Medicine

Country of Origin: China

Clinical Toxinology Resources website (www.toxinology.com-viewed 2012) lists post-synaptic neurotoxins and possibly cardiotoxins as present in the venom.

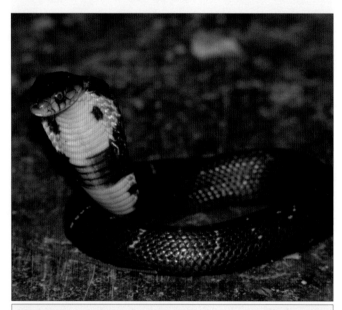

Photo 192. Chinese Cobra, *Naja atra*

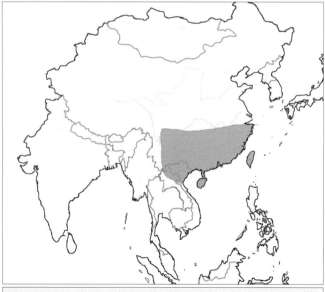

Map 224. Range of the Chinese Cobra, *Naja atra*.

Northern Philippine Cobra,
Naja philippinensis

Description and Identification: Average length is about 4.5 feet, but they may grow to 6 feet. In color these snakes are uniformly brown to light tan, but young snakes are much darker brown. Unlike many Asian cobras this species lacks hood markings.

Distribution, Habitat, and Biology: These snakes live in a variety of habitats but are generally restricted to elevations below 2,500 feet. They are terrestrial in habits, but are fond of areas near water. Loss of habitat and persecution by man has reduced the population of these snakes considerably from historical times when they were more common.

Venom and Bite: The venom of the Northern Philippine Cobra is reported to be highly toxic (some believe it is the most toxic of all the cobras). They are also known to be capable of spitting venom.

The World Health Organization (www.who.int/blood-products/snakeantivenoms), viewed 2012, lists the following antivenoms for this snake:

Product: Monovalent (Naja philippinensis) Cobra Antivenom

Manufacturer: Research Institute for Tropical Medicine, Biological Manufacturing Division

Country of Origin: Philippines

Post-synaptic neurotoxins and possibly cardiotoxins listed by Clinical Toxinology Resources (2012).

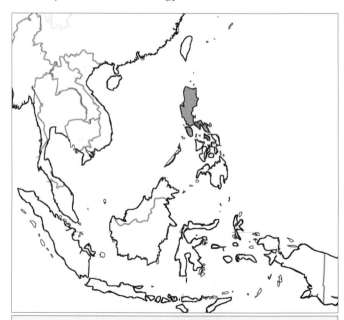

Map 225. Range of the Northern Philippine Cobra, *Naja philippinensis*.

Peters' Cobra,
Naja samarensis

Description and Identification: Also sometimes called the Southern Philippine Cobra. In sharp contrast to the Northern Philippine Cobra which is normally uniformly drab, this species is often vividly colored with a bright yellow throat, face, and edges of ventrals against a nearly black background.

Distribution, Habitat, and Biology: Found on the southern Philippine Islands of Mindanao, Samar, Bahal, and Leyte. Reportedly diurnal and common in human altered habitats while shunning deep forest (Smith 1993).

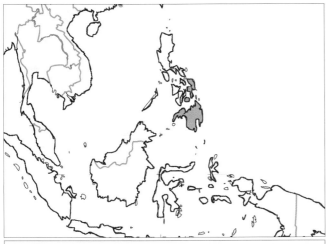

MAP 226. Range of the Peters' Cobra, *Naja samarensis.*

Venom and Bite: Like the preceding species (to which this snake was once assigned as a subspecies) these snakes are known to be capable of spitting venom. There seems to be very little information available on the venom of *samarensis*. It is probably a very dangerous snake.

The World Health Organization (www.who.int/blood-products/snakeantivenoms), viewed 2012, lists the same antivenom for this species as for the Northern Philippine Cobra.

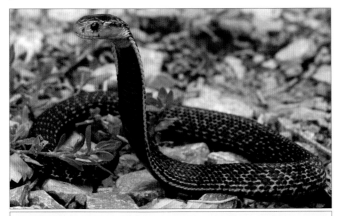

PHOTO 193. Peters' Cobra, *Naja samarensis*

Sumatran Spitting Cobra,
Naja sumatrana

Description and Identification: Ground color varies from light tan to black. Lighter specimens sometimes have darker scales contrasting with a light interstitial skin color, producing a dark speckled effect. Darker specimens may have a hint of light crossbars or be uniformly dark gray or black.

These snakes can exceed 5 feet and are relatively heavy bodied.

Distribution, Habitat, and Biology: Found on the islands of Sumatra, Borneo. Palawan and the southern end of the Malay Peninsula. Habitat includes dense tropical forests as well as areas of human disturbance (including urban areas).

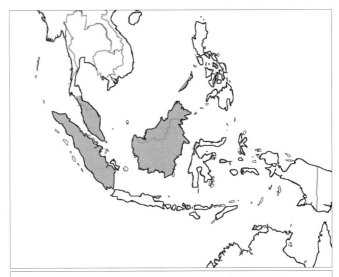

MAP 227. Range of the Sumatran Spitting Cobra, *Naja sumatrana.*

Venom and Bite: There is not much information on the venom of this species. It is probably a combination of neurotoxins and cytotoxins. Undoubtably this snake is capable of inflicting a fatal bite. Three antivenoms are listed by the World Health Organization. Two are produced by the Queen Saovabha Memorial Institute in Thailand (Cobra Antivenom and Neuro Polyvalent snake antivenom). Also listed is Monovalent (Naja philippinensis) Cobra Antivenom by Research Institute for Tropical Medicine in the Philippines. Information on the efficacy of this latter antivenom on *N. sumatrana* bites is unavailable.

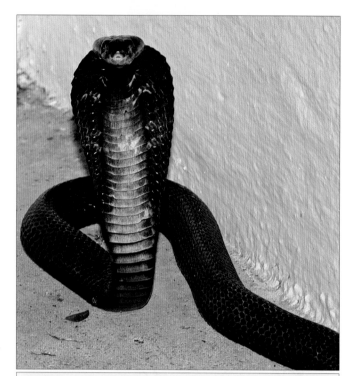

Photo 194. Sumatran Spitting Cobra, *Naja sumatrana* (black phase)

Indo-Chinese Spitting Cobra,
Naja siamensis

Description and Identification: The color of this cobra is variable. They can be light tan to gray brown or a mottled black and white. Many show a spectacle hood marking similar to the Common Cobra (*N. naja*).

Distribution, Habitat, and Biology: This cobra also goes by the name Thai Spitting Cobra and indeed most of its range is contained within the country of Thailand. It also ranges into parts of Laos, southern Cambodia, and extreme southern Vietnam.

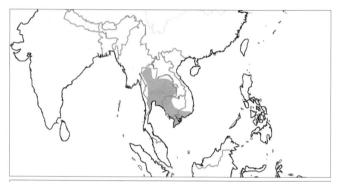

Map 229. Range of the Indo-Chinese Spitting Cobra, *Naja siamensis.*

Similar Species: The Indonesian Spitting Cobra (*Naja sputatrix*) is a very similar species that varies from uniform brown or yellowish to black. This species ranges across the southern Indonesian Island chain of Java in the west to Flores in the east. This is a dangerous snake that is capable of killing.

Venom and Bite: Bites by this snake are known to cause severe tissue damage and often, death. The World Health Organization website (viewed 2012) lists two antivenoms for this species. Both are produced in Thailand by the Queen Saovabha Memorial Institute. They are Cobra Antivenom and Neuro-polyvalent Snake Antivenom. In addition, the Munich Antivenom Index lists two other Antivenoms. Antivenin Polyvalent (Bio Farma, Indonesia), and Naja naja sputatrix (Twyford, Germany).

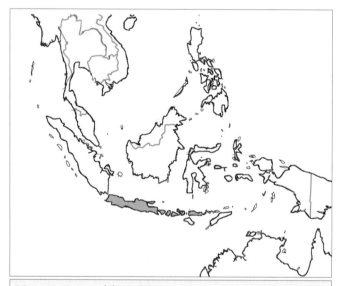

Map 228. Range of the Indonesian Spitting Cobra, *Naja sputatrix.*

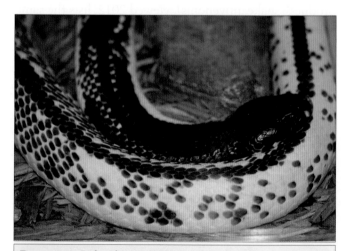

Photo 195. Indo-Chinese Spitting Cobra, *Naja siamensis*

Similar Species: The Burmese Spitting Cobra (*N. mandalayensis*) is probably closely related to the Siamese Spitting Cobra. Its small range in central Myanmar is sympatric with the Monacle Cobra and it may be confused with that species. But it can easily be distinguished from the Monocle Cobra by the lack of any type of hood markings on adult snakes. Young may have hood markings, but they are spectacle shaped rather than monocle shaped as in the Monocle Cobra (Slowinski & Wuster 2000).

These snakes have a rather small, restricted range and are apparently rare, less than a few dozen specimens have been collected to date.

Very little is known about its venom but it is most likely a dangerous snake. Clinical Toxinology Resources website (www.toxinology.com 2012) lists the following antivenoms for bites by this species.

    Product: Anti Cobra, Siamese Cobra

    Manufacturer: Pharmaceutical Industries Corp.

    Country of Origin: Myanmar

    Product: Bivalent

    Manufacturer: Pharmaceutical Industries Corp.

    Country of Origin: Myanmar

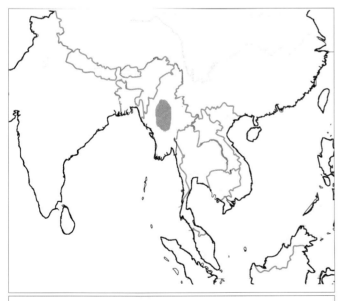

MAP 230. Range of the Burmese Spitting Cobra, *Naja mandalayensis.*

Family - Elapidae: Genus - Ophiophagus

King Cobra

At present, there is only a single, wide-ranging species within this genus. However, future studies may reveal several additional species. King Cobras are found throughout southeast Asia and most of Indonesia. This genus is endemic to the USPACOM (Part 1) region.

Definition: Head relatively short, flattened, moderately distinct from neck; snout broad, rounded, canthus indistinct. Body slender, tapering, neck region capable of expanding into a hood; tail long.

Eyes moderate in size; pupils round.

Head scales: The usual 9 on the crown, plus a pair of large occipitals in contact with one another behind the parietals. Laterally, nasal in narrow contact with one another behind the parietals. Laterally, nasal in narrow contact with elongate preocular.

Body Scales: Dorsals smooth, in 15 oblique rows at midbody and posteriorly, more (17-19) on neck. Ventrals 240-254; subcaudals 81-104, the anterior ones single, the remainder paired.

King Cobra,
Ophiophagus hannah

Description and Identification: This is the world's longest venomous snake, with a record length of over 18 feet. Most are fully grown at about 12 feet. Adults are usually uniformly colored dorsally, and the ground color is light yellow brown, tan, or olive brown. Young snakes are very dark brown or black with numerous narrow white bands around the back. This color fades with age, but young adults retain an increasingly indistinct banded pattern which often persists on mature snakes.

Distribution, Habitat and Biology: When threatened will raise as much as a third of the fore body off the ground and spread a narrow hood. A large specimen when hooded can literally "look a man in the eye." This snake has a peculiar gravelly hiss that sounds more like a growl than a hiss. These behaviors, coupled with a sometimes aggressive nature when cornered or protecting a nest full of eggs, produces a very impressive serpent!

Among zookeepers and venom lab professionals the King Cobra is known for its intelligence and fearlessness when cornered. In their natural habitat they are snakes of the forests and swamps and usually avoid areas of human activity. They feed mostly on other snakes. These snakes are found from India and Nepal all the way to the east coast of China. They also range southward throughout southeast Asia and Indonesia as far as the Philippines, Java, and the Celebes Islands.

Additional studies of the morphology, phylogeny, and distribution of the King Cobra may lead to the discovery of more than just a single, wide-ranging species.

Venom and Bite: Post-synaptic neurotoxins. Although their venom is less potent than the smaller cobras (genus-*Naja*), these huge snakes possess enormous quantities of venom. The venom glands of a large adult can yield enough venom to kill three dozen humans! A maximum envenomation by this snake is not survivable without antivenom and supportive therapy. Since this is a wide ranging snake that is found in many Asian countries there are a number of different antivenoms produced. Below is a partial list.

Product: King Cobra Antivenom
Manufacturer: Thai Red Cross
Country of Origin: Thailand
Product: Ophiophagus Antivenom
Manufacturer: University of Medicine & Pharmacy
Country of Origin: Vietnam
Product: Polyvalent Anti Snake Venom Serum
Manufacturer: Central Research Institute
Country of Origin: India

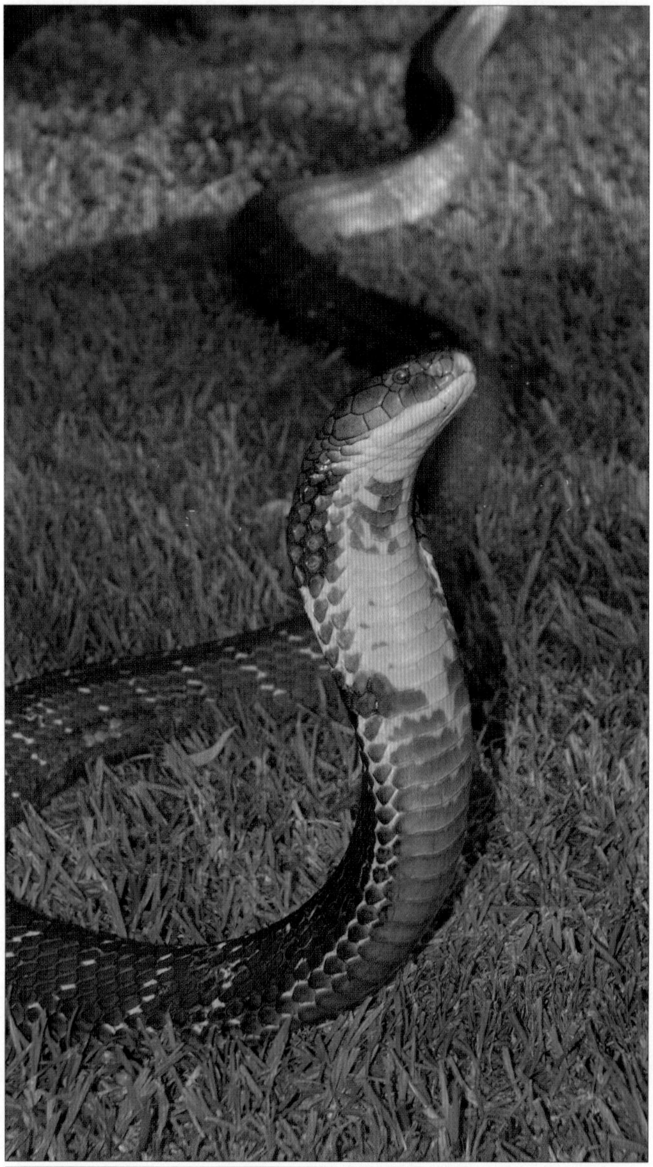

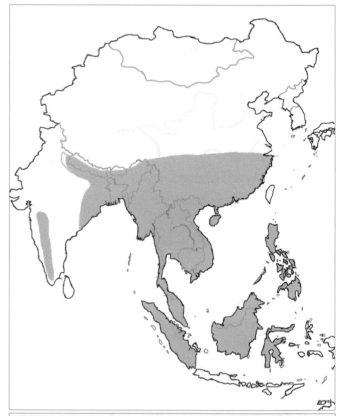

MAP 231. Range of the King Cobra, *Ophiophagus hannah*.

PHOTO 196. King Cobra, *Ophiophagus hannah*

Family - Elapidae: Genus - Bungarus

Kraits

Thirteen species are recognized; all inhabit Asia and most are found in southeastern Asia. Two species range westward into the USCENTCOM region in eastern Pakistan and eastern Afghanistan. All others are endemic to the USPACOM region. Kraits are innocuous looking snakes and are usually hesitant to bite, but their venom is a potent neurotoxin. Most species are of moderate (4 to 5 feet) length, but all are considered extremely dangerous. A few individuals reach lengths approaching 7 feet.

These are nocturnal snakes and when disturbed from their hiding places during daylight hours they usually react with a docile nature. At night however the become very active and alert and can be quick to bite. They have killed many people in the USPACOM region. One victim was Joseph B. Slowinski, a distinguished herpetologist from the United States, who was killed by a krait while doing field work in Asia in 2001.

Like the North American coral snakes, the kraits have many non-venomous mimics, and like coral snakes the bite of a krait produces no local effects and can lead to a false sense of security among victims. But their venom is a powerful neurotoxin and untreated envenomations result in a "short-circuiting" of the nerve impulses to vital organs like the diaphragm, leading to death by asphyxiation. In some species antivenom will not reverse symptoms after they have manifested, thus in treating bites by these snakes antivenom should be used aggressively. The venom of the kraits is purely neurotoxic and all species are extremely dangerous.

Antivenom is produced for the species which cause the most snakebites, but some species have no specific antivenom. Many Krait species are confusingly similar in appearance. Most have a pattern of light bands on a dark background, but on some the light bands are indistinct or entirely lacking.

Definition: Head small, flattened, slightly distinct from neck; no distinct canthus. Body moderately slender, cylindrical; tail short. Eyes small; pupils round or vertically subelliptical.

Head scales: The usual 9 on the crown; frontal broad. Laterally, nasal in broad contact with single preocular.

Body scales: Dorsals smooth, vertebral row enlarged and hexagonal (strongly so except in B. lividus) in 13-17 oblique rows at midbody. Ventrals 193-237; anal plate entire; subcaudals single or paired, 23-56.

Common Krait,
Bungarus caeruleus

Description and Identification: Very large individuals approach 6 feet in length. The Common Krait is typically a blueish gray to black snake with a series of narrow cream or white bands around the body. In some specimens the bands may be reduced or absent, producing a uniformly blue-black snake. They are often called "Blue Krait" in reference to their blueish gray or blue-black ground color. Another often used name for this species is "Indian Krait." Common Kraits have at least one non-venomous mimic, the Common Wolf Snake (*Lycodon*) of the family Colubridae.

Distribution, Habitat, and Biology: Ranges throughout the Indian subcontinent and the island of Sri Lanka. Strictly nocturnal, if encountered during the day this snake is usually quite docile and will hide its head beneath its coils rather than try to bite. Feeds on a wide variety of small vertebrates, with other snakes being a major food item. The habitat is most often areas of human activity/disturbance such as agricultural fields and pastures. Avoids dense forests.

Venom and Bite: Both pre-synaptic and post-synaptic neurotoxins present. Because this snake is common and widespread, and it prefers cultivated fields and human habitations (i.e., refuse, old buildings, etc.), it is a snake commonly encountered by humans. This is one of the "big four" among the dangerous snakes of India and it kills many humans each year throughout its range. Many victims are bitten at night in their homes while they sleep on the floor. The venom is a pure neurotoxin and quite

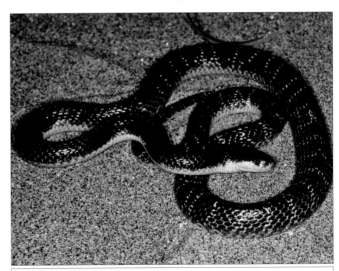

Photo 197. Common Krait, *Bungarus caeruleus*. See also page 156 Chapter 11 (USCENTCOM).

potent. In fact it is one of the most toxic venoms in the world, and though they do not possess a large quantity of venom, an adult snake has enough to kill up to 10 people.

World Health Organization list of antivenoms, (www.who.int/bloodproducts/snakeantivenoms) viewed 2012.

Product: Polyvalent Snake Antivenom (Asia)
Manufacturer: Biological E Limited
Country of Origin: India
Product: Polyvalent Snake Antivenom (Asia)
Manufacturer: Bharat Serums and Vaccines
Country of Origin: India
Product: Snake Antivenom IP (Asia)
Manufacturer: Haffkine Biopharmaceutical Corp.
Country of Origin: India
Product: Snake Venom Antiserum IP (Asia)
Manufacturer: VINS Bioproducts Ltd
Country of Origin: India
Product: Polyvalent Antisnake Venom
Manufacturer: National Institute of Health
Country of Origin: Pakistan

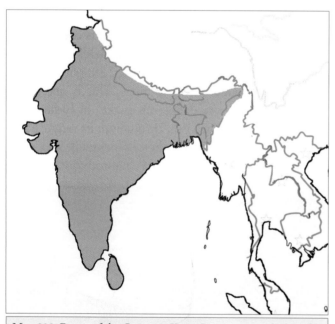

MAP 232. Range of the Common Krait, *Bungarus caeruleus*, in the USPACOM region.

Banded Krait,
Bungarus fasciatus

Description and Identification: This krait is characterized by alternating black and white (or black and yellow) bands. In some specimens the dark and light bands are nearly the same width, on others the light bands are slightly narrower. The appearance is more of a black and yellow (or black and white) banded snake rather than a black snake with light bands (as with many other kraits). The bands on this snake encircle the entire body. Its most diagnostic feature however is the shape of its body, which is triangular in cross section and has a pronounced vertebral ridge. The tip of the tail is noticeably blunt, another unique feature to this krait. Adults average about 5 feet but these large kraits can reach over 7 feet in length.

Distribution, Habitat, and Biology: Strictly nocturnal. Inoffensive by day but more active and alert and quicker to bite at night. Feeds mostly on other snakes. Found in forests, mangroves, dry woodland, and around areas of human disturbance and habitation. Endemic to the USPACOM region and widespread from India across southeast Asia and southern China and southward into Malaysia and Indonesia.

Venom and Bite: The venom of the Banded Krait is less toxic than that of the Common Krait, but it is a larger snake with larger venom glands. Though it kills fewer

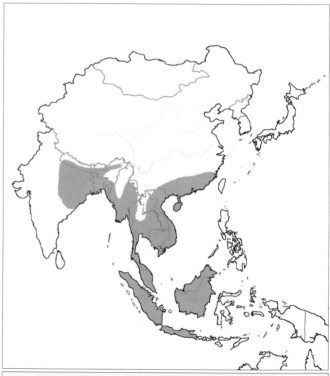

MAP 233. Range of the Banded Krait, *Bungarus fasciatus*.

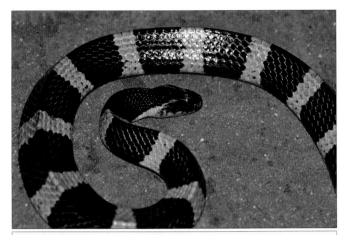

Photo 198. Banded Krait, *Bungarus fasciatus*

people than the Common Krait, it is a widespread and common snake and thus bites are frequent. Deaths are fairly common. It is estimated that this species can yield enough venom to kill several people.

World Health Organization list of antivenoms, (www. who.int/bloodproducts/snakeantivenoms) viewed 2012.

Product: Banded Krait Antivenin

Manufacturer: Queen Saovabha Memorial Inst.

Country of Origin: Thailand

Product: Neuro Polyvalent Snake Antivenom

Manufacturer: Queen Saovabha Memorial Inst.

Country of Origin: Thailand

Product: Polyvalent Anti Snake Venom

Manufacturer: Bio Farma

Country of Origin: Indonesia

Malayan Krait,

Bungarus candidus

Description and Identification: Very similar to the preceding species and occurring sympatrically with it in many areas. Differentiating between these two species can be tricky. Like the previous species, the Malayan Krait is a shiny, blue black snake with well defined white bands. In the Malayan Krait the body is more rounded in cross section.

Distribution, Habitat, and Biology: As it's name implies this species is found throughout the Malay Peninsula as well as much of southeast Asia and the islands of Sumatra and Java.

Venom and Bite: As with all members of the *Bungarus* genus, this species should be regarded as highly dangerous.

Antivenoms recommended by the World Health Organization are:

Product: Malayan Krait Antivenom (QSM)

Manufacturer: Queen Saovabha Memorial Institute

Country of Origin: Thailand

Product: Neuro-polyvalent Snake Antivenom

Manufacturer: Queen Saovabha Memorial Institute

Country of Origin: Thailand

From www.who.int/bloodproducts/snakeantivenoms/ database (viewed 2012).

As with other kraits, both pre-synaptic and post-synaptic toxins are present in the venom.

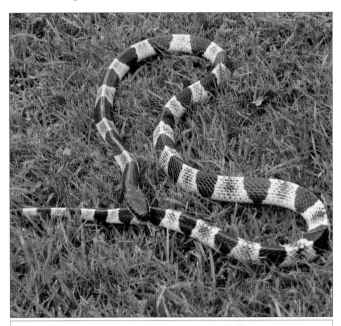

Photo 199. Malayan Krait, *Bungarus candidus*

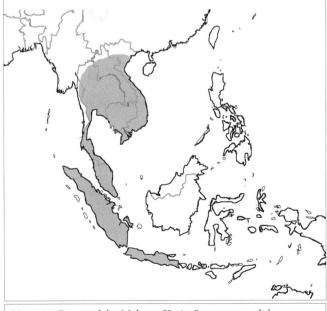

Map 234. Range of the Malayan Krait, *Bungarus candidus.*

Andaman Krait,
Bungarus andamanensis

Description and Identification: Very similar in appearance to the Common Krait (*B. caeruleus*) of the Indian subcontinent. Adult length is probably just over four feet.

Distribution, Habitat and Biology: Restricted to the Andaman Islands.

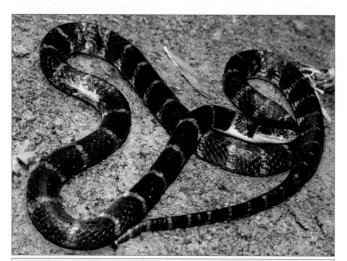

Photo 200. Andaman Krait, *Bungarus andamanensis*

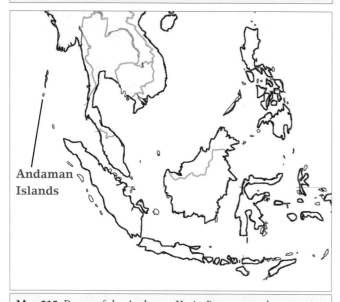

Map 235. Range of the Andaman Krait, *Bungarus andamanensis*.

Venom and Bite: There seems to be little known about this snake's venom or the effects of its bite. But it is a krait that grows to 4 feet, thus it is most likely a deadly species.

Many-banded Krait,
Bungarus multicinctus

Description and Identification: This species is typical of many kraits with a black and white banded pattern. This species is characterized by the large number of white bands, which is typically as many as 40 to 50. This species is very similar to the Malayan Krait, and the Banded Krait but those snakes typically have only about 30 light colored bands. These are fairly large snakes that can reach a maximum length of about 6 feet.

Distribution, Habitat, and Biology: In habits the Many-banded Krait is similar to all other kraits, being terrestrial, nocturnal, secretive and docile by day but quick to bite if molested at night. They are common snakes that inhabit a wide variety of habitats including dense forest and semi-open country in both upland and lowland areas.

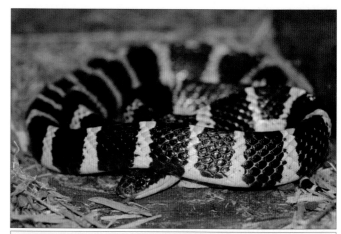

Photo 201. Many-banded Krait, *Bungarus multicinctus*

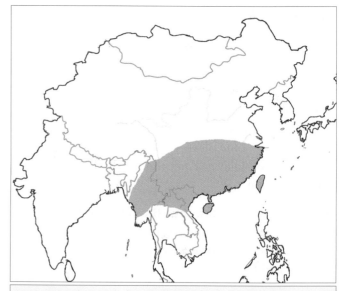

Map 236. Range of the Many-banded Krait, *Bungarus multicinctus*.

Venom and Bite: Very potent neurotoxin (pre and post-synaptic). Untreated bites have a very high fatality rate. These are common snakes and in southern China and Taiwan they are responsible for numerous snakebites.

Bungarus multicinctus antivenin by the Shanghai Institute Biological Technology (China) is a specific antivenom. Also available from the National Institute of Preventative Medicine in China is Bungarus antivenom and the bi-valent B. multicinctus/N.n.naja antivenom.

Red-headed Krait,
Bungarus flaviceps

Description and Identification: Very striking and distinctive coloring-head and tail bright red, body black with narrow bluish white stripe low on side and sometimes a narrow orange stripe or row of dots down middle of back.

Size about the same as the Banded Krait.

Distribution, Habitat, and Biology: Southern Burma to Vietnam and south through Malaysia and larger islands of Indonesia. Inhabits jungle mostly in hilly or mountainous country. A rare snake.

Venom and Bite: Little is known about the venom of the Red-headed Krait or the effects of a bite. No specific antivenom is listed by the World Health Organization but the Clinical Toxinology Resources website (www.toxinology.com-viewed 2012) lists Banded Krait Antivenin manufactured by Queen Saovabha Memorial Institute in Thailand.

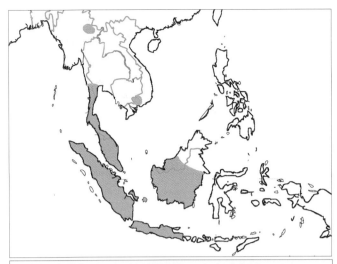

MAP 237. Range of the Red-headed Krait, *Bungarus flaviceps.*

Northeastern Hill Krait,
Bungarus bungaroides

Description and Identification: Blue-black with very narrow cream colored bars that may be reduced to transverse lines of small spots. Grows to about 4.5 feet.

Distribution, Habitat, and Biology: Occurs in several widely disjunct localities across southeast Asia.

Venom and Bite: Not much is known about the venom or bite of this snake. Most likely it is a dangerous species.

No antivenom is listed by the World Health Organization website, but Clinical Toxinology Resources website (www.toxinolgy.com) viewed 2012 lists the following:

Product: SII Polyvalent Antisnake Venom Serum
Manufacturer: Serum Institute of India
Country of Origin: India

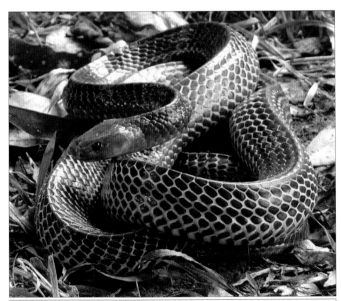

PHOTO 202. Red-headed Krait, *Bungarus flaviceps*

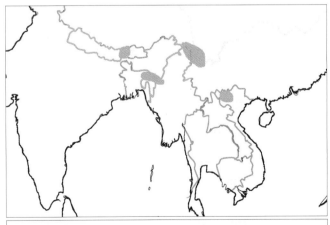

MAP 238. Range of the Northeastern Hill Krait, *Bungarus bungaroides.*

Ceylon Krait,

Bungarus ceylonicus

Description and Identification: A fairly typical "black & white" krait. White bands may be reduced on some specimens. Grows to about 4.5 feet.

Distribution, Habitat, and Biology: Endemic to the Island of Ceylon (Sri Lanka), where it occurs on the southern half of the island.

Venom and Bite: This is a deadly species. No specific antivenom is listed by the World Health Organization website, but Clinical Toxinology Resources website (viewed 2012) lists the following.

SII Polyvalent Antisnake Venom Serum

Manufactured by Serum Institute of India.

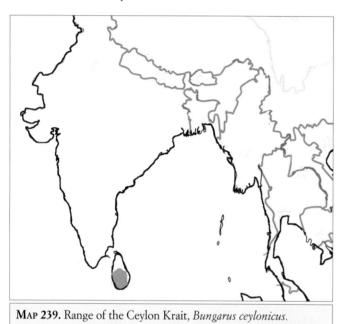

MAP 239. Range of the Ceylon Krait, *Bungarus ceylonicus*.

Black Krait,

Bungarus niger

Description and Identification: A nondescript drab colored snake. Usually uniformly gray-brown to black in color.

Distribution, Habitat, and Biology: Found in several widely dispersed regions from northern India, Nepal, and Bhutan to Bangladesh and parts of Myanmar.

Venom and Bite: Reportedly an inoffensive species that is hesitant to bite. Venom toxicity unknown but likely dangerous.

No specific antivenom is listed by the World Health Organization website, but Clinical Toxinology Resources website (viewed 2012) lists the following: SII Polyvalent Antisnake Venom Serum manufacturered by Serum Institute of India.

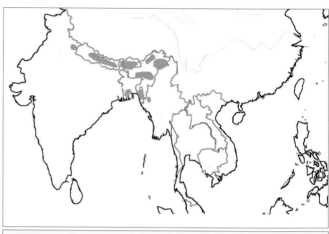

MAP 240. Range of the Black Krait, *Bungarus niger*.

Similar Species: The Lesser Black Krait, *B. lividus* is a smaller, less widely distributed version of the Black Krait that is found on the lower slopes of the Himalayas in western Nepal, northwest India and northern Bangladesh.

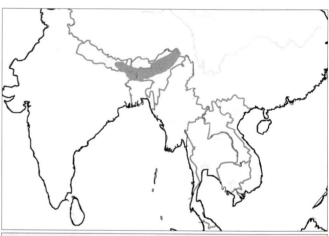

MAP 241. Range of the Lesser Black Krait, *Bungarus lividus*.

Sind Krait,

Bungarus sindanus

Description and Identification: Black with variable amount of white banding. White usually reduced. Edges of ventrals and labials may be pale yellow. A large krait that can reach 6 feet in length.

Distribution, Habitat and Biology: Also occurs in the USCENTCOM region. Range in the USPACOM region is restricted to India.

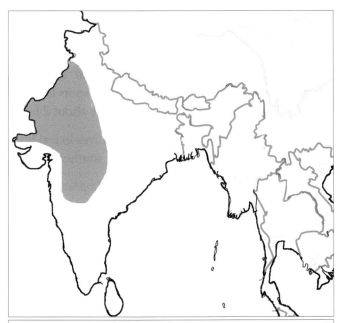

MAP 242. Range of the Sind Krait, *Bungarus sindanus*, in the USPACOM region.

Venom and Bite: Though inoffensive and reluctant to bite, this is a large krait that is quite dangerous. However, there is no specific antivenom listed by the World Health Organization website or the MAVIN Antivenom Index viewed 2012.

Clinical Toxinology Resources website (www.toxinology.com) viewed 2012, lists the following:

> Product: SII Polyvalent Antisnake Venom Serum
> Manufacturer: Serum Institute of India
> Country of Origin: India

Additional Species: The Burmese Krait (*B. magnimaculatus*) of central Myanmar (Burma), is similar to the Common Krait (*B. caeruleus*) and was formerly regarded as a subspecies of that krait.

Slowinski's Krait (*B. slowinskii*) endemic to Vietnam, was named in honor of American herpetologist Joseph Slowinski who was killed by a krait while doing field research in southeast Asia.

Family - Elapidae:

Genera - Calliophis, Sinomicrurus, and Hemibungarus

Oriental Coral Snakes

The most unique feature of this group of southeast Asia endemics is the presence in several species of extremely long venom glands which extend well down onto the snake's body (as much as one-third of their length). In fact, these snakes are also known by the name "Long Glanded Coral Snakes."

The *Calliophis* genus contains a total of 9 species, while *Sinomicrurus* consists of 5 species, and *Hemibungarus* is monospecific.

Like the *Micrurus* coral snakes of the western hemisphere, these snakes are shy and retiring in habits and rarely bite humans. Some species are regarded as virtually harmless, however, both *Calliophis* and *Sinomicrurus* contain species that have caused human deaths. Thus, all oriental coral snakes should be treated as potentially deadly.

Definition: Head small, not distinct from body. Body cylindrical, slender and elongated; tail short.

Eyes small to moderate in size; pupils round.

Head scales: The normal 9 on the crown; rostral broad and round, no canthus. Laterally, nasal in contact with single preocular or separated from it by prefrontal; preocular absent in C. bibroni. Dorsals smooth, in 13-17 nonoblique rows throughout body. Ventrals 190-328; anal plate entire or divided; subcaudals usually paired.

Barred Coral Snake,
Hemibungarus calligaster

Description and Identification: A small coral snake reaching only about 2 feet in length. Dorsal pattern black with narrow white rings, some red on head and tail.

Distribution, Habitat, and Biology: Endemic to the Philippines (except for Mindanao).

Venom and Bite: Little is known. This is a small snake and may not be deadly to man, but that remains unknown. No specific antivenom is produced.

Blue Malaysian Coral Snake,
Calliophis bivirgata

Description and Identification: Distinctive bright red head and tail contrasts sharply with uniformly blue-black dorsal pattern. Light colored lateral line runs down both sides the entire length of the body. Some specimens may also have paired, narrow, light mid-dorsal lines.

Distribution, Habitat, and Biology: Found throughout Malaysia from the Malay Peninsula to Java, including all of Sumatra and Borneo. A shy and secretive snake of leaf litter in tropical forests.

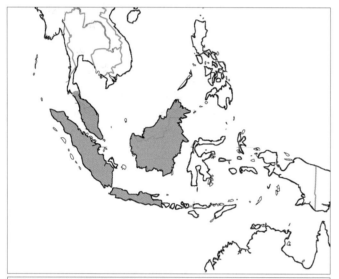

Map 243. Range of the Blue Malaysian Coral Snake, *Calliophis bivirgata.*

Venom and Bite: These secretive snakes are reluctant to bite and pose little threat under most circumstances. However, they may be quite dangerous. Herpetologist Mark O'Shea in his book *Venomous Snakes of the World* (2005) writes about this snake, "A Singapore man died five minutes after being bitten on the toe in the shower." No mention was made of whether the man died from an allergic reaction (anaphylaxis) or if the death resulted from the toxicity of the venom. No specific antivenom is produced. Clinical Toxinology Resources website (2012) and the Munich Antivenom Index (MAVIN) (2012) both list Polyvalent Anti Snake Venom Serum produced by Central Research Institute in India.

Speckled Coral Snake,
Calliophis maculiceps

Description and Identification: Dorsal coloration brown or reddish brown with small black spots laterally. Head and tip of tail black. Maximum size about 2 feet.

Distribution, Habitat, and Biology: Lives in leaf litter on the forest floor throughout much of southeast Asia.

Venom and Bite: Unknown. All *Calliophis* however should be considered as possibly dangerous. No specific antivenom available.

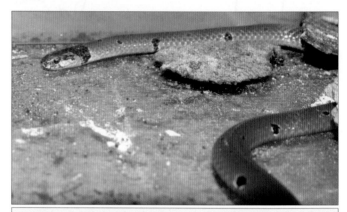

Photo 203. Speckled Coral Snake, *Calliophis maculiceps*

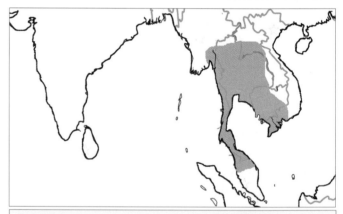

Map 244. Range of the Speckled Coral Snake, *Calliophis maculiceps.*

Indian Coral Snake,
Calliophis melanurus

Description and Identification: Dorsal coloration brown or reddish brown-sometimes with irregular dark spots. A small snake that is less than 20 inches in length.

Distribution, Habitat, and Biology: Found in India and Sri Lanka.

Venom and Bite: Unknown, but too small to be much of a threat.

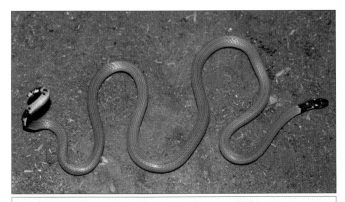

PHOTO 204. Indian Coral Snake, *Calliophis melanurus*

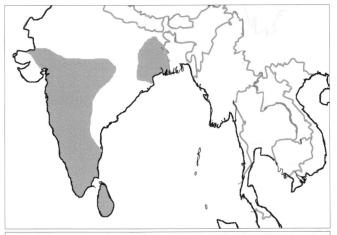

MAP 245. Range of the Indian Coral Snake, *Calliophis melanurus.*

Striped Coral Snake,
Calliophis intestinalis

Description and Identification: Dorsal coloration black, gray, or brown with a vertebral stripe that may be yellow, red, orange, or whitish. Venter often bright red with black bars. Maximum size about 2 feet.

Distribution, Habitat, and Biology: Sympatric with the previous species throughout Malaysia, but also found in the southern Philippines.

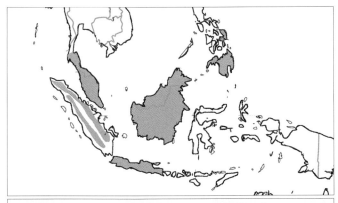

MAP 246. Range of the Striped Coral Snake, *Calliophis intestinalis.*

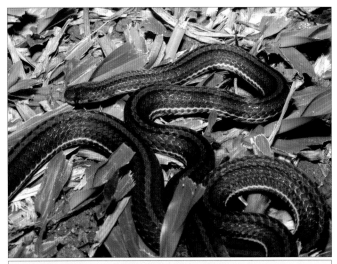

PHOTO 205. Striped Coral Snake, *Calliophis intestinalis*

Additional Species: There are 5 more Calliophis coral snakes endemic to southeast Asia and Indonesia. They are, Bibron's Coral Snake (*C. bibroni*), Beddome's Coral Snake (*C. beddomei*), Slender Coral Snake (*C. gracilis*), Black Coral Snake (*C. nigrescens*), and Blood-bellied Coral Snake (*C. haematoetron*). The range map below shows the respective ranges of these additional species.

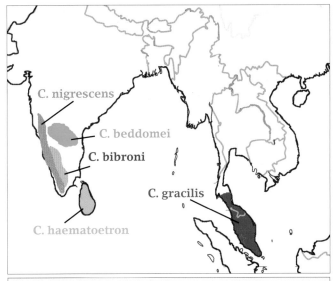

MAP 247. Range of additonal Coral Snake species. *C. bebroni, C. beddomei, C. gracilis, C. nigrescens,* and *C. haematoetron.*

MacClelland's Coral Snake,
Sinomicrurus macclellandi

Description and Identification: A red or reddish-brown snake with a series of narrow, widely spaced black bands across the back. The head is dark with a distinct broad white band behind the eyes. Grows to 30 inches.

Distribution, Habitat, and Biology: *S. macclellandi* is the most widely distributed of the *Sinomicrurus* coral snakes (see range map).

Venom and Bite: Unknown, but a herpetologist from Europe died from a bite by this species. No specific antivenom is available.

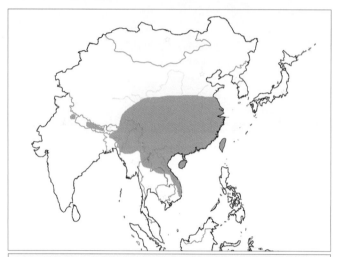

MAP 248. Range of MacClelland's Coral Snake, *Sinomicrurus macclellandi*.

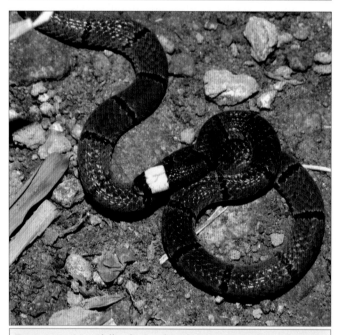

PHOTO 206. MacClelland's Coral Snake, *Sinomicrurus macclellandi*

Additional Species: Three of the four remaining species of *Sinomicrurus* native to Asia are island species. *S. sauteri* (no common name) and *S. hatori* (no common name) are both found on Taiwan. *S. japonicus* (Japanese Coral Snake) is endemic to Okinawa and the Ryukyu Islands. Finally, *S. kelloggi* (Kellog's Coral Snake) occurs in parts of southeastern China, Vietnam, and Laos.

Family - Viperidae

Subfamily - Azemiopinae - Fea Viper

Genus - Azemiops

Fea's Viper

A single species A. feae is known from the mountains of southeast Asia. It is a small species, less than 3 feet in length.

Definition: Head somewhat flattened, distinct from neck; snout broad and short, canthus obtuse. Body cylindrical, moderately slender; tail short.

Eyes moderate in size; pupils vertically elliptical.

Had scales: The usual 9 scutes on the crown; rostral broad, frontal broad. Laterally, eye in contact with supralabial row; nasal separated from preoculars by small squarish loreal.

Body scales: Dorsal smooth, in 17 nonoblique rows at midbody, few (15) posteriorly. Ventral rounded 180-189; subcaudal paired throughout or a few anterior ones single, 42-53.

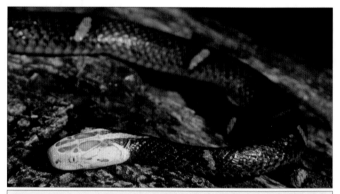

PHOTO 207. Fea's Viper, *Azemiops feae*

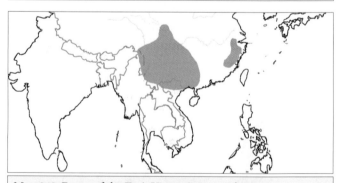

Map.249. Range of the Fea's Viper, *Azemiops feae*.

Venom and Bite: Herpetologist Mark O'Shea writes that the "venom is believed to be a neurotoxin and anticoagulant; mild human bites recorded."

No antivenom is produced.

Family - Viperidae

Subfamily - Viperinae - True Vipers

Genus - Vipera

True Adders

The genus *Vipera* contains a minimum of 20 species and some experts recognize up to 23. Most (18 species) are found in USEUCOM region. These are the "True Adders" of Europe, western Russia, and the Mediterranean region. With the exception of a few species they are restricted to those regions. However, at least one species ranges into the USPACOM region in parts of China and North Korea.

For more information regarding this genus see page 125, Chapter 10 (USEUCOM region).

Sakhalin Viper,
Vipera sakhalinensis

This species is found mostly in southeastern Russia and on Sakhalin Island (Russia). A disjunct population occurs in the USPACOM region along the China-North Korea border. For information on this species see page 125, Chapter 10, USEUCOM region.

Additional Species: *Vipera renardi,* the Steppe Viper ranges into the USPACOM region in a small part of northwest China. For photos and information on this species see Chapter 10, USEUCOM.

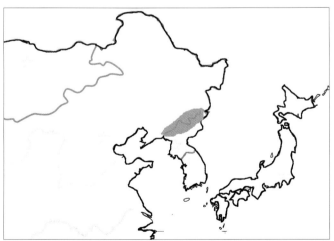

MAP 250. Range of the Sakhalin Viper, *Vipera sakhalinensis*, in the USPACOM region.

Family - Viperidae

Subfamily - Viperinae - True Vipers

Genus- Daboia

Large Middle East and Asian Vipers

The elongated, oval shaped head is distinctive of this genus. The *Daboia* genus contains only 3 species and all are large and dangerous snakes. Two species are found in the USPACOM region. One (*siamensis*) is endemic to this region but the other (*russelli*) is also found in the USCENTCOM region (in eastern Pakistan). A third species (*palestinae*) is endemic to the USCENTCOM region.

Definition: Pupil elliptical. Head distinct from the neck, broad; snout blunt or pointed, dorsum of head covered with small scales.

Body scales: Dorsal scales keeled in 24-33 rows at midbody. Ventrals 162-180; subcaudals paired 35-68; anal scute undivided.

Western Russell's Viper,
Daboia russelli

Description and Identification: Head wide, rather long; no enlarged plates on crown; no loreal pit; scales keeled. These features and the bold distinctive pattern readily distinguish this reptile from most other Asian snakes (except the closely related Eastern Russell's Viper, *D. siamensis*). It may be imitated by the harmless Russell's Sand Boa, however this species has narrow ventrals (less than the width of the belly) and a very short tail.

The color is brown, yellow-brown, or reddish-brown with 3 rows of large oval dark black-ringed spots which may be narrowly edged in white; the spots of the middle row often fuse on the latter half of the body; light V or X shaped mark on top of the head; belly pinkish brown to white with black spots.

These are fairly large vipers that average about 3 to 4 feet but can reach a maximum of 5 feet.

Distribution, Habitat, and Biology: This snake ranges from eastern Pakistan to Bangladesh, including nearly all of India and the island of Sri Lanka. A disjunct population is found on Java. Occurs in lowlands, but avoids permanently marshy areas. Primarily a hill or mountain snake in some areas and has been recorded at 7,000 feet elevation. Mainly nocturnal but active by day in cool weather. Hisses loudly when disturbed and strikes with great force and speed.

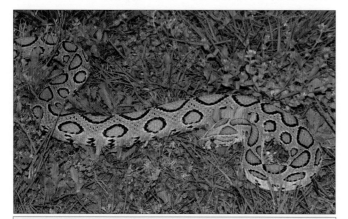

Photo 208. Western Russell's Viper, *Daboia russelli*

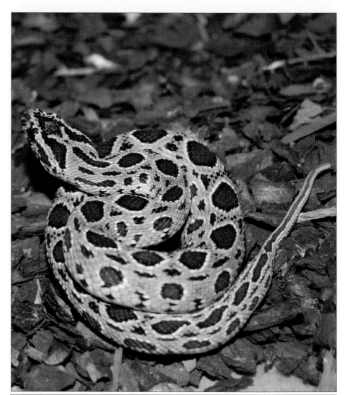

Photo 209. Eastern Russell's Viper, *Daboia siamensis*

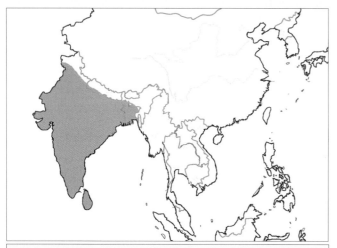

Map 251. Range of the Western Russell's Viper, *Daboia russelli* in the USPACOM region.

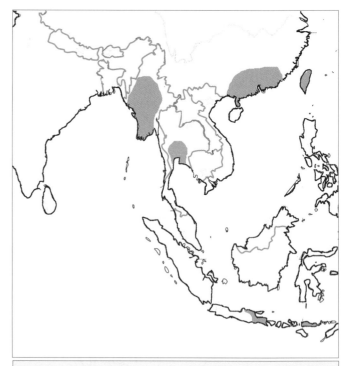

Map 252. Range of the Eastern Russell's Viper, *Daboia siamensis*.

Venom and Bite: These are very common snakes throughout their range and they can occur near human habitations. They are thus responsible for a large number of snakebites within their range with many fatalities. The venom is highly toxic. The book *Old World Vipers* (Phelps 2000) mentions that this snake's venom can vary from one geographical locale to another, and some antivenoms may or may not be effective in treating bites.

For a complete list of antivenoms the reader is referred to the following websites: www.who.int/bloodproducts/ snakeantivenoms (World Health Organization), www. toxinology.com (Clinical Toxicology Resources), and www.toxininfo.org (Munich Antivenom Index/MAVIN)

Similar Species: The nearly identical Eastern Russell's Viper (*D. siamensis*) is another highly dangerous snake that kills many of its victims. The biology of these two *Daboia* species is similar in most respects. This species ranges farther to the east into southeast Asia. See range map 252.

Family - Viperidae

Subfamily - Viperinae - True Vipers

Genus - Echis

Saw-scaled Vipers

In the 1965 edition of *Poisonous Snakes of the World*, 2 species of Saw-scaled Vipers were known. Today some experts recognize up to 12 species. Most are remarkably similar to one another and the exact taxonomic status of this group is still confusing and probably subject to future revision. Only one species is found in the USPA-COM region, (*Echis carinatus*) but it is fairly common within its range and is a significant health problem in the region. Although less than a length of 3 feet, it possesses a highly toxic venom and has been responsible for many deaths. When disturbed these snakes inflate the body and produce a hissing sound by rubbing the saw-edged lateral scales against one another. This same pattern of behavior is shown by the nonvenomous egg-eating snakes *Dasypeltis.*

Definition: Head broad, very distinct from narrow neck; canthus indistinct. Body cylindrical, moderately slender; tail short.

Eyes moderate in size. Pupils vertically elliptical.

Head Scales: A narrow supraocular sometimes present; otherwise crown covered with small scales, which may be smooth or keeled. Rostral and nasals distinct. Laterally, eye separated from labials by 1-4 rows of small scales; nasal in contact with rostral or separated from it by a row of small scales.

Body scales: Dorsals keeled, with apical pits, lateral scales smaller, with serrate keels, in 27-37 oblique rows at midbody. Ventrals rounded, 132-205; subcaudals single, 21-52.

Saw-scaled Viper,

Echis carinatus

Description and Identification: Head short and wide, snout blunt; body moderately stout; scales on top of head small, keeled; scales on side of body strongly oblique, the keels with minute serrations; subcaudals single.

Color pale buff or tan to olive brown, chestnut or reddish; midline row of whitish spots; side with narrow undulating white line; top of head usually shows light trident or arrowhead mark. Belly white to pinkish brown stippled with dark gray.

Average length 15 to 20 inches; maximum about 32 inches; sexes of about equal size.

Distribution, Habitat, and Biology: In the USPA-COM region this snake ranges across most of India and the island of Sri Lanka (Ceylon). Very adaptable, found from almost barren rocky or sandy desert to dry scrub forest and from seacoast to elevations of about 6,000 feet. The Saw-scaled Viper that is endemic to eastern India is the species *sochureki*. While some sources regard *sochureki* as a subspecies of *Echis carinatus*, most local experts within its range consider it to be a separate species (Harold Harlan, personal communication).

Primarily nocturnal. Will bury its body in the sand with only the top of head and eyes exposed. These are high strung snakes that are quick to strike if disturbed.

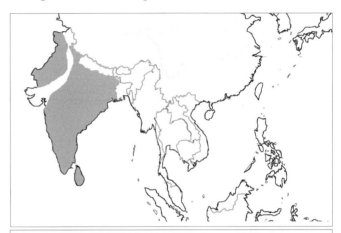

MAP 253. Range of the Saw-scaled Viper in the USPACOM region.

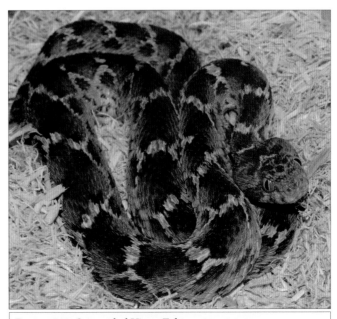

PHOTO 210. Saw-scaled Viper, *Echis carinatus*

Venom and Bite: Although this is a smallish snake, it is highly dangerous and is a significant cause of snakebite death throughout its range. Considered as group and based on the number of people killed, many experts consider the Saw-scaled Vipers to be among the world's deadliest snakes. The venom is strongly haemotoxic and almost entirely inhibits the blood's ability to clot.

List of Antivenoms: from (www.int/bloodproducts/snakeantivenoms/database-2012)

Product: Polyvalent Antisnake Venom

Manufacturer: National Institute of Health

Country of Origin: Pakistan

Product: Polyvalent Snake Antivenom (Asia)

Manufacturer: Biological Limited

Country of Origin: India

Product: Polyvalent Snake Antivenom.

Manufacturer: Razi Vaccine and Serum Research Institute

Country of Origin: Iran

Product: Snake antivenin I.P.

Manufacturer: Haffkine Biopharmaceutical Corporation Ltd.

Country of Origin: India

Family - Viperidae

Subfamily - Crotalinae - Pit Vipers

Genus- Calloselasma

Malayan Pit Viper

The genus Calloselasma contains a single species, the Malayan Pit Viper (*Calloselasma rhodostoma*). It is a terrestrial species that is highly cryptic and responsible for many snakebites.

Definition: Head broad, flattened , very distinct from neck; a sharply distinguished canthus. Body cylindrical or depressed, tapered, moderately stout to stout; tail short to moderately long.

Eyes moderate in size, pupils vertically elliptical.

Head scales: 9 on the crown. Loreal pit present.

Body scales: Dorsals smooth with apical pits.

Dorsal scale rows at midbody 19-25.

Malayan Pit Viper,
Calloselasma rhodostoma

Description and Identification: Head triangular, snout pointed, facial pit present. The only Asian pit viper with large scales on the crown and smooth body scales.

Middle of back reddish or purplish brown, sides pale with dark speckling; series of dark brown crossbands, narrow in midline, wider on sides, edged with white or buff; belly pinkish white mottled with brown; top of head dark brown, sides light pinkish brown, the colors separated by a white stripe that passes just above the eye.

Average length 23-32 inches. Maximum 3.5 feet.

Distribution, Habitat, and Biology: Thailand, northern Malaysia, Cambodia, Laos, Vietnam, Java, Sumatra. Apparently requires climate with well-marked wet and dry seasons. Frequents forests generally at low elevations; common on rubber plantations. In a departure from the reproductive habits of most pit vipers, the Malayan Pit Viper is an egg-layer.

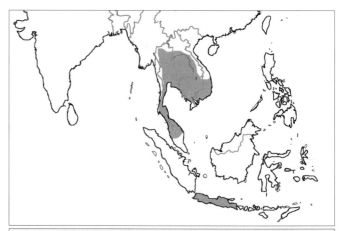

MAP 254. Range of the Malayan Pit Viper, *Calloselasma rhodostoma.*

Venom and Bite: A bad tempered snake, quick to strike if disturbed. In northern Malaysia it causes approximately 700 snakebites annually with a death rate of about 2 percent. Weeders and tappers on rubber estates are most frequently bitten. This snake is remarkably sedentary and has often been found at the site of an accident after several hours.

The venom contains enzymes that impact on the blood's clotting ability, These enzymes have been used for medical purposes.

A number of specific antivenoms have been produced in several countries where this species is found. Listed next are two of these antivenoms.

Product: Malayan Pit Viper Antivenom

Manufacturer: Queen Saovabha Memorial Institute

Country of Origin: Thailand

Product: Malayan Pit Viper Antivenom

Manufacturer: Venom Research Unit, Univ. of Medicine and Pharmacy

Country of Origin: Vietnam

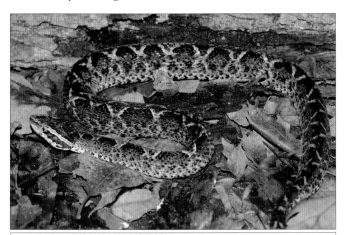

PHOTO 211. Malayan Pit Viper, *Calloselasma rhodostoma*

Family - Viperidae

Subfamily - Crotalinae - Pit Vipers

Genus- Hypnale

Hump-nosed Pit Vipers

Description and Identification: This genus is comprised of 3 species of small, terrestrial pit vipers that are very reminiscent of the South American Hog-nosed Pit Vipers (*Porthidium*). This is only one example of the wide range of similarities that exist in many species of Asian pit vipers and new world pit vipers which provides a classic example of "convergent evolution."

The slightly upturned snout is characteristic in this genus. All are cryptically patterned with a "leaf litter brown" dorsal color interrupted with darker brown triangular blotches along the vertebral line. Blotches may be alternate or slightly offset. The top of the face from the nose to the back of the jaw usually shows a lighter color sometimes in the form of a broad, light line.

Definition: Head broad and flattened, snout somewhat pointed and slightly upturned. Head disinct from neck. Loreal pit present.

Eyes moderate in size, pupils vertically elliptical.

Dorsals weakly keeled in 17-19 rows.

Hump-nosed Pit Viper,
Hypnale hypnale

Description and Identification: Of typical viperine build with stout body and wide head with facial pit; snout pointed and turned up; large frontal and parietal shields but shields of snout small and irregular.

Ground color reddish, tan or gray-brown with a series of small angular, paired, dark blotches on each side of the vertebra. Light postocular stripe sometimes present.

Average length 112-18 inches.

Distribution, Habitat, and Biology: Restricted to a small region on southern India and all of Sri Lanka. These snakes are terrestrial in habits and live among leaf litter where they are well camouflaged.

Venom and Bite: Despite their small size, fatalities have been recorded from bites by members of this genus. They are apparently quite common within their range and accidents are frequent.

No specific antivenom is produced. Clinical Toxinology Resources (viewed 2012) lists two antivenoms for this species. SII Polyvalent Antisnake Venom Serum and SII Bivalent Antisnake Venom Serum. Both produced by Serum Institute of India Ltd.

Similar Species: There are at least two other species of Hump-nosed Vipers and both are endemic to Sri Lanka where they occur in very small populations. Those species are *Hypnale nepa* (Sri Lankan Hump-nosed Viper) and *Hypnale walli* (Wall's Hump-nosed Viper).

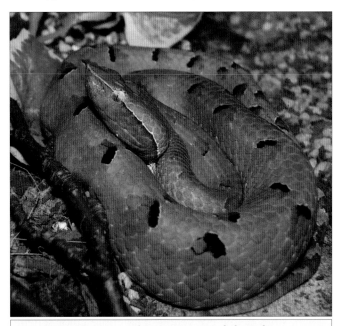

PHOTO 212. Hump-nosed Pit Viper, *Hypnale hypnale*

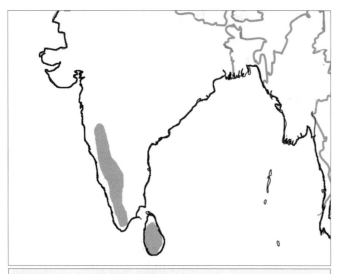

MAP 255. Range of the Hump-nosed Pit Viper, *Hypnale hypnale.*

Family - Viperidae

Subfamily - Crotalinae - Pit Vipers

Genus - Deinagkistrodon

Sharp-nosed Pit Viper

This genus contains a single species which is known by a variety of common names including the Sharp-nosed Pit Viper, Chinese Copperhead, and Hundred Pace Snake. The latter name is derived from the belief that bitten victims will die after one hundred paces.

Definition: Head broad, flattened, very distinct from neck; a sharply distinguished canthus, snout sharply pointed and strongly upturned on the tip. Body stout, tail short. Loreal pit present.

Eyes moderate in size, pupils vertically elliptical.

Body scales: Dorsals tubercularly keeled, in 21-23 rows.

Sharp-nosed Pit Viper,
Deinagkistrodon acutus

Description and Identification: A pit viper with the snout ending in an upturned pointed appendage and large shields on the crown.

Ground color gray or brown with dark brown crossbands narrow at the center of the back, wide on the sides, wide parts often tinged with dull orange; belly cream with large black spots that extend onto the sides; top of head dark brown, sides below eye yellow. The entire color scheme suggests that of the United States Copperhead.

Average length 35-45 inches; maximum about 5 feet.

Distribution, Habitat, and Biology: Southern China, northern Vietnam, Hainan, Taiwan. Found mostly in rocky, wooded hilly country.

Feeds on a variety of small vertebrate prey. Reproduction is by egg-laying. This snake's resemblance to the North American Copperhead is remarkable and in the 1965 edition of *Poisonous Snakes of the World*, this snake was placed in the same genus (*Agkistrodon*).

Venom and Bite: *D. acutus* venom is almost entirely haemotoxic and contains haemorraghic enzymes. Extracts of these venom components have been used medicinally for treating blood disorders.

Large individuals of this snake are potentially deadly to humans. Two specific antivenoms are produced for this snake, both in China.

> Product: Agkistrodon Acutus Antivenom
> Manufacturer: Shanghai Institute Biological Technology Co. Ltd.
> Product: Monvalent Antivenom Snorkel Viper
> Manufacturer: Natonal Institute of Preventative Medicine

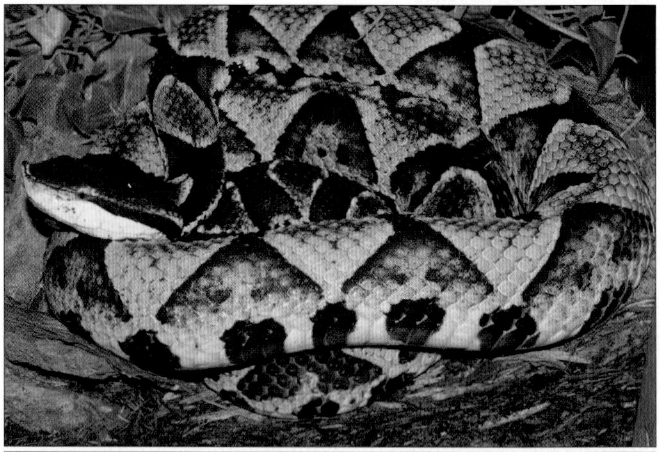

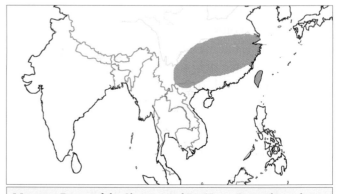

PHOTO 213. Sharp-nosed Pit Viper, *Deinagkistrodon acutus*

MAP 256. Range of the Sharp-nosed Pit Viper, *Deinagkistrodon acutus.*

Family - Viperidae

Subfamily - Crotalinae - Pit Vipers

Genus - Gloydius

Asian Moccasins

At least 12 species are recognized. These pit vipers are primarily Asian in origin and all but one can be found in the USPACOM region. One species can be found in the USEUCOM and at least one (maybe two) in the US-CENTCOM region.

These snakes are usually called "Asian Moccasins" because they were once included in the genus *Agkistrodon* with the North American Copperheads and Cottonmouths. They are also known by the name "Mamushi," which is the Japanese name for the *Gloydius* species that is native to Japan (*G. blomhoffi*).

Definition: Head broad, flattened, very distinct from narrow neck; a sharply distinguished canthus.

Eyes moderate in size, pupils vertically elliptical.

Head scales: 9 large plates on the crown.

Body scales: Dorsal scales keeled in 20-23 rows at midbody.

The exact taxonomic status of this genus is still somewhat confusing, and the precise ranges of a number of species is not fully understood. The species list used here is created from the Reptile Database (www.reptile-database.org) viewed 2012. Other sources may show a different species list. These are a diverse, wide-ranging group and they are the most northerly distributed pit vipers in the old world.

One species *G. himalayanus* (Himalayan Pit Viper) holds the distinction of being the world's highest ranging snake, having been found at altitudes above 14,000 feet (from *Venomous Snakes of the World* by Mark O'Shea, 2005).

For additional photos of members of this genus see Chapter 11 (USCENTCOM) and Chapter 10 (USEUCOM).

Mamushi,

Gloydius blomhoffii (Japanese)
Gloydius brevicaudus (Short-tailed)
Gloydius ussuriensis (Ussurian)

These three snakes are very similar in appearance and biology and they are treated here in a single account.

Description and Identification: Dorsal coloration is brown, reddish, or grayish with a series of paired dark blotches on each side of the vertebra. These blotches usually have a light center. The head typically viperine, flat on top, pronounced canthus, loreal pit, and a dark postocular stripe bordered above by a narrower light stripe. The upper labials are also a lighter color, usually matching the dorsal color present between the dark blotches. There are 23 scale rows at midbody.

Distribution, Habitat, and Biology: These 3 species have ranges that are more or less contiguous (except that *A. blomhoffii* is found on the islands of Japan). All 3 species were once regarded as one species.

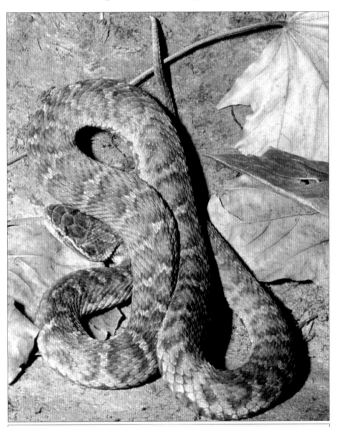

PHOTO 214. Ussurian Mamushi, *Gloydius ussuriensis*

Venom and Bite: The venoms of several *Gloydius* species have been shown to have some neurotoxic properties, and one study revealed that some are many times more potent in mice than that of *Deinagkistrodon acutus*, the Sharp-nosed Viper (Chen et.al. 1992). All three of the above species have caused deaths.

Antivenom listed by World Health Organization for *G. blomhoffii* and *G. brevicaudus*.

Product: Mamushi Antivenom "Kaketsuken"

Manufacturer: The Chemo-SAero-Therapeutic Research Institute (Kaketsuken)

Country of Origin: Japan

Antivenom listed by World Health Organization for *G. brevicaudus* and *G. ussuriensis*.

Product: Agkistrodon (Salmusa) Antivenom

Manufacturer: Korea Vaccine Co., Ltd.

Country of Origin: Republic of Korea

Additional Species: There are at least 8 additonal species of Gloydius found in the USPACOM region. Those species are listed below.

Rock Mamushi - *G. saxatalis*

Central Asian Pit Viper - *G. intermedius*

Likiang Pit Viper - *G. monticola*

Tibetan Pit Viper - *G. strauchi*

Himalayan Pit Viper - *G. himalayanus*

Snake Island Mamushi - *G. sheadoensis*

G. lijianlii

Tsushima Mamushi - *G. tsushimaensis*

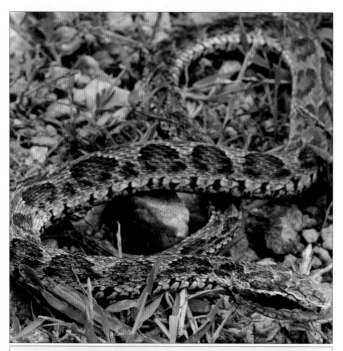

PHOTO 215. Short-tailed Mamushi, *Gloydius brevicaudus*

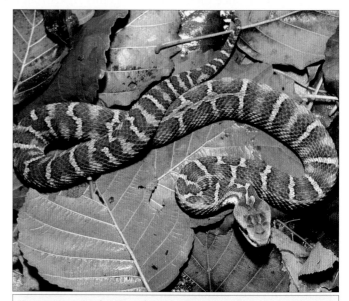

PHOTO 216. Rock Mamushi, *Gloydius saxatilis*

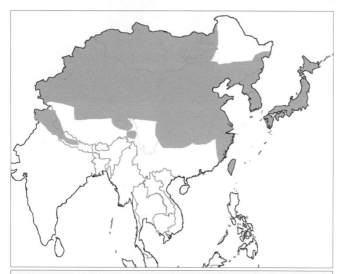

MAP 257. Presumed range of the *Gloydius* genus in the USPACOM region.

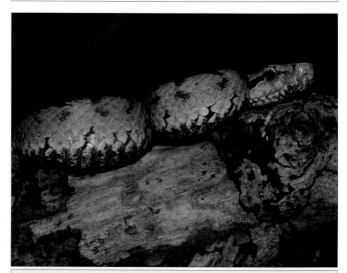

PHOTO 217. Snake Island Mamushi, *Gloydius sheadoensis*

Family - Viperidae

Subfamily - Crotalinae - Pit Vipers

Genus - Ovophis

Asian Mountain Vipers

This is another wide-ranging genus that has undergone significant revisions since the first publication of *Poisonous Snakes of the World* in 1965 when they were regarded as members of the *Trimeresurus* genus. The arrangement of species and their respective distribution is probably still subject to further investigation. There are 4 species listed in the Reptile Database (viewed 2012), but recent studies suggest a significant change in the taxonomy and distribution of members of this genus, (Malhotra et al. 2011). There are 5 species pictured here. All are endemic to Asia.

Definition: The head is large, chunky and flat on top. Distinct from the neck; snout short. The body is quite stout and the tail is short.

Eyes small to moderate in size, pupil elliptical.

Body scales: Dorsal scales weakly keeled along the vertebra, smooth laterally, in 23-25 rows.

Mountain Pit Vipers,
Ovophis species

The 4 species being treated here in a single account are those listed in the Reptile Database (viewed 2012). This arrangement of species may not reflect the true picture of the taxonomy and distribution of species within this genus (see Malhotra et. al 2011.)

Description and Identification: One of the more widespread species is the Chinese Mountain Pit Viper (*O. monticola*). This species is variable in color and may be brownish, grayish, or reddish with a series of dark vertebral blotches that sometimes form bands across the back. The Hemihabu (*O. okinavensis*) tends to be brown with blotches indistinct. The Tonkin Mountain Pit Viper (*O. tonkinensis*) is usually vividly marked with distinct dark blotches on a yellowish, grayish, or reddish ground color. Meanwhile the Tibetan Mountain Pit Viper (*O. zayuensis*) is inclined to exhibit a more faded pattern on a reddish ground color.

Distribution, Habitat, and Biology: They are terrestrial and are egg layers, though the young snakes sometimes hatch very soon after eggs are deposited.

Despite their name they can sometimes be found in lowlands as well as mountains and plateaus. Primarily forest snakes but also found in agricultural areas. *O. monticola*, (Chinese Mountain Pit Viper) is the most widespread and is found throughout much of China and southeast Asia. *O. okinavensis* (Hemihabu) is an island species, while *O. zayuensis*, (Tibetan Mountain Pit Viper) inhabits a small area of southeastern Tibet.

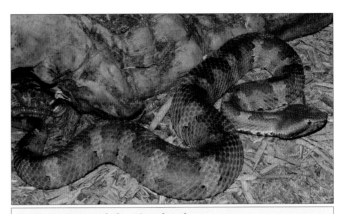

PHOTO 218. Hemihabu, *Ovophis okinavensis*

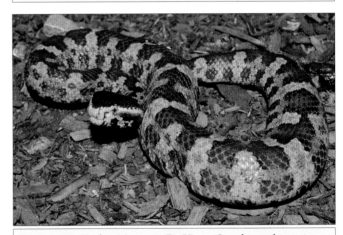

PHOTO 219. Tonkin Mountain Pit Viper, *Ovophis tonkinensis*

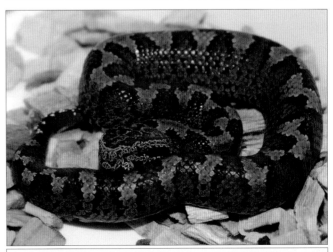

PHOTO 220. Oriental Mountain Pit Viper, *Ovophis orientalis*

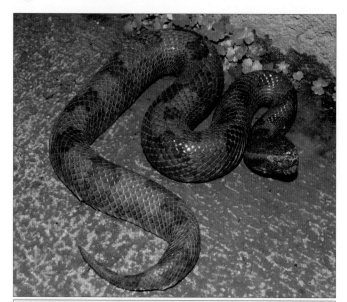

PHOTO 221. Indo-Malayan Mountain Pit Viper, *Ovophis convictus*

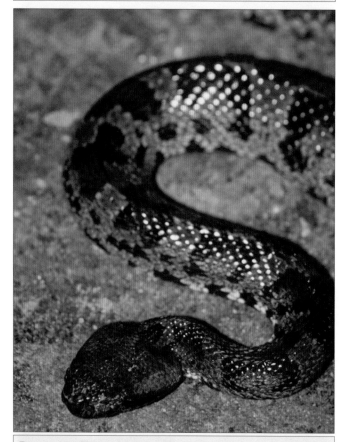

PHOTO 222. Taiwan Mountain Pit Viper, *Ovophis makazayazaya*

Venom and Bite: Deaths have been recorded from the bite of *O. monticola,* and all species are probably capable of killing. No specific antivenoms are available for this genus.

Clinical Toxinology Resources lists three antivenoms for *Ovophis monticola.*

Product: Polyvalent Antisnake Venom Serum

Manufacturer: Central Research Institute

Country of origin: India

Product: Green Pitviper Antivenom

Manufacturer: Thai Red Cross Society

Country of origin: Thailand

Product: Bivalent Antivenom Pit Viper, Trimeresurus Antivenom

Manufacturer: National Institute of Preventative Medicine

Country of origin: Taiwan

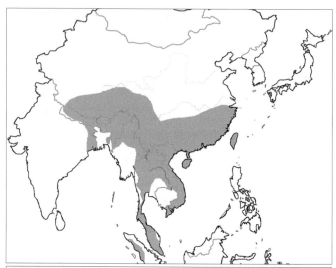

MAP 258. Combined range of the Asian Mountain Pit Vipers, *Ovophis* species.

Family - Viperidae

Subfamily - Crotalinae - Pit Vipers

Genus - Garthius

Mount Kinabalu Pit Viper

There is little information regarding this rare genus. There is only one species. It is a large headed, heavy bodied pit viper that can reach at least 2 feet in length. This genus superficially resembles the previous genus (*Ovophis*) and it was once regarded as belonging to that genus. Some still suggest that the two are synonymous.

Mount Kinabalu Pit Viper,
Garthius chaseni

Description and Identification: Coloration is an alternating series of dark brown and light brown bands across the body.

Distribution, Habitat, and Biology: Known only from the vicinity of Mount Kinabalu on the northern end of the island of Borneo. Only a handful of specimens have been examined.

Venom and Bite: Nothing known. No antivenom.

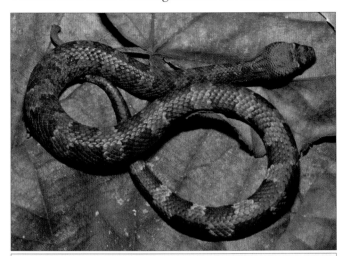

Photo 223. Mount Kinabalu Pit Viper, *Garthius chaseni*

Family - Viperidae

Subfamily - Crotalinae - Pit Vipers

Genus - Protobothrops

Habu Pit Vipers

An Asian pit viper genus that in the 1965 edition of *Poisonous Snakes of the World* was considered to be a part of the *Trimeresurus* genus. These snakes are endemic to the USPACOM (Part 1) region. They are long snakes (some exceed 7 feet) but slim bodied. All are mainly terrestrial.

Defintion: Triangular shaped head very distinct from narrow neck. Snout pointed. Body slender, tail long.

Head elongate with top of head covered with small scales. Eyes moderate in size. Pupils vertically elliptical.

Dorsals keeled in 19-39 rows.

Chinese Habu,
Protobothrops mucrosquamatus

Description and Identification: A long, slim bodied pit viper that can grow to 7.5 feet. The head is distinctly triangular and very distinct from the narrow neck. The ground color is usually some shade of brown or reddish brown with darker brown or charcoal dorsal blotches.

The top of the head is unmarked and matches the ground color. A thin, dark postocular strip is evident.

Distribution, Habitat, and Biology: The most wide-ranging member of its genus, found in most of southern China and the islands of Taiwan and Hainan. Also found in portions of Vietnam, Laos, and Myanmar.

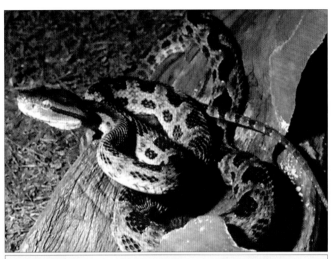

Photo 224. Chinese Habu, *Protobothrops mucrosquamatus*

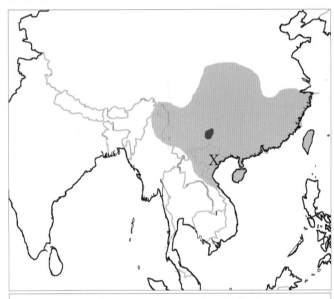

Map 259. Range of the Chinese Habu, *Protobothrops mucrosquamatus*, the Trungkhan Pit Viper, *P. trungkhanensis* (X), and the Mao-lan Habu, *P. maolanensis* (red).

Venom and Bite: The Chinese Habu is a dangerous species that has caused deaths. Several antivenoms are listed by the Clinical Toxinology Resources.

Product: Polyvalent Anti Snake Venom Serum
Manufacturer: Central Research Institute
Country of Origin: India
Product: SII Polyvalent Antisnake Venom Serum
Manufacturer: Serum Institute of India
Country of Origin: India

A single antivenom is listed by the World Health Organization.

Product: Antivenom Tr. mucrosquamatus/stegnegeri

Manufacturer: National Institute of Preventative Medicine

Country of Origin: China

Similar Species: Two newly described species, the Mao-lan Pit Viper (*P. maolanensis*) and the Trungkhanh Pit Viper (*P. trungkhanhensis*) are both smaller species and both have very limited ranges (see map 259). Meanwhile, the Elegant Pit Viper, *Protobothrops elegans,* is endemic to Japan's Ryuku Islands.

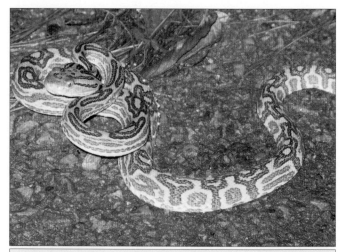

PHOTO 226. Okinawa Habu, *Protobothrops flavoviridis*

Distribution, Habitat, and Biology: Found only on Japan's Ryuku Islands. Limited to the larger islands, including Okinawa. Here it occupies nearly all habitats, including at times human dwellings. Habu wine is made by placing the body of this species into a jar of distilled spirits.

Venom and Bite: This species is famous for having been a very important health hazard until recent times. Fifty years ago it had the distinction of being the source of the highest snakebite incidence per capita of any other venomous snake in the world. Today, eradication programs on the islands it inhabits and effective antivenom therapy have greatly reduced the number of fatalities.

These are large snakes with a long striking range and they may bite at the slightest provocation. Thankfully an effective specific antivenom (Habu Antivenom) by the Chemo-Sero-Therapeutic Research Institute in Japan, has greatly reduced the danger posed by this species.

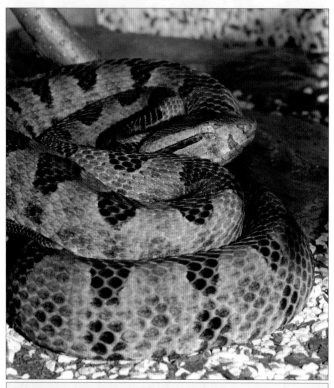

PHOTO 225. Elegant Pit Viper, *Protobothrops elegans*

Okinawa Habu,
Protobothrops flavoviridis

Description and Identification: The specific name, *flavoviridis* literally means yellow-green. In color the Okinawa Habu is pale yellow and olive with markings of darker olive or brown on the dorsal surface. The sides of the face are pale olive and the labial scales yellowish. The top of the head is strongly marked with irregular dark lines and there is a pronounced, dark postocular stripe. Though rather slender bodied, these are large snakes that can reach a length approaching 8 feet, the longest of any pit viper in the USPACOM region. Average size is about 4 to 5 feet.

Tokara Habu,
Protobothrops tokarensis

Description and Identification: Ground color varies from very pale brown to dark chocolate. Dorsal blotches are usually small and sometimes noticeably faded. Can reach a maximum length of about 5 feet.

Distribution, Habitat, and Biology: Limited to two small islands in northern end of the Ryuku Island chain. Mainly terrestrial but will often ascend into bushes and trees. Occupies most any habitat on the islands, including close proximity to human habitations.

Venom and Bite: Little is known about the venom or the bite, and no specific antivenom is produced. Presumably similar to the Okinawa Habu.

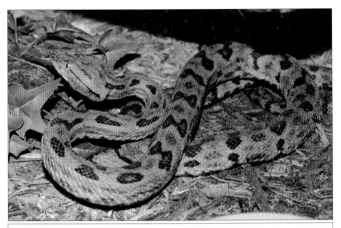

Photo 227. Tokara Habu, *Protobothrops tokarensis*

Red-spotted Pit Viper,
Protobothrops jerdonii

Description and Identification: Despite the name, not all Red-spotted Pit Vipers have red spots.

These are variable snakes and several subspecies are recognized. The ground color may be yellow or greenish yellow and there are a series of dorsal blotches that can be black, red edged in black, brownish edged in white, or olive brown. The spaces between the blotches and the lateral surfaces are heavily diffused with dark & light speckling. There is a dark inverted V-shaped marking on the top of head (begins at snout and forms a broad dark stripe down each side of the top of head). Grows to just over 3 feet in length.

Distribution, Habitat, and Biology: From Nepal to northern Vietnam including a large swath of southern China. More arboreal and less nocturnal than other members of its genus.

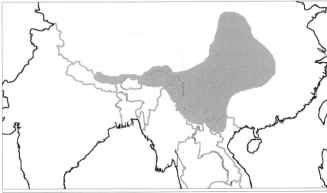

Map 260. Range of the Red-spotted Pit Viper, *Protobothrops jerdonii*.

Venom and Bite: Although there are no known fatalities from its bite, little is known about the venom potency. Potential for inflicting a lethal bite cannot be ruled out.

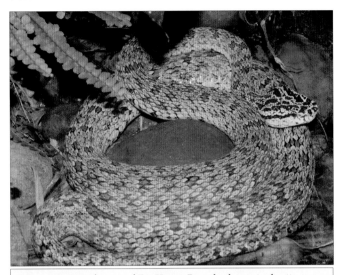

Photo 228. Red-spotted Pit Viper, *Protobothrops jerdonii*

Horned Pit Viper,
Protobothrops cornutus

Description and Identification: Among the smallest of the *Protobothrops*, these snakes are fully grown at about 18-20 inches. The scales above the eye are elongate and raised into a horn-like structure. The body is moderately slender. Color is brownish with a series of darker brown dorsal blotches.

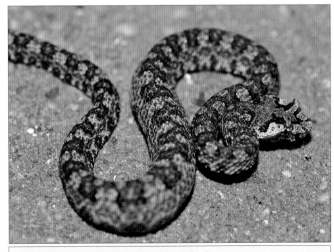

Photo 229. Horned Pit Viper, *Protobothrops cornutus*

Distribution, Habitat, and Biology: A woodland species that associates with rocky outcroppings. Apparently terrestrial.

Venom and Bite: Nothing is known about the venom or effects of its bite. There is no specific antivenom.

Similar Species: The Three-horned Scaled Pit Viper (*P. sieversorum*) is similar to the Horned Pit Viper. This species was until recently relegated to a monotypic genus (*Triceratolepidophis*).

Author's Note: Though both species are found in locales in Vietnam, they occur in disjunct and isolated populations and the exact areas of their range is poorly known.

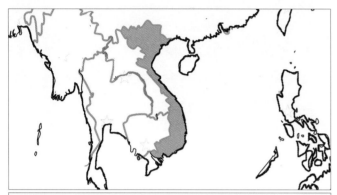

MAP 261. Presumed range of the Horned Pit Viper, *Protobothrops cornutus* and the Three-horned Scaled Pit Viper, *Protobothrops sieversorum*.

Mangshan Pit Viper,
Protobothrops mangshanensis

Description and Identification: Intricately marked with a highly cryptic lichen-like pattern of greens and browns. Large and heavy-bodied, these snakes can reach a maximum of at least 6.5 feet.

Distribution, Habitat, and Biology: Known only from the Mount Mang region of China. Some experts consider this snake to be the only member of the genus *Zhaoermia.*

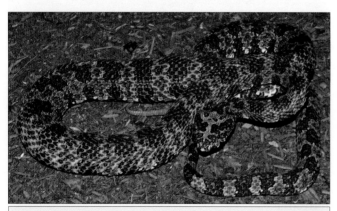

PHOTO 230. Mangshan Pit Viper, *Protobothrops mangshanensis*

Venom and Bite: Little known. No specific antivenom available.

Additional Species: Along with the aforementioned species, there are 2 other members of this genus. Kaulback's Lance-headed Pit Viper *P. kaulbacki*) is found in northern Myanmar and a small area of southeast Tibet and barely ranges into southern China along the Tibet, Myanmar border. The Szechwan Pit Viper (*P. xiangchengensis)* occupies a rather small range within the Sichuan Province of China.

Family - Viperidae

Subfamily - Crotalinae - Pit Vipers

Genus - Trimeresurus

Arboreal Asian Pit Vipers

With 48 species currently recognized this is the most diverse pit viper genus in the world. They are mostly arboreal and all are endemic to the USPACOM region.

Definition: Head large and very distinct from the neck; canthus sharp. Body slender to moderately stout; *tail prehensile.*

Eyes moderate to large; pupils vertically elliptical.

Head scales: Top of head covered with numerous small scales.

Body scales: Dorsals keeled; in 19-25 rows at midbody.

When the original edition of *Poisonous Snakes of the World, A Manual for Use by U.S. Amphibious Forces* was first published back in 1965, nearly all of the pit vipers in Asia that were not placed in the *Agkistrodon* genus were included in the genus *Trimeresurus.* In more recent times many new genera have been named along with scores of new species.

This genus has always been problematical for herpetologists and still presents some real challenges in regards to proper identification, and some experts have divided *Trimeresurus* into several additional genera. Here the author has followed The Reptile Database, www.reptile-database.org (viewed 2012), which does not recognize the following additional genera that may be in use by others: *Cryptelytrops, Sinovipera, Popeia, Peltopelor, Himalayophis,* and *Parias.*

Author's Note: The decision to follow the Reptile Database in regards to the classification of the *Trimeresurus* genus is in no way an individual statement of opinion concerning the correct taxonomy of this group of Asian pit vipers. Such presumption is well beyond the expertise of this author. Rather, I have chosen to use the Reptile Database because that source is widely used by the Armed Forces Pest Management Board in constructing their website "Living Hazards Database." As this book is primarily a manual for U.S. Military forces, I felt it prudent to defer to the same source used by the U.S. military (see the second page of this book's Introduction on page viii). I have deviated from the Reptile Database in regards to one small group of the "Trimeresurus complex," and that is in regards to the newly recognized genus of *Viridovipera*. Again, this designation represents an attempt to maintain congruency with the nomenclature used by the Armed Forces Pest Management Board's Living Hazards Database.

New species of *Trimeresurus* are being described regularly, and some are being described as members of the new genera mentioned earlier, that is, *Cryptelytrops* etc., (as in Malhotra et al. Zootaxa 2011). There will no doubt be continued debate regarding the taxonomy of this genus well into the future. The body of knowledge regarding these snakes is far from complete, and further taxonomic changes within this genus and descriptions of new species are likely.

In the species accounts which follow, two genus names will frequently appear. One will be the name *Trimeresurus*. The other will be the name (in parentheses) of the newer genus used by many experts. Example: Pope's Pit Viper, *Trimeresurus (Popeia) popeiorum.*

In regards to their potential for danger to humans, several species of Trimeresurus are known to have killed. But as a group they are less dangerous than many other venomous snakes within their range. The venom potency of individual species in not well understood. Many species within this genus are commonly referred to as "Bamboo Vipers."

Green Tree "Bamboo" Pit Vipers

Author's Note: This grouping is based on similar morphological features (i.e., color), rather than on phylogeny. Included in this group are members of the genus *Viridovipera*, which were until recently regarded as members of the *Trimeresurus* genus.

Description and Identification: Among the *Trimeresurus,* the species that pose the biggest identification issues are those that exhibit a uniformly green color. There are as many as 20 species of Green Tree Pit Vipers, sometimes referred to as "Bamboo Vipers" that are mostly green and very closely resemble one another. A quick glance at the series of photographs which follow will provide ample evidence of the confusing similarities of these species.

Most of these snakes are separated from one another by such subtle morphological features as scalation, hemipene structure, shape of the head, relative size of the eye, iris color, etc.

Further complicating the identification challenge is the fact that many exhibit some degree of sexual dimorphism as well as ontogenic (age-related) color changes. Males of many species may (or may not), have a ventro-lateral series of spots or a ventro-lateral lines that are white bordered or red. The presence and color of the lines or spots may relate to sex or age. Adult females are often uniformly green and frustratingly similar in appearance.

As if all this weren't confusing enough, there are some normally green species that can sometimes occur in a color phase that is uniformly yellow!

Thus, from a practical standpoint an in-depth discussion of the morphological characters which define each species would be exasperatingly detailed for a volume such as this one, and better left to authors with greater expertise in dealing with this genus. These snakes average about 2 feet in length. Large adults can reach 3 feet, a few can reach 4.

Distribution, Habitat, and Biology: As far as the biology of these snakes is concerned, once again all are very much alike. They are arboreal snakes that inhabit forested regions. They tend to be nocturnal in habits and some prowl the forest floor at night, retreating to the bushes and trees by day.

Foods listed include birds, rodents, lizards, and tree frogs.

All are endemic to southern Asia, Malaysia, and the islands of Indonesia (including the Philippines).

White-lipped Bamboo Pit Viper,

Trimeresurus (Cryptelytrops) albolabris

Venom and Bite: Symptoms are usually relatively mild but a few deaths have been recorded.

Antivenoms listed by www.who.int/bloodproducts/antivenoms-viewed 2012:

Product: Green Pit Viper Antivenom

Manufacturer: Queen Saovabhava Memorial Inst.

Country of Origin: Thailand

Product: SAV-Tri

Manufacturer: Institute of Vaccines and Biological Substances

Country of Origin: Vietnam

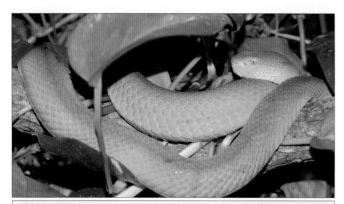

Photo 231. White-lipped Pit Viper, *Trimeresurus (Cryptelytrops) albolabris*

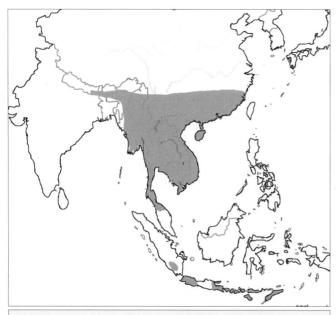

Map 262. Range of the White-lipped Pit Viper, *Trimeresurus (Cryptelytrops) albolabris*.

Red-tailed Bamboo Pit Viper,

Trimeresurus (Cryptelytrops) erythrurus

Venom and Bite: Little known. Antivenom listed are by the Serum Instituet of India include, SII Bivalent Anti Snake Venom Serum and SII Polyvalent Anti Snake Venom Serum.

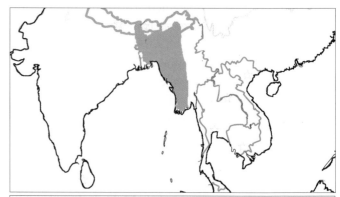

Map 263. Range of the Red-tailed Bamboo Viper, *Trimeresurus (Cryptelytrops) erythrurus*.

White-lipped Island Bamboo Pit Viper,

Trimeresurus (Cryptelytrops) insularis

Venom and Bite: Little known. Probably not highly dangerous but potential for lethal bite cannot be ruled out.

World Health Organization antivenom list:

Product: Green Pit Viper Antivenom

Manufacturer: Queen Saovabhava Memorial Inst.

Country of Origin: Thailand

Product: Haemato-polyvalent Antivenom

Manufacturer: Queen Saovabhava Memorial Inst.

Country of Origin: Thailand

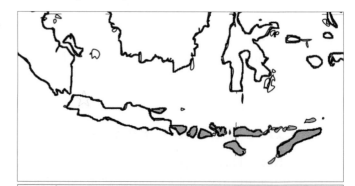

Map 264. Range of the White-lipped Island Pit Viper, *Trimeresurus (Cryptelytrops) insularis*.

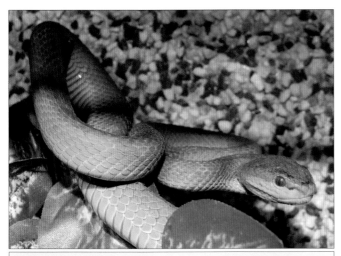

Photo 232. White-lipped Island Pit Viper, *Trimeresurus (Cryptelytrops) insularis*

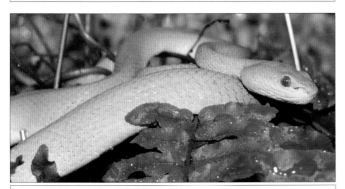

Photo 233. White-lipped Island Pit Viper, yellow morph, *Trimeresurus (Cryptelytrops) insularis*

Kramer's Bamboo Pit Viper,

Trimeresurus (Cryptelytrops) macrops

Venom and Bite: Unknown. Possibly capable of killing. Antivenom listed by www.toxinology.com-viewed 2012.

   Product: Green Pit Viper Antivenom
   Manufacturer: Queen Saovabhava Memorial Inst.
   Country of Origin: Thailand

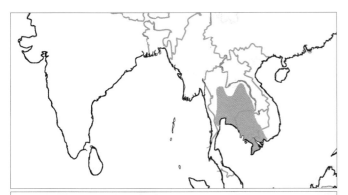

Map 265. Range of the Kramer's Pit Viper, *Trimeresurus (Cryptelytrops) macrop*s.

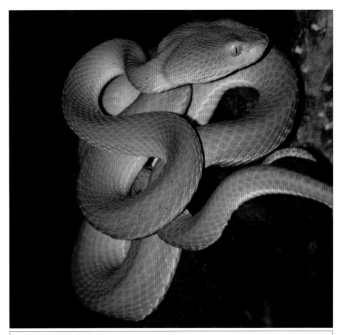

Photo 234. Kramer's Pit Viper, *Trimeresurus (Cryptelytrops) macrops*

Cardamom Mountains Bamboo Pit Viper,

Trimeresurus (Cryptelytrops) cardamomensis

This new species was described as recently as 2011 (Malhotra, et al. Zootaxa). It was previously confused with the Kramer's Pit Viper, *T. macrops* (see preceding species). This snake occupies a small range in southeastern Thailand and southwest Cambodia. Its name is derived from the Cardamom Mountains.

Venom and Bite: Unknown. Presumably similar to the Kramer's Pit Viper.

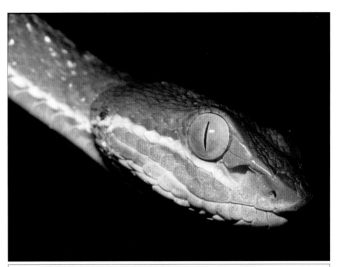

Photo 235. Cardamom Mountains Bamboo Pit Viper, *Trimeresurus (Cryptelytrops) cardamomensis*

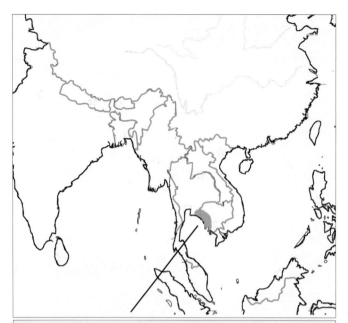

MAP 266. Range of the Cardamom Mountians Bamboo Pit Viper, *Trimeresurus (Cryptelytrops) cardamomensi*s.

Pope's Bamboo Pit Viper,

Trimeresurus (Popeia) popeiorum

Venom and Bite: Little information is avaiable.

Antivenom listed by www.toxinology.com-viewed 2012. Green Pit Viper Antivenom by Queen Saovabhava Memorial Institute (Thailand), Polyvalent Anti Snake Venom Serum by Central Research Institute (India), and SII Polyvalent Anti Snake Venom Serum from the Serum Institute of India.

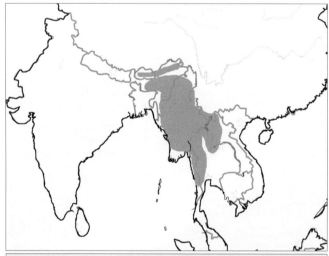

MAP 267. Range of the Pope's Bamboo Tree Viper, *Trimeresurus (Popeia) popeiorum.*

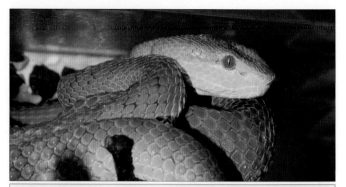

PHOTO 236. Pope's Bamboo Pit Viper, *Trimeresurus (Popeia) popeiorum* (male)

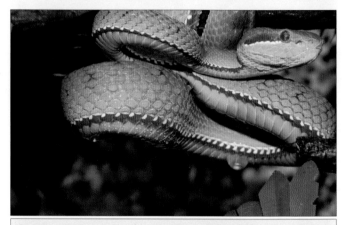

PHOTO 237. Pope's Bamboo Pit Viper, *Trimeresurus (Popeia) popeiorum* (female)

Sabah Bamboo Pit Viper,

Trimeresurus (Popeia) sabahi

Venom and Bite: Unknown. Antivenoms listed by www.toxinology.com (viewed 2012), are the same as for the previous species.

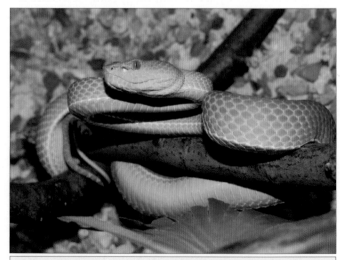

PHOTO 238. Sabah Bamboo Pit Viper, *Trimeresurus (Popeia) sabahi* (female)

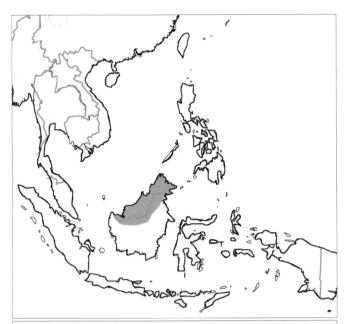

MAP 268. Range of the Sabah Bamboo Pit Viper, *Trimeresurus (Popeia) sabahi*

Cameron Highlands Bamboo Pit Viper,
Trimeresurus (Popeia) nebularis

Venom and Bite: Little known. Antivenoms listed by www.toxinology.com (viewed 2012), are the same as for the previous species.

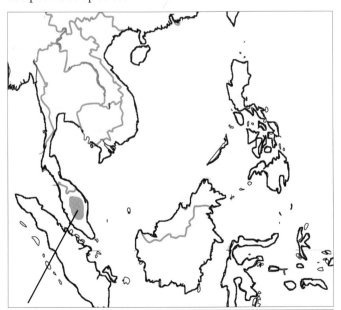

MAP 269. Range of the Cameron Highlands Pit Viper, *Trimeresurus (Popeia) nebularis*

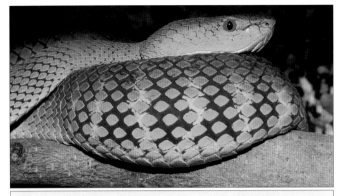

PHOTO 239. Cameron Highlands Bamboo Pit Viper, *Trimeresurus (Popeia) nebularis* (female)

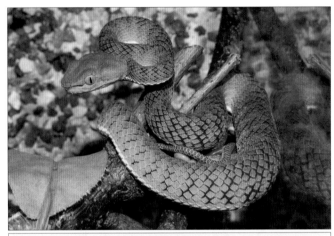

PHOTO 240. Cameron Highlands Bamboo Pit Viper, *Trimeresurus (Popeia) nebularis* (male

Siamese Peninsula Pit Viper,
Trimeresurus (Popeia) fucatus

Venom and Bite: Little known. Antivenoms listed by www.toxinology.com (viewed 2012), are the same as for the previous species.

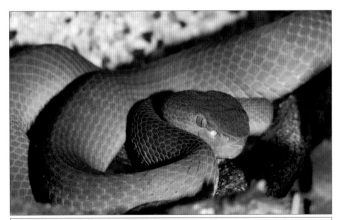

PHOTO 241. Siamese Peninsula Bamboo Pit Viper, *Trimeresurus (Popeia) fucatus* (female)

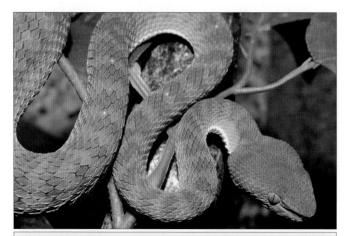

PHOTO 242. Siamese Peninsula Bamboo Pit Viper, *Trimeresurus (Popeia) fucatus* (male)

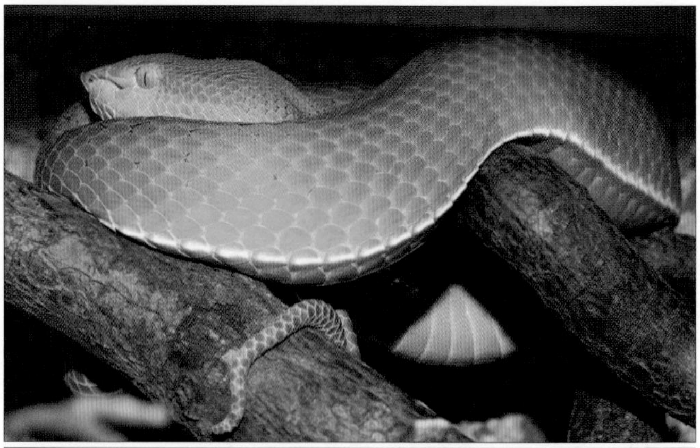

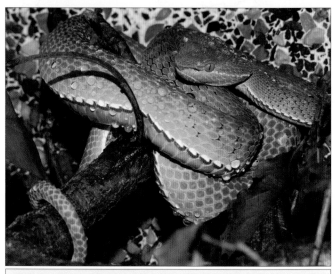

PHOTO 243. Vogel's Green Tree Pit Viper, *Viridovipera (Trimeresurus) vogeli* (female)

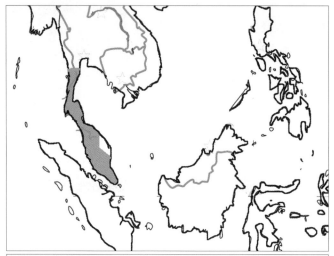

MAP 270. Range of the Siamese Peninsula Pit Viper, *Trimeresurus (Popeia) fucatus.*

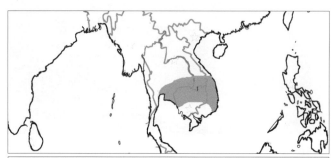

PHOTO 244. Vogel's Green Tree Pit Viper, *Viridovipera (Trimeresurus) vogeli* (male)

Vogel's Green Tree Pit Viper,
Viridovipera (Trimeresurus) vogeli

Venom and Bite: Unknown. Possibly capable of inflicting a lethal bite. Listed antivenom is Green Pit Viper Antivenom Queen Saovabhava Memorial Inst. (Thai Red Cross Society) in Thailand.

MAP 271. Range of the Vogel's Green Tree Pit Viper, *Viridovipera (Trimeresurus) vogeli.*

Chinese Green Tree Bamboo Pit Viper,
Viridovipera (Trimeresurus) stejnegeri

Venom and Bite: Procoagulants, possible anticoagulants and possible haemorragins. Has caused deaths. Partial antivenom list from www.toxinology.com-viewed 2012 includes the following.

Product: Green Pit Viper Antivenom
Manufacturer: Queen Saovabhava Memorial Inst.
Country of Origin: Thailand
Product: Polyvalent Antisnake Venom Serum
Manufacturer: Central Research Institute
Country of Origin: India

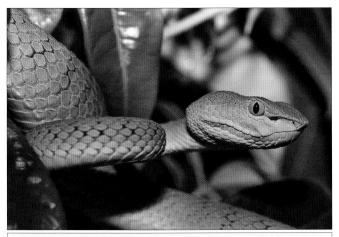

Photo 245. Chinese Green Tree Pit Viper, *Viridovipera (Trimeresurus) stejnegeri*

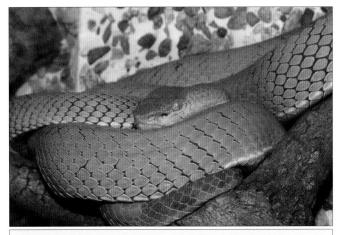

Photo 246. Gumprecht's Green Tree Viper, *Viridovipera (Trimeresurus) gumprechti* (female)

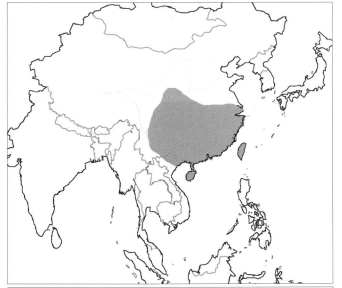

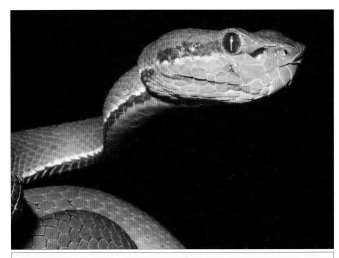

Photo 247. Gumprecht's Green Tree Viper, *Viridovipera (Trimeresurus) gumprechti* (male)

Map 272. Range of the Chinese Green Tree Viper, *Viridovipera (Trimeresurus) stejnegeri.*

Gumprecht's Green Pit Viper,

Viridovipera (Trimeresurus) gumprechti

Venom and Bite: Unknown. Antivenoms are the same as those listed for other Bamboo Pit Vipers.

Indian (Common) Bamboo Viper,

Trimeresurus gramineus

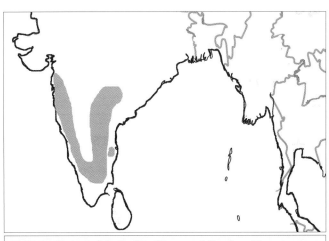

Map 274. Range of the Indian (Common) Bamboo Viper, *Trimeresurus gramineus.*

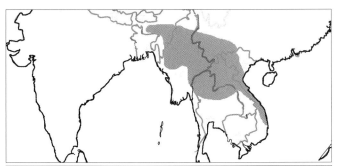

Map 273. Range of the Gumprecht's Pit Viper, *Trimeresurus gumprechti.*

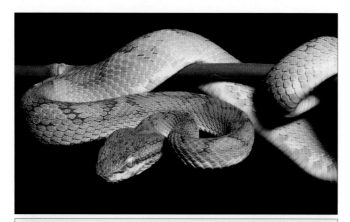

PHOTO 248. Indian (Common) Bamboo Viper, *Trimeresurus gramineus*

Venom and Bite: Procoagulants, myotoxins, and haemorragins. Potential for fatal bite unlikely but cannot be ruled out. Polyvalent Antivenoms listed by www.toxinology.com (viewed 2012) are produced by the Serum Institute of India (see previous species).

Similar Species: In addition to the species already discussed, several other mostly green colored "Bamboo Vipers" occur in the USPACOM (Part 1) region. Those that are currently known listed below.

Barat's Pit Viper - *T. barati* (Sumatra)

Large-scaled Pit Viper - *T. macrolepis* (southern India)

Matuo Bamboo Pit Viper - *T. medoensis* (northeastern India and northern Myanmar)

Ruby-eyed Green Pit Viper *T. rubeus* (Cambodia and Vietnam)

Nepal Bamboo Pit Viper *T. septentrionalis* (Nepal, northern India)

Sichuan Pit Viper - *T. sichuanensis* (Sichuan Province of China)

Tibetan Bamboo Pit Viper - *T. tibetanus* (Nepal, Tibet)

Yunnan Bamboo Pit Viper - *T. yunnanensis* (northeast India, southern China, northern Myanmar)

Brown "Bamboo" Pit Vipers

Author's Note: This grouping is based on similar morphological features (i.e., color), rather than on phylogeny.

Description and Identification: In this group of "Bamboo Vipers" the predominant colors are browns and grays rather than green. In body form and head shape they are identical to the Green Tree group, that is, moderately stout bodied, head large and very distinct from the neck. As with the previous group, sexual dimorphism is not uncommon.

In size they are about the same as the Green Tree group with most averaging 2.5 feet, with a maximum of around 3 feet in most species. One (*T. cantori*) can reach nearly 4.

Distribution, Habitat, and Biology: As might be guessed from the dominant colors of brown and gray, these snakes tend to be more terrestrial and semi-arboreal in habits. Like the preceding group they are mostly nocturnal. These are mostly island species, and all are found only in Part One of the USPACOM region.

Banded Pit Viper,
Trimeresurus (Cryptelytrops) fasciatus

Venom and Bite: Unknown. No antivenoms listed.

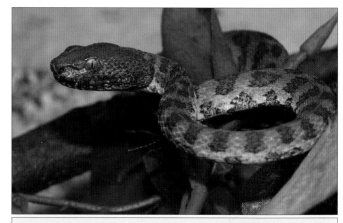

PHOTO 249. Banded Pit Viper (male), *Trimeresurus (Cryptelytrops) fasciatus*

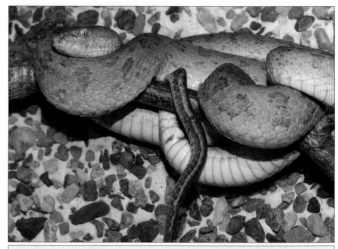

PHOTO 250. Banded Pit Viper (female), *Trimeresurus (Cryptelytrops) fasciatus*

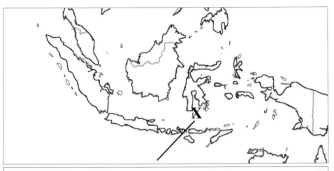

Map 275. Range of the Banded Pit Viper, *Trimeresurus (Cryptelytrops) fasciatus.*

Ashy Pit Viper,
Trimeresurus puniceus

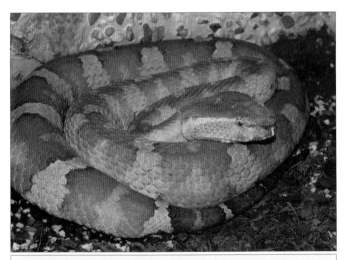

Photo 251. Ashy Pit Viper (female), *Trimeresurus puniceus*

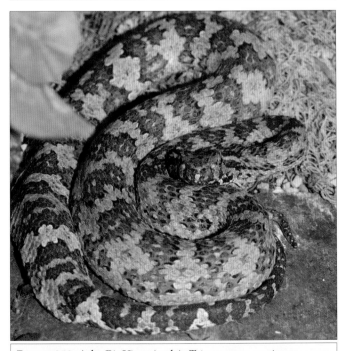

Photo 252. Ashy Pit Viper (male), *Trimeresurus puniceus*

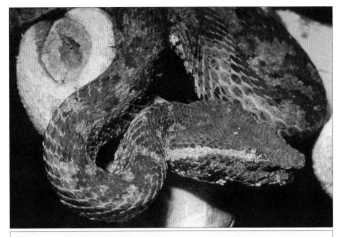

Photo 253. Ashy Pit Viper, *Trimeresurus puniceus*

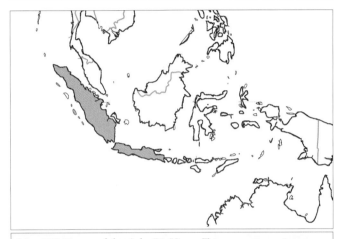

Map 276. Range of the Ashy Pit Viper, *Trimeresurus puniceus.*

Venom and Bite: Not believed to be highly dangerous but effects of bite unknown. Antivenom listed by Clinical Toxinology Resources is Green Pit Viper Antivenin by Thai Red Cross Society in Thailand.

Wirot's Pit Viper,
Trimeresurus wiroti

Venom and Bite: Unknown. No antivenoms listed.

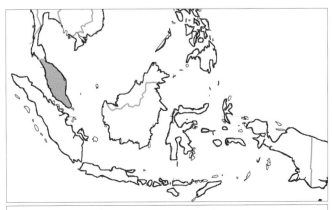

Map 277. Range of the Wirot's Pit Viper, *Trimeresurus wiroti.*

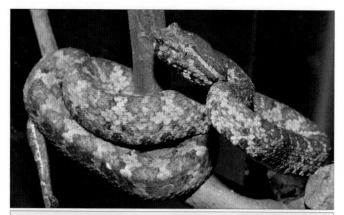

Photo 254. Wirot's Pit Viper (male), *Trimeresurus wiroti*

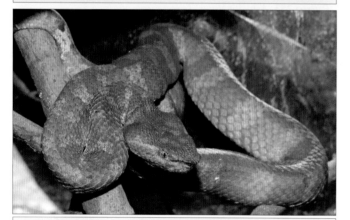

Photo 255. Wirot's Pit Viper (female), *Trimeresurus wiroti*

Andaman and Nicobar Islands Bamboo Pit Vipers

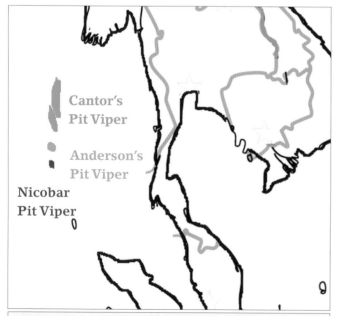

Cantor's Pit Viper

Anderson's Pit Viper

Nicobar Pit Viper

Map 278. Range of the Cantor's Pit Viper, *T. cantori*; Anderson's Pit Viper, *T. andersoni*; and the Nicobar Island Pit Viper, *T. labialis*.

Nicobar Island Pit Viper,
Trimeresurus (Cryptelytrops) labialis

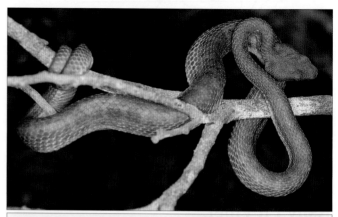

Photo 256. Nicobar Island Pit Viper, *Trimeresurus (Cryptelytrops) labialis*

Cantor's Pit Viper,
Trimeresurus (Cryptelytrops) cantori

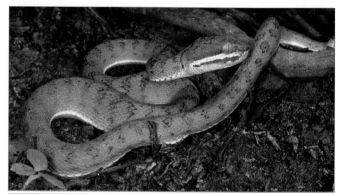

Photo 257. Cantor's Pit Viper, *Trimeresurus (Cryptelytrops) cantori*

Anderson's Pit Viper,
Trimeresurus (Cryptelytrops) andersoni

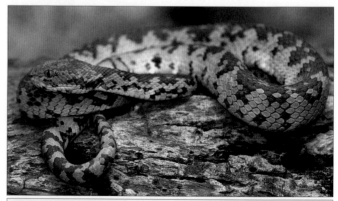

Photo 258. Anderson's Pit Viper, *Trimeresurus (Cryptelytrops) andersoni*

Similar Species: In addition to the species shown, there are at least 4 additional brownish pit vipers that make up this group. Listed below are their names and where they can be found.

T. andalasensis- No common name (Sumatra)

T. borneensis - Borneo Pit Viper (Borneo)

T. gracilis - Slender Pit Viper (Taiwan)

T. strigatus - Horse-shoe Pit Viper (south India)

Miscellaneous "Bamboo" Pit Vipers

Author's Note: This grouping not based on phylogeny.

In this group has been lumped all the remaining *Trimeresurus* pit vipers. A few are variable enough so that some color phases may be confused with members of either of the other two groups, but for the most part the species in this grouping are usually readily identified by color and pattern.

Beautiful Pit Viper,
Trimeresurus (Cryptelytrops) venustus

Kanburi Pit Viper,
Trimeresurus (Cryptelytrops) kanburiensis

Description and Identification: These two snakes are very similar in appearance, both being pale green with reddish brown or purplish markings that form bands more or less. The Beautiful Pit Viper may be the more variable of the two, and its ground color can vary from pale green to bluish.

Average length around 2 feet.

Distribution, Habitat, and Biology: Both species are native to Thailand. *T. kanburiensis* occupies a small area near the northern portion of the Malay Peninsula, while *T. venustus* lives in a similarly small region in the middle of the peninsula. Both are mainly arboreal, nocturnal species. Both reportedly inhabit bamboo forests.

Venom and Bite: Unknown. Probably neither is highly dangerous, but potential to inflict a fatal bite cannot be ruled out.

Antivenom listed by www.toxinology.com-viewed 2012.

   Product: Green Pit Viper Antivenom

   Manufacturer: Queen Saovabhava Memorial Inst.

   Country of Origin: Thailand

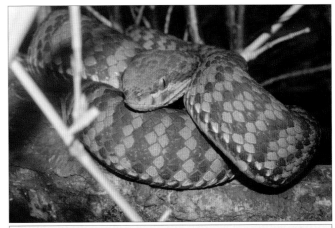

PHOTO 259. Beautiful Pit Viper, *Trimeresurus (Cryptelytrops) venustus*

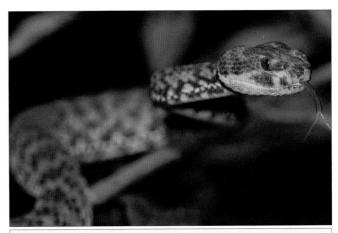

PHOTO 260. Kanburi Pit Viper, *Trimeresurus (Cryptelytrops) kanburiensis*

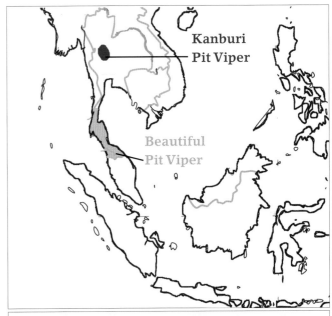

MAP 279. Range of the Beautiful Pit Viper, *T. venustus* and Kanburi Pit Viper, *T. kanburiensis*.

Mangrove Viper,

Trimeresurus (Cryptyletrops) purpureomaculatus

Description and Identification: This is one of the few species of *Trimeresurus* for which the taxonomic status has remained the same since the original publication of this volume back in 1965 (although some now place it in the genus *Cryptelytrops*). General body build about the same as that of the Green Tree Vipers; usually 25-27 scale rows at midbody.

Color variable. One common variety purplish brown with or without a whitish lateral line and with or without green spots. Another color phase is olive or gray without green spots. Tail uniformly brown or spotted gray and brown; belly white more or less clouded with brown.

Average length 30-35 inches; maximum about 40 inches.

Distribution, Habitat, and Biology: East Bengal, southern Burma, Malay Peninsula, Sumatra, and Andaman Islands. Largely restricted to the seacoast and to islands; particularly common in mangrove swamps. Also found inland in jungle up to 6,000 feet elevation. Usually found in low vegetation or among rocks.

Venom and Bite: A fairly common cause of snakebite in coastal Malaya. Fatalities are rare but have been recorded. Antivenoms listed by Clinical Toxinology Resources are the same as those for the various Green Tree Pit Vipers.

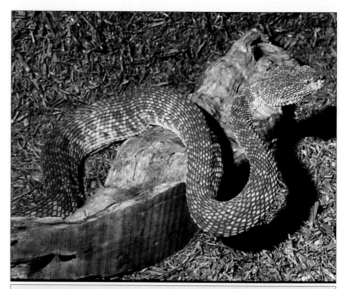

Photo 262. Mangrove Viper, *Trimeresurus (Cryptelytrops) purpureomaculatus*

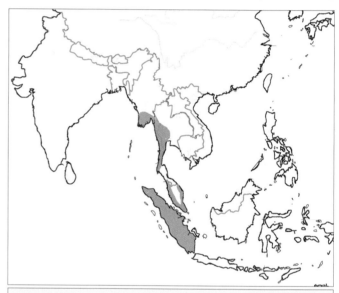

Map 280. Range of the Mangrove Viper, *Trimeresurus (Cryptelytrops) purpureomaculatus*.

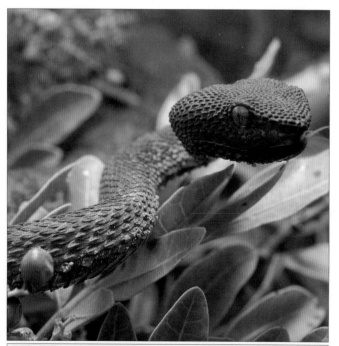

Photo 261. Mangrove Viper (dark morph), *Trimeresurus (Cryptelytrops) purpureomaculatus*

Philippine Bamboo Pit Viper,

Trimeresurus (Parias) flavomaculatus

Description and Identification: This species shows considerable variation and not all are as strikingly colored as the specimen shown below. Some shade of green with reddish or orange blotches is common. Brown color morphs also apparently occur. Grows to maximum of about 3 feet.

Distribution, Habitat, and Biology: Another mainly arboreal species. Inhabits low-lying tropical jungle. Small vertebrates like frogs and lizards are its main prey.

Venom and Bite: Unknown. No antivenoms listed. Antivenoms listed for other "Bamboo Vipers" may be useful in treating bites.

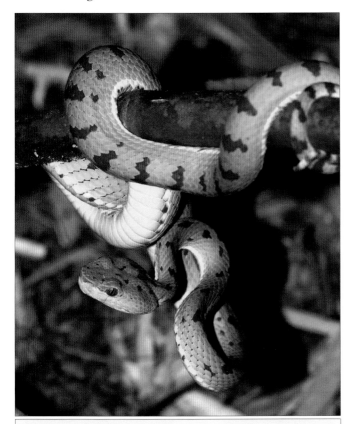

PHOTO 263. Philippine Pit Viper, *Trimeresurus (Parias) flavomaculatus*

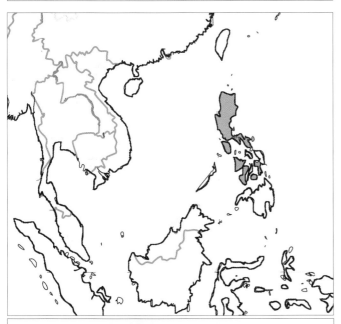

MAP 281. Range of the Philippine Pit Viper, *Trimeresurus flavomaculatus.*

Sumatran Pit Viper,
Trimeresurus (Parias) sumatranus

Description and Identification: Ground color ranges from bright green to very pale greenish-white. There are numerous black bars across the dorsum and the interstitial spaces are jet black. The head is also heavily marked with black.

Distribution, Habitat, and Biology: Inhabits forests of the Malay Peninsula, Sumatra, and Borneo. Reportedly common on cocoa plantations.

Venom and Bite: Unknown. Lethal potential cannot be ruled out. Antivenom is Green Pit Viper Antivenom by Science Division of the Thai Red Cross Society.

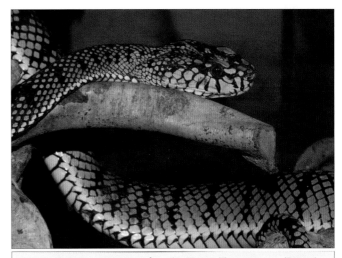

PHOTO 264. Sumatran Bamboo Pit Viper, *Trimeresurus (Parias) sumatranus*

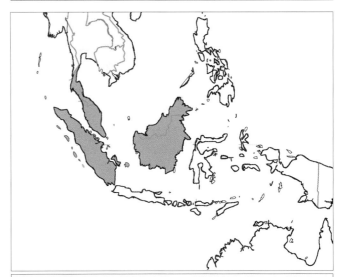

MAP 282. Range of the Sumatran Pit Viper, *Trimeresurus (Parias) sumatranus.*

Indonesian Pit Viper,
Trimeresurus (Parias) hageni

Venom and Bite: Unknown. Possibly capable of inflicting a lethal bite. Has a reputation for being quick to strike if threatened. Antivenom is Green Pit Viper Antivenom by Science Division of the Thai Red Cross Society.

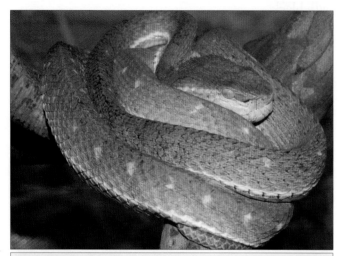

PHOTO 265. Indonesian Bamboo Pit Viper, *Trimeresurus (Parias) hageni*

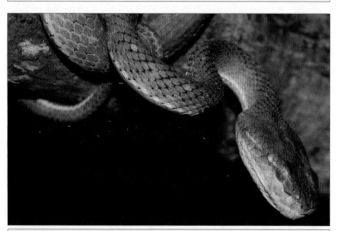

PHOTO 266. Indonesian Bamboo Pit Viper, *Trimeresurus (Parias) hageni*

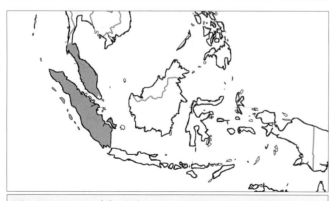

MAP 283. Range of the Indonesian Pit Viper, *Trimeresurus (Parias) sumatranus.*

McGregor's Pit Viper,
Trimeresurus (Parias) mcgregori

Description and Identification: Formerly considered a subspecies of the Philippine Pit Viper (*T. flavomaculatus*). The distinct yellow color of the McGregor's Pit Viper makes for easy recognition. Some specimens may be uniformly yellow, others will have dark dorsal blotches or bands that vary in intensity from being very distinct to somewhat faded. A white color phase also occurs (a very unusual color for snakes), which may be age related.

These snakes can attain a length of just over 3 feet.

Distribution, Habitat, and Biology: Found only on the tiny islands of Batan and Sabtang in the northern Philippines. They are apparently more terrestrial in habits than many other "Bamboo Vipers." Their bright yellow color is synonymous with that of some members of the *Bothriechis* (i.e., Eyelash Viper) genus in the new world.

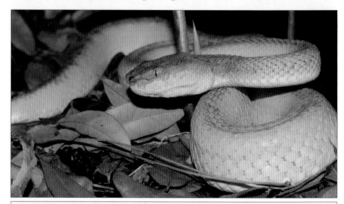

PHOTO 267. McGregor's Pit Viper, *Trimeresurus (Parias) mcgregori*

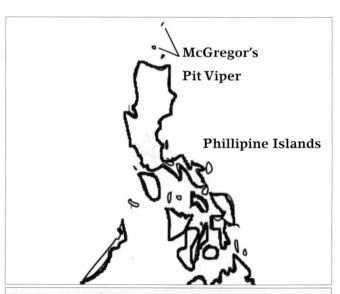

MAP 284. Range of McGregor's Pit Viper, *Trimeresurus mcgregori.*

Schultze's Pit Viper,
Trimeresurus (Parias) schultzei

Description and Identification: A large *Trimeresurus* that can exceed 4 feet. Green with yellow or white lateral stripe and reddish tail. Angular black dorsal markings and black interstitial spaces.

Distribution, Habitat, and Biology: Arboreal and nocturnal denizen of tropical jungles on the Philippine island of Palawan.

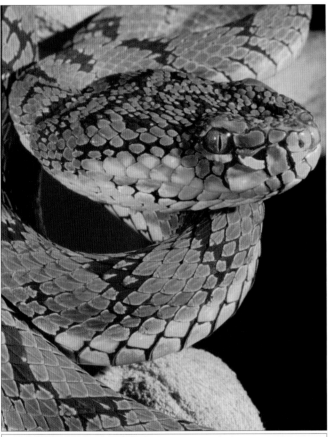

PHOTO 268. Schultze's Pit Viper, *Trimeresurus (Parias) schultzei*

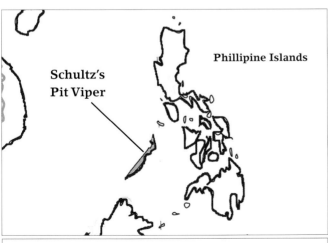

MAP 285. Range of Schultze's Pit Viper, *Trimeresuruss schultzei.*

Sri Lankan Bamboo Pit Viper,
Trimeresurus trigonocephalus

Description and Identification: Pale blue-green ground color with black circles on the dorsum and black interstitial skin is the color phase most often seen in zoos. Can also occur in a green or gray-green ground color. Average length about 2.5 feet but can reach a length of over 4 feet.

Distribution, Habitat, and Biology: Range restricted to the Island of Sri Lanka (Ceylon). An arboreal forest species primarily, but adaptable to human disturbed habitats. May be found in both low bushes and treetops. All types of small vertebrates are listed as food items.

Venom and Bite: Its presence in agricultural areas often leads to human encounters. However, bites are rare and there are apparently no known fatalities.

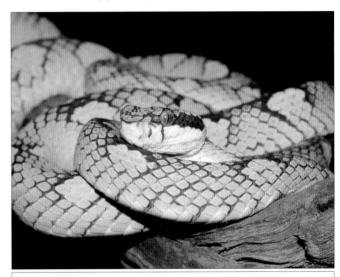

PHOTO 269. Sri Lankan Bamboo Pit Viper, *Trimeresurus trigonocephalus*

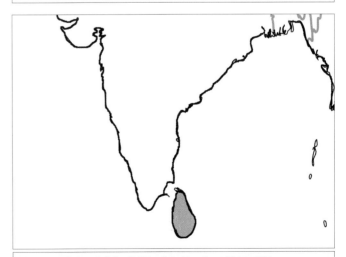

MAP 286. Range of the Sri Lankan Bamboo Viper, *Trimeresurus trigonocephalus*

Malabarian Pit Viper,
Trimeresurus malabaricus

Description and Identification: The ground color of this snake is highly variable, ranging from pale green to olive, blueish-green, greenish yellow, or even reddish. The dorsal surface is consistently marked with large irregular blotches that are brown to reddish.

Distribution, Habitat, and Biology: This species is endemic to southwestern India. It is found in the forests of the Western Ghats (an upland region that parallels the southwestern coast of India).

Venom and Bite: Venom potency and effects of bites unknown. No specific antivenom.

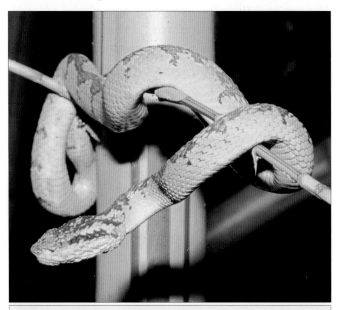

Photo 270. Malabarian Pit Viper, *Trimeresurus malabaricus*

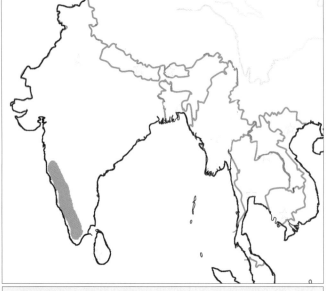

Map 287. Range of the Malabarian Pit Viper, *Trimeresurus malabaricus.*

Additional Species: In addition the *Trimeresurus* species mentioned thus far, there are 8 others that collectively range across much of the southern portions of the USPACOM region (Part 1). Those additional species and regions where they can be found are listed below.

T. brongersmai - Brongersma's Pit Viper (Mentawei Islands-Sumatra)

T. buniana - Fairy Pit Viper (West Malaysia)

T. fasciatus - Banded Pit Viper (Tanahdjampea Island-Indonesia)

T. honsonensis - No common name (southern Vietnam)

T. malcomi - Malcom's Pit Viper (Borneo)

T. phuketensis - No common name (Phuket Island-Malaysia)

T. toba - Toba Pit Viper (Sumatra)

T. truongsonensis - Quang Binh Pit Viper (Vietnam)

Family - Viperidae

Subfamily - Crotalinae - Pit Vipers

Genus - Tropidolaemus

Temple Pit Vipers

This genus is very similar to the previous genus (*Trimeresurus*) and these snakes were once included in that grouping. There are only 5 species in this small genus, and all are found in Part 1 of the USPACOM region. Like the previous genus, the Temple Pit Vipers are subject to ontogenic and sexually related morphologies and can present some difficulties in regards to proper identification. Locality can be a very useful tool in proper identification. The common name "Temple Vipers" is derived from the best known species in the group, the Wagler's or "Temple" Pit Viper. A thriving population of this species lives within the confines of The Snake Temple in Penang, Malaysia where they have become a tourist attraction.

Definition: Head large and very distinct from the neck; canthus sharp. Body slender to moderately stout; *tail prehensile.*

Eyes moderate to large; pupils vertically elliptical.

Head scales: Top of head covered with numerous small scales which are keeled.

Body scales: Dorsals keeled; in 127-148 rows at midbody. Subcaudals 40-54.

Wagler's Temple Viper,
Tropidolaemus wagleri

Description and Identification: Morphologically, this species exhibits both sexual dimorphism (color and size differences) and ontogenic color variation. Females are noticeably larger than males.

Young snakes are green, usually (but not always) changing color as they mature. Adult males may retain the green ground color, while, adult females are black with yellow, white or greenish markings.

Distribution, Habitat, and Biology: Wagler's Temple Viper is famous for its presence within a Buddhist temple in Penang, Malaysia where a number of these snakes live inside an old temple that has become a popular tourist attraction. Like all other members of its genus this is an arboreal species. It inhabits jungle and forest from sea level to about two thousand feet elevation.

Venom and Bite: These snakes seem quite placid and bites are rare. There are no known fatalities from its bite, although they may be capable of killing. No specific antivenom is available for this species but Clinical Toxinology Resources website (www.toxinology.com-viewed 2012) does list Green Pit Viper Antivenom by Queen Saovabha Memorial Institute in Thailand.

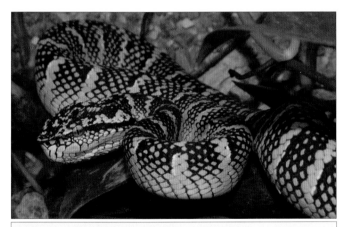

Photo 271. Wagler's Temple Viper, *Tropidolaemus wagleri*

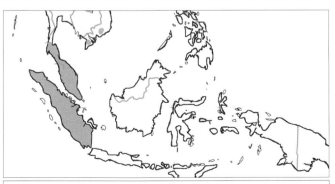

Map 288. Range of the Wagler's Temple Viper, *Tropidolaemus wagleri.*

Borneo Temple Viper,
Tropidolaemus subannulatus

Description and Identification: Highly variable. Bright green with thin crossbars of red, white, or dark green is a common color morph. Ground color may also be blue or blue-green. Postocular stripe red, white, black, or red bordered by white. Exhibits both sexual and ontogenic color variations.

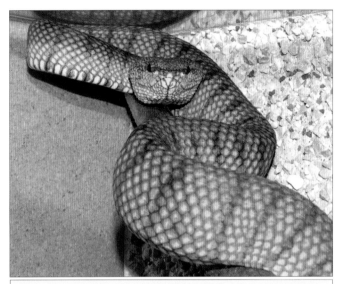

Photo 272. Borneo Temple Viper, *Tropidolaemus subannulatus* (adult female)

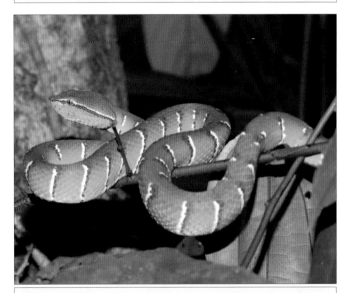

Photo 273. Borneo Temple Viper, *Tropidolaemus subannulatus* (immature)

Philippine Temple Viper,
Tropidolaemus philippensis

Description and Identification: Ground color blueish-green to turquoise blue. Thin crossbands on back black or dark blue; postocular stripe black or white.

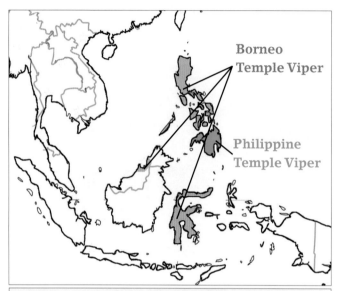

Borneo
Temple Viper

Philippine
Temple Viper

MAP 289. Range of the Borneo Temple Viper, *Tropidolaemus subannulatus*, and the Philippine Temple Viper, *Tropidolaemus philippensis*.

Additional Species: The Hutton's Temple Viper (*T. huttoni*) is a rare species restricted to southern India, while the Broad-banded Temple Viper *T. laticinctus*, is likewise a rare species found in a small region of the island of Celebes (Sulawesi).

Current References

Books

Dowling, Herndon G., Sherman A. Minton, and Findlay E. Russell. 1965. *Poisonous Snakes of the World.* Department of the Navy Bureau of Medicine and Surgery. Washington, DC.

Gopalakrishnakone, P. and L.M. Chou. 1990. *Snakes of Medical Importance (Asia-Pacific Region).* Venom and Toxin Research Group, National University of Singapore.

Mirtschin, Peter and Richard Davis. 1992. *Dangerous Snakes of Australia.* New Holland Ltd. London, England.

O'Shea, Mark. 2005. *Venomous Snakes of the World.* Princeton University Press. Princeton, NJ.

Phelps, Tony. 2010. *Old World Vipers, A Natural History of the Azemoipinae and Viperinae.* Edition Chimaira. Frankfort, Germany.

Journals

Chen, Y.; Zhang, D.; Jiang, K. & Wang, Z. 1992. "Evaluation of Snake Venoms among Agkistrodon Species in China". Asiatic Herpetological Research 4: 58-61.

David, Patrick, Gernot Vogel, & Alan Dubois. 2011. "On the need to follow rigorously the Rules of the Code for subsequent designation of a nucleospecies (type species) for a nominal genus which lacked one: the case of the nominal genus Trimeresurus Lacepede", 1804 (Reptilia: Squamata: Viperidae). Zootaxa 2292 1-51.

Levitan, Alan E. et al. 2003. "The Dangerously Venomous Snakes of Myanmar". Proceedings of the California Academy of Sciences Vol 54(24) 407-462.

Malhotra, Anita, Karen Dawson, Peng Guo, & Roger S. Thorpe. 2011. "Phylogenetic structure and species in the mountain pitviper *Ovophis monticola* (Serpentes: Viperidae: Crotalinae) in Asia". Molecular Genetics and Evolution 59 444-457.

Malhotra, Anita, and Roger S. Thorpe 2004. "A phylogeny of four mitochondrial gene regions suggests a revised taxonomy for Asian pitvipers". Molecular Genetics and Evoution 32 83-100.

Orlov, N.; Anajeva, A.; Ryabov, S. & Rao, D.-Q. 2003. "Venomous Snakes of Southern China". Reptilia (GB) (31) :22-29.

Smith, Brian. 1993. "Notes on a collection of squamate reptiles from eastern Mindanao, Philippine Islands part 2: Serpentes". Asiatic Herpetological Research 5: 96-102.

Slowinski, Joseph B. and Wolfgang Wuster. 2000. "A New Cobra (Elapidae: Naja) From Myanmar (Burma)". Herpetologica 56(2) 257-270.

Slowinski, J. B. 1994. "A phylogenetic anaylysis of Bungarus (Elapidae) based on morphological characters". Journal of Herpetology 28 (4): 440-446.

Maduwage, Kalana; Anjana Silva, Kelum Manamendra-Arachchi & Rohan Pethiyagoda. 2009. "A taxonomic revision of the South Asian hump-nosed pit vipers (Squamata: Viperidae: Hypnale)". Zootaxa 2232: 1-28.

David, Patrick, Nicolas Vidal, & Oliver S.G. Pauwels. 2001. "A Morphological Study of Stejneger's Pit Viper Trimeresurus stegnegeri (Serpentes, Viperidae, Crotalinae) with description of a new species from Thailand". Russian Journal of Herpetology Vol. 8 (3) 205-222.

Yang, Jian-Huan; Nikolai L. Orlov & Yin Yong Wang. 2011. "A new species of pit viper of the genus Protobothrops from China (Squamata: Viperidae)". Zootaxa 2936: 59-68.

Vogel, G.; David, P.; Lutz, M.; van Rooijen,J. & Vidal, N. 2007. "Revision of the Tropidolaemus wagleri complex (Serpentes, Viperidae, Crotalinae). I. Definition of included taxa and redescription of Tropidolaemus wagleri". Zootaxa 1644:1-40.

Yan XU; Quin, LIU; Edward A. MYERS; Lian WANG; Song HUANG; Yun HE; Peihao PENG, and Png GUO. 2012. "Molecular Phylogeny of the Genus Gloydius (Serpentes: Crotalinae)". Asian Herpetological Research 3 (2) 127-132.

Prasarnpun S., Walsh j., Awad S.S., and Harris J.B. 2005. "Envenoming by kraits: the biological basis of treatment resistant neuromuscular paralysis". Brain 128(pt12): 2987-96.

Websites

Global Snakebite Initiative - www.snakebiteinitiative.org

Munich Antivenom Index (MAVIN) - www.toxinfo.org/antivenoms

University of Adelaide, Clinical Toxinology Resources Wesbsite (2012) - www.toxinology.com

World Health Organization - www.who.int/bloodproducts/snakeantivenoms/database

The Reptile Database - http//www.reptiledata-base.org

Catalogue of Life - www.catalogueoflife.org

Armed Forces Pest Managment Board - www.afpmb.org/content/living-hazards-database

www.andamannicobarsnakes.com

www.naturemalaysia.com

www.snakesoftaiwan.com

www.iucnredlist.org

Original References

KUNTZ, Robert E. 1963. Snakes of Taiwan. U.S. Naval Medical Research Unit No. 2: Taipei, Taiwan, pp. 1–79, color pls., text figs. (not numbered).

LEVITON, Alan E. 1961. Keys to the Dangerously Venomous Terrestrial Snakes of the Philippine Islands. Silliman Jour., vol. 8, pp. 98–106, figs. 1–2.

POPE, Clifford. 1935. The Reptiles of China. Nat. Hist. Cent. Asia, vol. 10 New York, pp. i–iii + 1–604, 27 pls. figs., map.

STEJNEGER, L. 1907. Herpetology of Japan and Adjacent Territory. Bull. U.S. Nat. Mus., vol. 58, pp. i–xx, 1–577, 35 pls.

WERLER, John E. and Hugh L. KEEGAN. 1963. Venomous Snakes of the Pacific Area. In Venomous and Poisonous Animals and Noxious Plants of the Pacific Region. (H. L. Keegan and W. V. MacFarlane, eds.) Pergamon Press: Oxford, pp. 219–325, figs. 1–78.

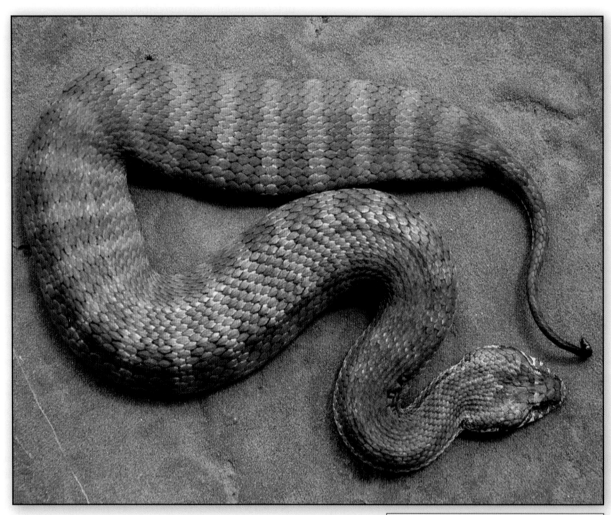

New Guinea Death Adder,
Acanthophis laevis

CHAPTER **14**

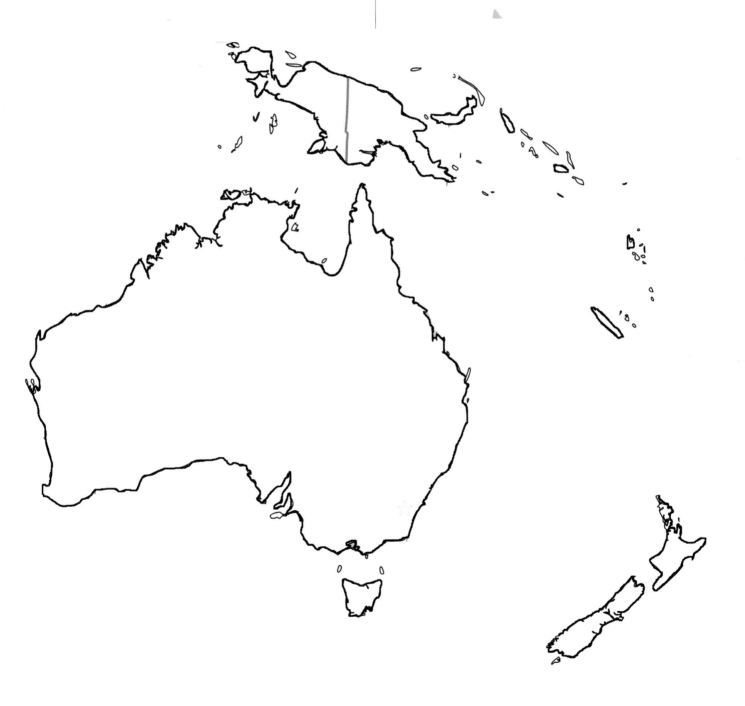

MAP 290. Region 6, Part Two United States Pacific Command. Australia and South Pacific Islands.

Family - Elapidae Genus - Acanthophis

Death Adders

There are now 7 species of Death Adders known to science (some experts say several more). Hoser (1998) lists a total of 12 species. That number is up from what was only 2 when the original edition of *Poisonous Snakes of the World* was published in 1965.

There are no vipers or pit vipers found within the range of the Death Adders, but these members of the cobra family have evolved to occupy an empty niche in the ecosystem of the region where they live. Not only do they act like vipers, adopting a "sit and wait" ambush strategy for prey, they also are viper-like in appearance with short stout bodies and broad triangular heads that are distinct from the neck. They even have vertically elliptical pupils and keeled scales.

Death Adders are found throughout most of Australia and parts of New Guinea.

Definition: Head broad, flattened and distinct form neck; a distinct canthus rostralis. Body thick and depressed; tail short with a long terminal spine

Eyes moderate in size; pupils vertically elliptical..

Head Scales: The usual 9 on the crown, somewhat roughened with raised edges; supraoculars broad, overhanging eye. Eye separated from supralabials by a row of small suboculars.

Body Scales: Dorsals keeled and pointed, in 21-23 rows at midbody. Ventrals 113-135; anal plate entire; subcaudals mostly single, some terminal ones paired, 40-52. Tail with a terminal spine made up of several scales.

Though quite heavy bodied, Death Adders are short snakes that are less than 3 feet in length. In another example of convergent evolution with the Viperidae, many Death Adders have bright yellow tail tips which they use for caudal luring.

All species of Death Adder are readily identified in the field by their viper-like appearance (short-thick body, head very distinct from neck, tail short, pupils elliptical). These are the only snakes within their range which resemble the Viperidae in overall appearance.

The Death Adders possess extremely potent neurotoxic venom in the form of both pre-snyaptic and post-synaptic neurotoxins.

Common Death Adder,
Acanthophis antarcticus

Description and Identification: Ground color variable from gray or brown to reddish. A series of light and dark transverse bands alternate the entire length. Although typically distinct they may rarely be less evident. This is one of the largest Death Adders and can grow to a maximum of about 40 inches.

Distribution, Habitat, and Biology: Ranges across much of western and southern Australia and a few islands in Indonesia. Also apparently occurs in Papua New Guinea but distribution maps for that region are unavailable. A terrestrial snake of leaf litter in vegetated brush lands and forests. Apparently declining as a result of human alteration of habitat. Food is frogs, lizards, and some small mammals.

Venom and Bite: Extremely potent pre-synaptic and post-synaptic neurotoxins. This species also has anticoagulant toxins. Prior to the development of a specific antivenom as many as 50 percent of snakebites by this species resulted in death.

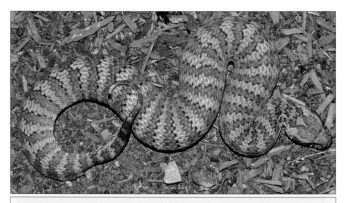

PHOTO 274. Common Death Adder, *Acanthophis antarcticus*

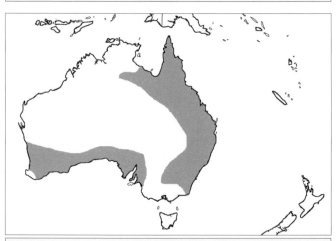

MAP 291. Range of the Common Death Adder, *Acanthophis antarcticus*

Death Adder Antivenom by Commonwealth Serum Laboratories in Australia is the specific antivenom for treating bites by this species. Also produced by the same manufacturer is CSL Polyvalent Snake Antivenom.

Desert Death Adder,
Acanthophis pyrrus

Description and Identification: Similar to the preceding species, but more slender bodied. Most specimens are decidedly reddish in color. Somewhat smaller than *A. antarcticus* with a maximum length of about 30 inches.

Distribution, Habitat, and Biology: Inhabits the arid regions of central and western Australia. Nocturnal. Food chiefly lizards.

Venom and Bite: Presumably similar to the preceding species. Antivenoms are the same as for the Common Death Adder.

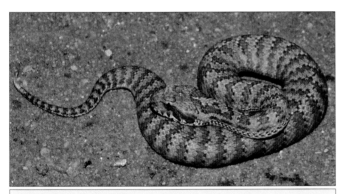

PHOTO 275. Desert Death Adder, *Acanthophis pyrrus*

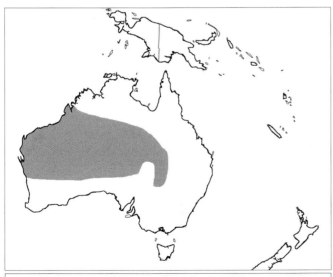

MAP 292. Range of the Desert Death Adder, *Acanthophis pyrrus*

New Guinea Death Adder,
Acanthophis laevis

Description and Identification: Typical Death Adder body-short, very stout. Tends to brownish or grayish in color. Grows to nearly 3 feet.

Distribution, Habitat, and Biology: New Guinea and some adjacent small islands. Occupies nearly all habitats.

Venom and Bite: Presumably similar to the Common Death Adder. Antivenoms are the same as for the Common Death Adder.

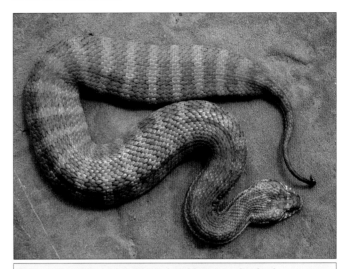

PHOTO 276. New Guinea Death Adder, *Acanthophis laevis*

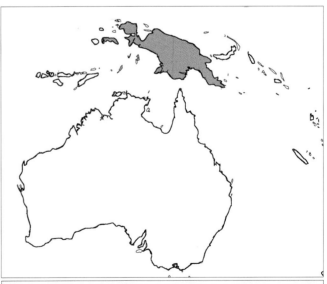

MAP 293. Range of the New Guinea Death Adder, *Acanthophis laevis*

Rough-scaled Death Adder,
Acanthophis rugosus

Description and Identification: This species is recognized from other Death Adders by the markedly rough scales on the head and neck region.

Distribution, Habitat, and Biology: Endemic to the southernmost part of the island of New Guinea.

Habitat is described as "grassland and savanna." Overall color usually dark.

Venom and Bite: Clinical Toxinology Resources website (viewed 2012) list pre- and post-synaptic neurotoxins, myotoxins, and anticoagulants. Only the neurotoxins appear to be clinically significant. Antivenoms are the same as for the Common Death Adder.

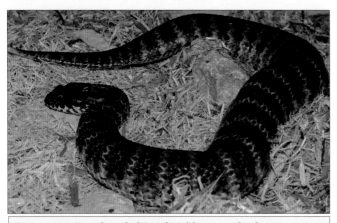

PHOTO 277. Rough-scaled Death Adder, *Acanthophis rugosus*

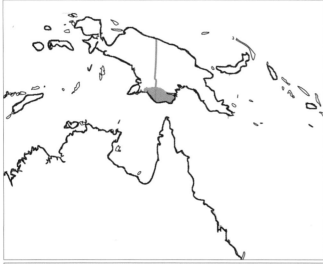

MAP 294. Range of the Rough-scaled Death Adder, *Acanthophis rugosus*.

Northern Death Adder,
Acanthophis praelongus

Description and Identification: As with other Death Adders. Overall color is variable.

Distribution, Habitat, and Biology: Restricted to the more humid tropical areas in the north of Australia.

Venom and Bite: Presumably similar to the other Death Adder species. Antivenoms are the same as for the Common Death Adder.

Additional Species: There are at least 2 more species of Death Adder (Hoser 1998 describes a total of 12) and there may be several more that are either newly described or yet to be described. *A. hawkei*, the Barkly Tableland Death Adder and the Pilbara Death Adder are both endemic to Australia.

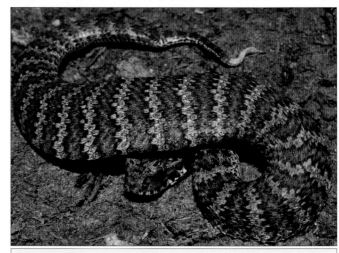

PHOTO 278. Northern Death Adder, *Acanthophis praelongus*

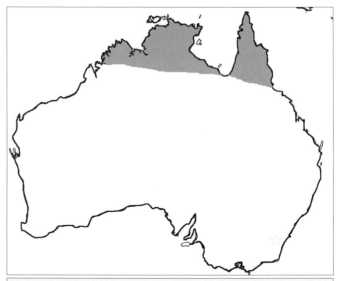

MAP 295. Range of the Northern Death Adder, *Acanthophis praelongus*.

Family - Elapidae Genus - Notechis

Tiger Snake

Some experts recognize only a single species with several subspecies. Here two are recognized.

Definition: Head relatively broad, flattened, and moderately distinct from the neck. A distinct canthus rostralis. Body relatively stout, flattened dorso-ventrally; tail rather short.

Eyes moderated in size; pupils round.

Head scales: The usual 9 on the crown; frontal wide and shield shaped. Laterally, nasal in contact with preocular.

Body scales: Dorsals smooth in 17-20 oblique rows at midbody; fewer posteriorly. Ventrals 160-184; anal plate entire; subcaudals single, 43-59.

This genus is endemic to Australia.

Eastern Tiger Snake,
Notechis scutatus

Description and Identification: Ground color highly variable from olive-green to gray or brown. There is typically a series of yellowish to cream colored bands across the back. Occasional specimens are uniformly unbanded. These are large snakes that can exceed 6 feet in length.

Distribution, Habitat, and Biology: Some source of water is a habitat requirement for these snakes as they feed heavily on frogs. They are thus found in the vicinity of streams, lakes, and swamps. When threatened this snake flattens the body into a ribbon-like shape. Presumably this makes the snake look larger and more menacing to a potential threat.

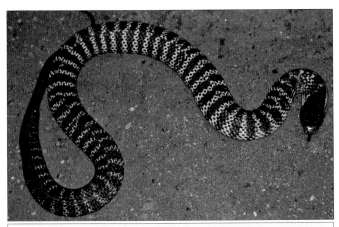

PHOTO 279. Eastern Tiger Snake, *Notechis scutatus*

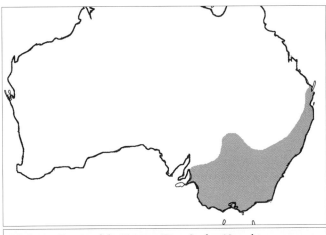

MAP 296. Range of the Eastern Tiger Snake, *Notechis scutatus.*

Venom and Bite: Venom is a very potent neurotoxin (both pre- and post-synaptic) which also has some haemotoxic, cytotoxic, and myotoxic properties. The death rate for untreated bites is estimated at 40-50 percent. Considering that many venomous snakebites result in only slight envenomations, this must be considered as one of the world's deadliest snakes. Fortunately, there is a specific antivenom for bites by this species.

> Product: Tiger Snake Antivenom
> Manufacturer: CSL Limited
> Country of Origin: Australia

Also listed for this species by Clinical Toxicology Resources website (viewed 2012) is:

> Product: Polyvalent Snake Antivenom
> Manufacturer: CSL Limited
> Country of Origin: Australia

Western Tiger Snake,
Notechis ater

Description and Identification: Very similar to the preceding species and difficult to distinguish. For the layman, range is the most reliable means of differentiating the two species. If anything, this species is more variable than the Eastern Tiger Snake. Many specimens have distinct yellow to whitish bands but some populations may be mostly solid black. Reaches 6 feet in length.

Distribution, Habitat, and Biology: Similar in biology and habitat to the Eastern Tiger Snake, feeding mostly on frogs and tadpoles in the vicinity of wetlands and drainages.

Venom and Bite: Even deadlier than the Eastern Tiger Snake. Antivenoms are the same as for that species.

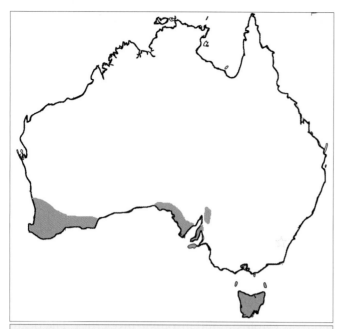

Map 297. Range of the Western Tiger Snake, *Notechis ater.*

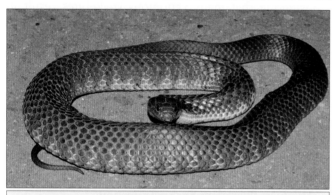

Photo 280. Western Tiger Snake, *Notechis ater*

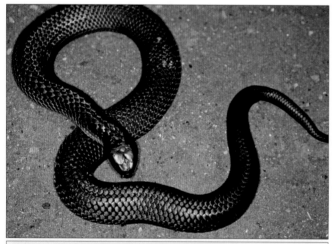

Photo 281. Western Tiger Snake, *Notechis ater*

Family - Elapidae Genus - Pseudonaja

Brown Snakes

At least 9 species are currently recognized (some say 10). All are endemic to Australia. Some members of the genus may exceed the Tiger Snake in dangerousness. The genus name *Pseudonaja* literally means "false cobra." The name "Brown Snakes" is descriptive of many members of this genus, but most are highly variable in color.

Definition: Body slender, head elongate and only slightly distinct from neck.

Eyes moderate in size, pupils round.

Body scales: Dorsals smooth, 17-21 rows at mid body; ventrals 185-235; subcaudals 45-75 (divided), anal scute divided.

At least some species are swift moving, easily agitated snakes that are quick to bite if cornered.

Identifying the Brown Snakes can be a nightmare for the layman, as nearly all species exhibit a wide array of color morphs. In addition, each color morph appears in many species. A uniformly brown or tan snake, or one with blotches, may be a Western Brown Snake or an Eastern Brown Snake.

Fortunately for snakebite victims identifying the Brown Snakes down to species is not critical as the antivenom used is universal for all members of this genus. What is critical is seeking immediate treatment for any *Pseudonaja* bite, as local symptoms may be absent even in the case of a lethal envenomation. In the 1965 edition of this volume these snakes were placed in the genus *Demansia* with the Whipsnakes.

Eastern Brown Snake,
Pseudonaja textilis

Description and Identification: Varies in color from light tan to dark brown. Can be uniformly brown dorsally or lightly mottled with obscure lighter tans and/or darker browns. Large specimens can exceed 7 feet.

Distribution, Habitat, and Biology: Found both in Australia and Papua New Guinea. Unlike most venomous snakes which strike their prey, inject their venom and pull back and wait for the prey to succumb, feeding Brown Snakes grasp their prey and constrict in the manner of many harmless snakes. They also employ their venom while constricting.

Venom and Bite: This species is fast moving and can be quick to bite if molested. The venom is a potent cocktail of both pre- and post-synaptic neurotoxins and powerful procoagulants. The Eastern Brown snake kills more people than any other snake in Australia.

Considering that Australia is home to many of the world's deadliest species, that is a significant statistic.

CSL Limited of Australia produces a specific antivenom, Brown Snake Antivenom. Also available is CSL Limited's Polyvalent Snake Antivenom.

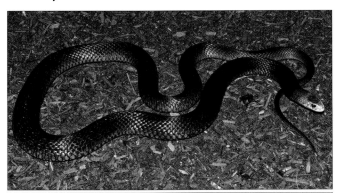

PHOTO 282. Eastern Brown Snake, *Pseudonaja textilis*

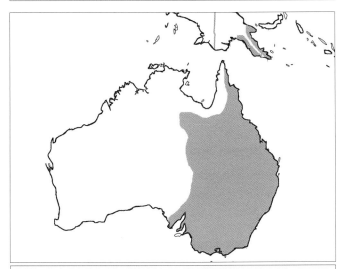

MAP 298. Range of the Eastern Brown Snake, *Pseudonaja textilis.*

Western Brown Snake,
Pseudonaja mengdeni

Description and Identification: The color is extremely variable and may be light brown, yellowish, or jet black. Some specimens are light brown with a blackish "collar", others may be light brown with dark bands. Another large species (record 6 feet 8 inches). Most adults are about 5 feet in length.

Distribution, Habitat, and Biology: Wide-ranging across all of western and central Australia, where it occupies a variety of habitats from woodlands to desert.

Venom and Bite: Another highly dangerous snake with as many as 20 percent of untreated bites resulting in death (from www.toxinology.com-viewed 2012). Antivenoms are the same as for other Brown Snakes, that is, Brown Snake Antivenom and Polyvalent Snake Antivenom from Commonwealth Serum Laboratories in Victoria, Australia.

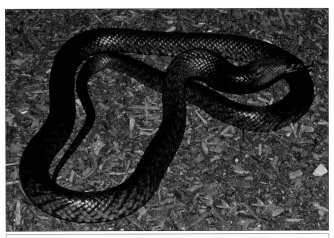

PHOTO 283. Western Brown Snake, *Pseudonaja mengdeni*

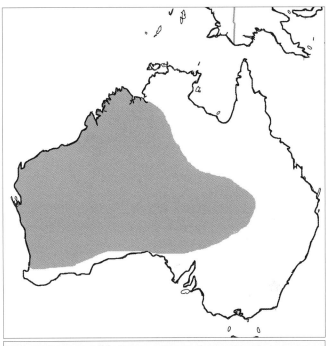

MAP 299. Range of the Western Brown Snake, *Pseudonaja mengdeni.*

Dugite,
Pseudonaja affinis

Description and Identification: Most easily identified by range, although it may overlap with the Eastern Brown Snake along the northern edges of its range.

Distribution, Habitat, and Biology: As with other *Pseudonaja*, this is a diurnal, terrestrial snake that is alert, active and swift. In hot weather they may become more nocturnal. Lizards, mice, and other snakes are food items.

Venom and Bite: Another large and dangerously venomous snake. Antivenoms are the same as for other *Pseudonaja*.

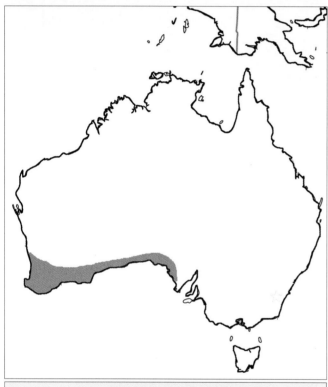

MAP 300. Range of the Dugite, *Pseudonaja affinis*.

Northern Brown Snake,
Pseudonaja nuchalis

Description and Identification: A typical Brown Snake in regards to body size and shape. As many as 16 different color morphs makes attempts at a written description of color and pattern fruitless. Range can be a useful factor in making a proper identification, although it does overlap with the Eastern Brown snake on the eastern edge of its range. Grows to a maximum of 6 feet.

Distribution, Habitat, and Biology: As with other *Pseudonaja*. Lizards, mice, birds, and other snakes are listed as food items.

Venom and Bite: Another large and dangerously venomous snake with a high potential for inflicting a lethal bite. Antivenoms are the same as for other *Pseudonaja*.

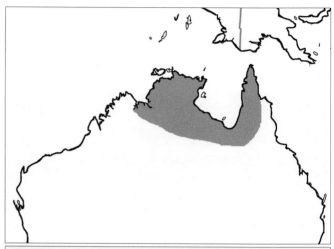

MAP 301. Range of the Northern Brown Snake, *Pseudonaja nuchalis*.

Additional Species:

Ingram's Brown Snake - *P. ingrami*

Found in the vicinity of the Barkly Tablelands in north central Australia. Grows to 5.5 feet and is a highly dangerous species.

Peninsula Brown Snake - *P. inframacula*

Found in coastal regions of South Australia. Grows to about 5 feet and is a deadly species.

Speckled Brown Snake - *P. guttata*

Fairly widespread in the Northern Territory and Queensland (Australia). Maximum length nearly 5 feet. Deadly.

Shield-snouted Brown Snake - *P. aspidoryncha*

Found in parts of in South Australia, New South Wales, and the northern tip of Victoria. High potential for lethal bite.

Ringed Brown Snake - *P. modesta*

Ranges throughout western and central Australia. Range is nearly synonymous with the Western Brown Snake. This species is a smaller (3 ft.), less dangerous member of the *Pseudonaja* genus. Its bite, though potentially dangerous, is unlikely to produce a fatal effect.

Antivenoms for the above species are the same as for other *Pseudonaja*.

Family - Elapidae Genus - Oxyuranus

Taipans

If you took a poll of herpetologists who work with venomous snakes and ask them to name the five deadliest snakes in the world, the Taipans would appear on everyone's list. Many would place them right at the top. There are 3 species and all are endemic to the USPACOM (Part 2) region.

The following description is from the 1965 edition of *Poisonous Snakes of the World.* Back then only one species was recognized.

Definition: Head elongate and narrow but distinct from neck; a distinct canthus rostralis. Body elongate and cylindrical; a moderately long tapering tail.

Eyes large, pupil round.

Head scales: The usual 9 on the crown. Laterally, nasal in contact with preocular.

Body scales: Dorsals with low but distinct keels, in 21-23 rows at midbody, reduced to 17 posteriorly.

Ventrals 230-247. Anal plate entire; subcaudals 50-72 all paired.

Coastal Taipan,
Oxyuranus scutellatus

Description and Identification: Dorsum uniformly brown and usually unmarked, shades vary from light to dark brown. The head is noticeably lighter than the body, especially along the labials. Specimens from the Papua New Guinea populations (subspecies *canni*) are distinctly different, with darker bodies, dark heads and usually an orange vertebral stripe. These are long, relatively slender snakes that can grow up to 10 feet in length (longest venomous snake in the Australia-New Guinea region). Most specimens are 7 to 8 feet as adults.

Distribution, Habitat, and Biology: Ranges along the northern coastal regions of Australia Queensland,

Northern Territory, and Western Australia. Also in the coastal lowlands of southern Papua New Guinea. These are slender, alert, and fast moving serpents that hunt both rodents and small marsupial mammals. A lighting strike and then withdrawal to wait for the venoms effect keeps them from suffering injury from sharp teeth and claws.

Venom and Bite: Long fangs for an elapid and an extremely potent pre-synaptic and post-synaptic neurotoxic venom with procoagulants and systemic myotoxins. They will usually flee when approached but if forced to fight back they will do so with vigor, their speed allowing them to sometimes inflict multiple bites. In Australia deaths are rare but New Guinea populations are a significant source of snakebite mortality in the southern portions of that island. This is unquestionably one of the world's most dangerous snake species and a significant envenomation is not survivable without proper treatment.

Antivenoms:

Taipan Antivenom and Polyvalent Snake Antivenom by Commonwealth Serum Laboratories of Australia.

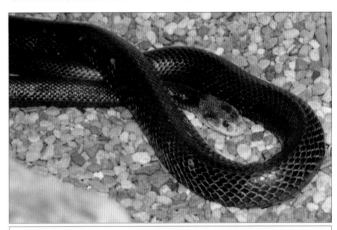

PHOTO 284. Coastal Taipan, *Oxyuranus scutellatus*

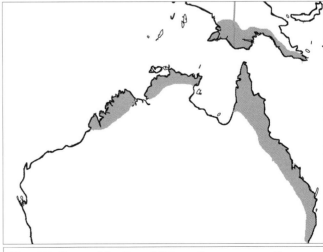

MAP 302. Range of the Coastal Taipan, *Oxyuranus scutellatus.*

Inland Taipan,
Oxyuranus microlepidotus

Description and Identification: Dorsum light to dark brown. Dark flecking often present on the dorsum, sometimes forming faint dark bands, especially towards the tail. The ventral scutes are a pale yellowish or pale orange which laterally may invade the first row or two of dorsal scales. The head is usually dark brown or black, though some specimens may show light brown head color. These are large snakes, but not as big as the Coastal Taipan. Maximum length for the Inland Taipan is just over 8 feet.

Distribution, Habitat, and Biology: Found in arid central Australia. Hunts rodents along dried river beds (O'Shea 2005). This species also goes by the name Fierce Snake.

Venom and Bite: The Inland Taipan lives in an area where the human population is low and bites are extremely rare. This is a fortunate situation, as this snake has the *most toxic venom of any snake on earth*. Mark O'Shea in his book "*Venomous Snakes of the World*" (2005) states that the Inland Taipan has enough venom to kill 62 adult humans!

Antivenom is the same as that for the Coastal Taipan.

Additional Species: A third Taipan species, the Western Desert Taipan (*O. temporalis*) is found in arid regions of south western Australia, including portions of Western Australia, South Australia and the Northern Territory.

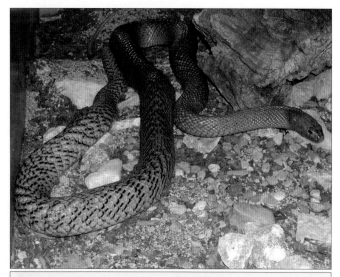

PHOTO 285. Inland Taipan, *Oxyuranus microlepidotus*

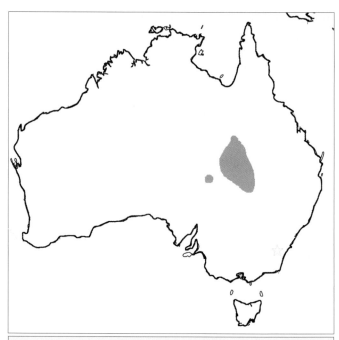

MAP 303. Range of the Inland Taipan, *Oxyuranus microlepidotus.*

Family - Elapidae Genus - Pseudechis
Australian Blacksnakes

Despite the common name Blacksnakes, many species of *Pseudechis* are actually brown. Others are red and black or yellow and black. Some sources list 7 species in this genus, although some list 8, while still others now recognize 9. The 7 species examined here are widely accepted as valid. Although most are found in Australia, at least one species (maybe more) occurs on the island of New Guinea.

Although several species have caused human fatalities, these snakes are not as deadly from a standpoint of venom toxicity as many other snakes within the USPACOM (Part 2) region. The exception being the Papuan Blacksnake (*P. papuanus*) which may be the most dangerous member of the genus. Though the toxicity of their venom is not as high as many other species, these snakes do have a large amount of venom. The most widespread species (*P. australis*) is responsible for many bites in Australia.

Definition: Head small and not distinct from neck; no canthus rostralis; snout conspicuously blunted. Body cylindrical and moderately slender; tail short.

Eyes very small, pupils round.

Head scales: The usual 9 on the crown; frontal and prefrontals very broad; rostral broad. Laterally, preocular present of fused with prefrontal; if present preocular in contact with nasal or separated from it by prefrontal.

Body scales: Dorsals smooth in 17-21 rows.

Ventrals 159-235; anal plate divided or entire; subcaudals 40-75; single or paired, often both.

Papuan Blacksnake,
Pseudechis papuanus

Description and Identification: One of the few Australian Blacksnakes that is actually black, but not found in Australia! Dorsal color is typically jet black, though it may rarely be brownish. There can be some cream on the throat and/or nose. Venter is also quite dark. A large, heavy bodied snake that can grow to 8 feet.

Distribution, Habitat, and Biology: Endemic to the island of New Guinea. Inhabits swamps and marshes in coastal lowlands and also rainforest. Feeds mainly on frogs. There is concern among biologists that this species (and other frog eaters) on the island of New Guinea may be threatened by the invasion of the poisonous Cane Toad (*Bufo marinus*) whose toxic secretions can kill animals that ingest it.

Venom and Bite: Probably the most dangerous member of the genus, with a high potential for lethality.

Antivenom: Papuan Blacksnake Antivenom
Producer: Commonwealth Serum Laboratories
Country of Origin: Australia

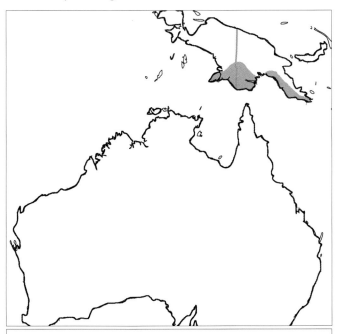

MAP 304. Range of the Papuan Blacksnake, *Pseudechis papuanus.*

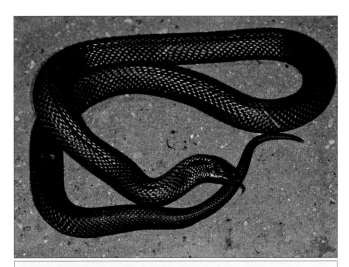

PHOTO 286. Papuan Blacksnake, *Pseudechis papuanus*

King Brown Snake,
Pseudechis australis

Description and Identification: Confusing with the true Brownsnakes (*Pseudonaja*, page 268) is common. In spite of the name, the King Brown snake is a member of the Australian Blacksnake genus (*Pseudechis*). This Blacksnake happens to be brown in color, and also quite large (maximum length just over 8 feet). It is the largest of the genus. The color is variable but usually some shade of brown. Can be reddish or yellowish.

Distribution, Habitat, and Biology: The most widespread member of the Australian Blacksnake genus. King Browns are found throughout nearly all of Australia except for the southernmost portion of the continent. They also occur in southern New Guinea. New Guinea populations are considered by many to be a distinct species, *P. rossignoli*, the Papuan Dwarf King Brown Snake. King Browns occur in nearly all habitats in Australia except permanent wetlands.

Venom and Bite: Being widespread and fairly common, the King Brown is responsible for a significant number of snakebites in Australia. The venom is less toxic than many other elapids in the region, but it possesses large amounts of venom. The Queensland Museum's "dangerousness index" ranks this species as the second most dangerous snake in Australia (Mirtschin & Davis, *Dangerous Snakes of Australia*, 1992). It should be noted that the index used to make that determination incorporated a total five factors, including venom toxicity, venom yield, fang length, temperament, and frequency of bite. Fatalities today are rare due mainly to advancements in snakebite therapy.

The Antivenom for treating bites is Blacksnake Antivenom by Commonwealth Serum Laboratories (CSL Limited) in Australia. Also listed is Polyvalent Snake Antivenom by the same producer.

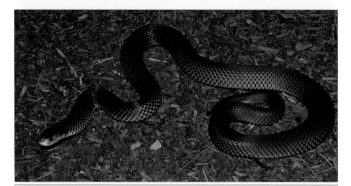

PHOTO 287. King Brown Snake, *Pseudechis australis*

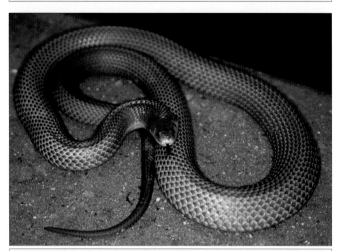

PHOTO 288. King Brown Snake, *Pseudechis australis*

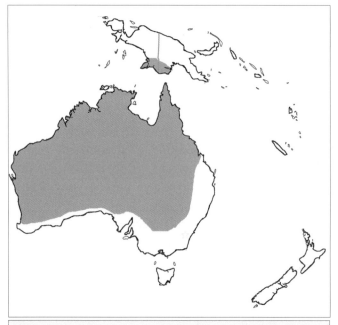

MAP 305. Range of the King Brown Snake, *Pseudechis australis.*

Red-bellied Blacksnake,
Pseudechis porphyriacus

Description and Identification: A large, shiny black snake with a bright red belly. Red pigment extends laterally onto the first few dorsal scale rows. Snout light brown. Maximum length just over 8 feet.

Distribution, Habitat, and Biology: Found in eastern Australia. Habitat is wetlands and mesic woodlands. Food mostly frogs but will opportunistically feed on any small vertebrate, including fish.

Venom and Bite: The venom has a relatively low potency and the yield is much less than the preceding species. Still, this is a dangerous snake and the potential for a lethal bite (especially in children) cannot be ruled out. Antivenom is Blacksnake Antivenom or Polyvalent Snake Antivenom by CSL Limited in Australia.

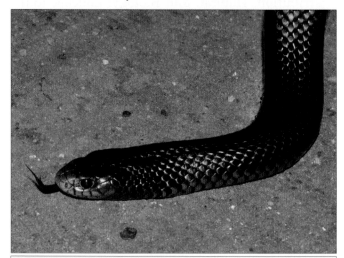

PHOTO 289. Red-bellied Blacksnake, *Pseudechis porphyriacus*

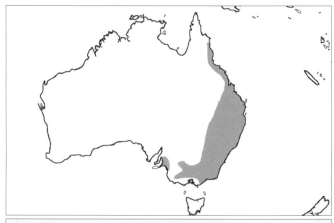

MAP 306. Range of the Red-bellied Blacksnake, *Pseudechis porphyriacus.*

Collett's Blacksnake,
Pseudechis colletti

Description and Identification: Adults average about 5 feet. Maximum length just over 6 feet. This is one of the most recognizable venomous snakes in the region. Color is black (rarely brown) with bright red or orange laterally that may extend across the top of the back to form red/orange bands.

Distribution, Habitat, and Biology: Endemic to Australia where it occupies a rather small range in central Queensland. Prefers dry habitats.

Venom and Bite: Both toxicity and yield are relatively low compared to other species in the region. Must still be regarded as potentially a deadly species. Antivenom is the same as for other Australian Blacksnakes.

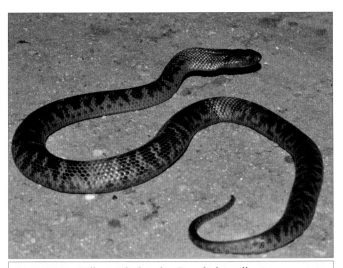

PHOTO 290. Collett's Blacksnake, *Pseudechis colletti*

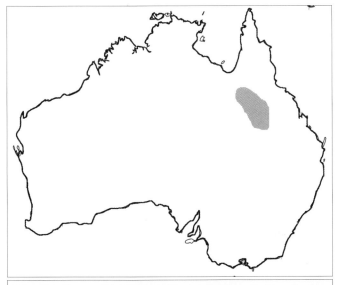

MAP 307. Range of the Collett's Blacksnake, *Pseudechis colletti.*

Additional Species: At least three other members of this genus occur. They are the Spotted Mulga Snake, *P. butleri*, the Spotted Black Snake, *P. guttatus*, and Weigel's Black Snake *P. weigeli.*

The ranges of these additional species is shown below.

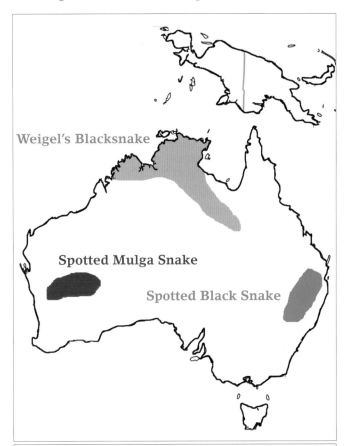

MAP 308. Range of the additional Australian Blacksnakes, *Pseudechis* species.

Family - Elapidae Genus - Salmonelaps

Solomons Coral Snake

In the 1965 edition of this book this snake was placed in the genus *Denisonia* (pg. 281) and was known as the Solomons Copperhead. Can grow to 4 feet but most are smaller. Dark gray to brown or reddish with faint whitish crossbands and white ventrals. Endemic to the Solomon Islands only.

Venom unknown. No Antivenom.

Family - Elapidae Genus - Austrelaps

Australian Copperheads

There are 3 species and all are native to Australia. One is also found in Tasmania. In 1965 a single species was recognized but it was then included in the genus *Denisonia*. Copperheads are heavy bodied snakes with small pointed heads and no distinct neck. Unlike most elapids, the Australian Copperheads are Viviparous.

Definition: Head small and not distinct from neck. Snout pointed.

Eyes moderately large, pupils round.

Body scales: Dorsals smooth in 15-17 (rarely 19) rows. First row of dorsal scales enlarged. Ventrals 140-165; subcaudals 35-55 single.

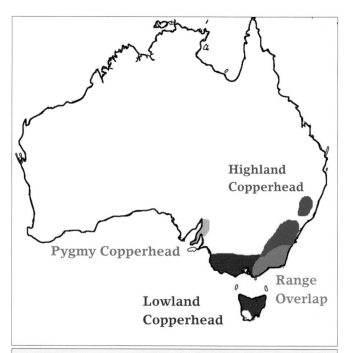

MAP 309. Range of the Australian Copperheads, *Australaps* species.

Common Copperhead,

Australaps superbus

Description and Identification: Averages about 4.5 feet. Can grow to nearly 6 feet. The most striking morphological feature of the copperheads is the noticeably powerful body. A 5 foot specimen is a rather large and heavy snake. Uniformly brown in color, varying from light tan to coppery to nearly black.

Distribution, Habitat, and Biology: The Common Copperhead, also goes by the name Lowland Copperhead a reference to its preferred habitat. Eats lizards, frogs, mammals, and other snakes.

Venom and Bite: Copperhead venom is a neurotoxin and the potential for inflicting a fatal bite is high with larger specimens. Early use of antivenom is imperative, as some neurotoxic effects may be irreversible past a certain point (Marcon and Nicholson, 2011). No specific antivenom is produced. Tiger Snake Antivenom or Polyvalent Snake Antivenom (both by CSL Limited in Australia) are listed as effective in treating bites by *Austrelaps* species.

Additional Species: The two other Australian Copperhead species are very similar. The Highland Copperhead (*A. ramsayi*) is more at home in upland areas, while the Pygmy Copperhead (*A. labialis*) is smaller (average 2 feet, maximum 3 feet).

Family - Elapidae Genus - Denisonia

Ornamental Snakes

Represented by 2 species of small (18-24 inches) heavy bodied, smooth scaled dark brown or black snakes that are endemic to Queensland and New South Wales (Australia). Neither species is considered dangerous to man but they are included here because the genus *Denisonia* was included in the original edition of *Poisonous Snakes of the World.* Ironically, in that original volume the genus *Denisonia* was made up of the Australian Copperheads (*Austrelaps*) and the Solomons Coral Snake (*Salmonelaps*).

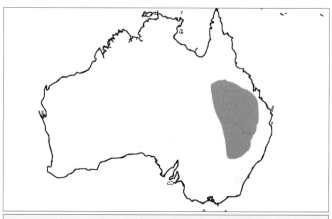

MAP 310. Range of the Ornamental Snakes, *Denisonia* species.

Family - Elapidae Genus - Demansia

Whipsnakes

There are 13 species of Whipsnakes native to Australia and New Guinea. These alert, slender, and fast moving snakes remind American herpetologists of the harmless racers and coachwhips of southern North America. *Demansia* however are front fanged elapids (cobra family). The venom is relatively mild and bites by these snakes are not generally considered to be life threatening. Some species however may be more dangerous.

The uniform dorsal coloration is some shade of brown or black. Some specimens have distinctive light and dark rings on the neck or head. Overall they resemble both the Brown Snakes and the Australian Blacksnakes and they are frequently confused with those more dangerous species. Most species average about 3-4 feet. The largest can reach 6 feet.

List of Whipsnake Species:

Olive Whipsnake - *D. olivacea*

Greater Black Whipsnake - *D. papuensis*

Narrow-headed Whipsnake - *D. angusticeps*

Black-necked Whipsnake - *D. calodera*

Carpentaria Whipsnake - *D. flagellatio*

Yellow-faced Whipsnake - *D. psammophis*

Sombre Whipsnake - *D. queasitor*

Crack-dwelling Whipsnake - *D. rimicola*

Rufous Whipsnake - *D. rufescens*

Shine's Whipsnake *D. shinei*

Gray Whipsnake - *D. simplex*

Collared Whipsnake - *D. torquata*

Lesser Black Whipsnake - *D. vestigiata*

Venom and Bite: There are some unknowns regarding the venom and its effects in humans. Many known bites have resulted in only minor, localized symptoms. There has apparently been at least one death from the bite of *D. vestigiata* (Australian Venom Research Institute - www.avru.org, viewed 2012). Also, Clinical Toxinology Resources website (www.toxinology.com, viewed 2012) lists *D. rufescens* as possibly dangerously venomous.

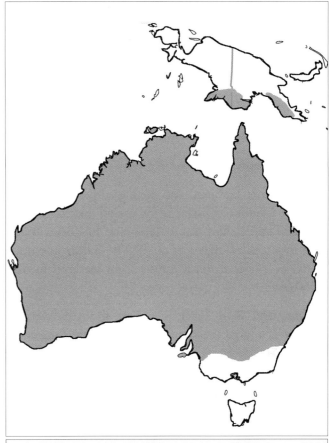

MAP 311. Combined range of the Whipsnakes, *Demansia* species.

Family - Elapidae Genus - Micropechis

New Guinea Small-eyed Snake

A single species is recognized.

Definition: Head fairly distinct from neck; snout pointed. Body moderately stout, cylindrical; tail short.

Eyes very small; pupils round.

Head scales: There usual 9 on the crown; rostral broad and obtusely pointed. Laterally, nasal in contact with preocular.

Body scales: Dorsals smooth in 15 oblique rows throughout body. Ventrals 178-225; anal plate divided; subcaudals 36-55 paired.

New Guinea Small-eyed Snake,
Micropechis ikaheka

Description and Identification: Adults average between 3 and 4 feet. Occasional individuals attain lengths in excess of 5 feet; record 7 feet (Williams, et al., 2004).

Body coloration made up of yellow (or tan) and black (or brown) scales. Black scales roughly arranged in irregular crossbands but each is edged with yellow- sometimes to the extent that the pattern is lost. In specimens from eastern New Guinea the pattern may be lost on the anterior one-third of the body which is brown, but the crossbands persist posteriorly. Belly color yellow with some scutes edged with black.

Dorsals smooth and glossy, in 15 rows at midbody.

Distribution, Habitat, and Biology: New Guinea and the Aru Islands. Thought to be mainly terrestrial with fossorial tendencies, but at least one has been found high in a tree (Williams et al., 2004). Mainly nocturnal in habits. Mesic tropical forests from sea level to over 4,000 feet.

Venom and Bite: Little is known about the venom, but this is a large snake and probably quite dangerous. Deaths from its bite have been recorded.

Family - Elapidae Genus - Loveridgelaps

Solomon Small-eyed Snake

Another genus containing a single species, *L. elapoides*, the Solomon Small-eyed Snake. In many respects very similar to the New Guinea Small-eyed snake and the two were once considered to be congeneric. Endemic to the Solomon Islands (presence confirmed on Guadalcanal, Gizo, Santa Isabel, and Florida islands). No antivenom.

Family - Elapidae Genus - Tropidechis

Rough-scaled Snake

In 1965 two species were recognized. Today *T. sadlier* is regarded as synonomous with *T. carinatus,* the Rough-scaled Snake by most sources.

Definition: Head distinct from neck; a distinct canthus rostralis. Body moderately stout and cylindrical; tail moderately long.

Eyes moderate in size; pupils round.

Head scales: The usual 9 on the crown. Laterally, nasally in contact with preocular.

Body scales: Dorsals heavily keeled in 23 rows at midbody. Ventrals 160-185, anal plate entire; subcaudals 50-60 undivided.

Can grow to about 40 inches. Coloration is brown with irregular dark spots that may form crossbands dorso-anteriorly.

Venom and Bite: Regarded as dangerously venomous. Has caused at least one fatality. No specific antivenom is available but Clinical Toxinology Resources of Australia lists Tiger Snake Antivenom by CSL Limited of Australia for treating bites.

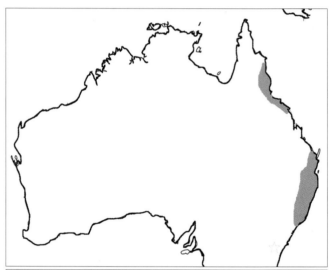

MAP 312. Range of the Rough-scaled Snake, *Tropedechis carinatus.*

Family - Elapidae Genus-Rhinoplocephalus

Square-nosed Snake

Some sources today list 5 species. Others believe that additional species added since the 1965 edition of this book belong in the genus *Cryptohis*. That determination is being followed here. In 1965 this snake was called Mueller's Snake.

A single species, *R. bicolor* is known from southern Western Australia. It is small, up to about 16 inches in length. It is a nocturnal, fossorial snake.

Definition: Head small and only slightly distinct from neck; snout broad and flattened. Body cylindrical and moderately slender; tail short.

Eyes small; pupils round.

Head scales: Internasals absent, giving 78 instead of the usual 9 scales on the crown. Rostral very broad and only slightly free from other scales on the sides. Laterally, nasal in contact with preocular (with the lower preocular when there are two).

Body scales: Dorsals smooth, in 15 rows at midbody; reduced to 13 posteriorly. Ventrals 149-159; anal plate entrie; subcaudals single, 28-34.

Venom and Bite: In 1965 the original authors of this book did not regard this as a dangerous species. It is now suspected to possibly caused at least one death. Their is no antivenom available.

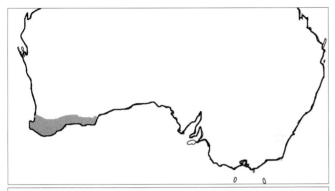

Map 313. Range of the Square-nosed Snake, *Rhinoplocephalus bicolor.*

Family - Elapidae Genus - Hoplocephalus
Broad-headed Snakes

Three species are currently recognized; all are Australian. They appear to be the only Australian elapid snakes that are specialized for an arboreal life. Only one of the species, *H. bungaroides*, attains a large enough size to be a danger, though probably the others also can deliver a painful bite.

Definition: Head broad and distinct from the slender neck; no canthus rostralis. Body relatively slender; tail moderately long.

Eyes moderate in size; pupils round.

Head scales: The normal 9 on the crown; frontal rather long. Laterally, nasal in contact with preocular.

Body scales: Dorsals smooth, in 21 rows at midbody, fewer posteriorly. Ventrals laterally angulate and notched (a typical indication of a treesnake), 221-227; anal plate entire; subcaudals single, 40-60.

Three genera of harmless tree snakes also occur in Australia. All may be distinguished from *Hoplocephalus* by a loreal scale, (giving 3 scales between the nostril and eye) and a longer tail (more than 80 subcaudals).

Broad-headed Snake,
Hoplocephalus bungaroides

Description and Identification: In the 1965 edition of *Poisonous Snakes of the World*, this snake was referred to as the Australian Yellow-spotted Snake. The broad head and eyes with round pupils; angulated, keeled, and notched ventral scutes, and moderately long tail distinguish this snake. Adults average 3 to 4 feet in length; some individuals attain a length of 5 feet.

Ground color black or dark brown. Numerous conspicous yellow spots form irregular crossbands or a broken network over the body. Tail solid black or almost so.

Dorsal scales in 21 rows at midbody; 2114-221 ventrals; 40-60 subcaudals.

Distribution, Habitat, and Biology: With the smallest range of any of the three *Hoplocephalus* species, *bungaroides* is restricted to a specialized habitat of sandstone outcroppings in the vicinity of the city of Sydney (Australia) and is now regarded as an endangered species.

Venom and Bite: No known fatalities, but some bites have produced serious symptoms. Venom mainly procoagulants. Possibly capable of inflicting a lethal bite.

Additonal Species: *H. stephensi,* Stephen's Banded Snake is black with pale gray bands. The Pale-headed Snake, *H. bitorquatus* is a slaty gray or black snake with a pale gray to whitish head that is distinctly marked with irregular black spots.

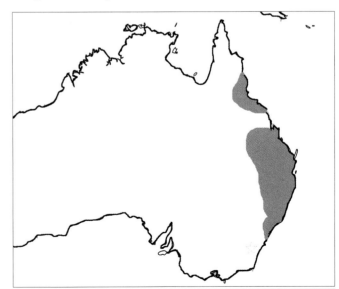

Map 314. Combined range of the Broad-headed Snakes, *Hoplocephalus* species.

Author's Note: The following genus and species accounts are of a conglomerate of small, front-fanged elapids native to the USPACOM-Part 2 region. Though these are technically venomous snakes, they are not generally regarded as dangerous to man. In that manner they are of little significance as a snakebite threat and thus their inclusion here deviates from the format of the other chapters in this book (where only those species known to be dangerous to man are included).

However, the original authors of this book elected to include several of the following Australia/New Guinea genera and species that were known to science in 1965. In keeping with that tradition, I have included those that were in the original edition as well as the newer genera and species that have become known since 1965.

Family - Elapidae Genus - Elapognathus

Little Brown Snakes

This genus contains two species (*E. cornutus* and *E. minor*). They grow to about 16 inches. They are found only in the southwestern section of Western Australia and are not considered dangerous.

Definition: Head small and only slightly distinct from neck. Body cylindrical and moderately stout; tail moderate in length.

Eyes rather large; pupils round.

Head scales: The usual 9 on the crown. Laterally, the long nasal is in contact with the single preocular.

Body scales: Dorsals smooth but finely striated, in 15 rows at midbody; fewer (13) posteriorly. Ventrals 120-130; anal plate entire; subcaudals single, 52-68.

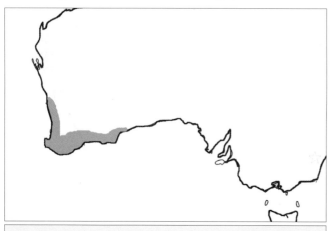

MAP 315. Combined range of the Little Brown Snakes, *Elapognathus* species.

Family - Elapidae Genus-Parapistocalmus

Bougainville Coral Snake

In the 1965 edition of this volume this species went by the common name Hediger's Snake.

A single species, *P. hedigeri*, is known from Bougainville Island, Solomons group. It is a small burrowing snake; the largest known specimen is about 20 inches in length. It is not believed to be a dangerous species.

Definition: Head small and not distinct from neck; no canthus rostralis; snout conspicuously blunted. Body cylindrical and moderately slender; tail short.

Eyes very small; pupils round.

Head scales: The usual 9 on the crown; frontal and prefrontals very broad; rostral broad. Laterally, preocular present or fused with prefrontal; if present preocular in contact with nasal or separated from it by prefrontal.

Body scales: Dorsals smooth, in 15 rows throughout body. Ventrals 159-169; anal plate divided or entire; subcaudals paired, 32-35.

Family - Elapidae Genus - Aspidomorphus

Crown Snakes

Three species are known. All are endemic to New Guinea. These are small snakes less than 2 feet in length. Though technically venomous, they are not known to be dangerous to man. No Antivenom.

List of Species:

    Striped Crown Snake - *A. lineaticollis*
    Mueller's Crowned Snake - *A. muelleri*
    Schlegel's Crowned Snake - *A. schlegeli*

Family - Elapidae Genus - Echiopsis

Bardick

This genus contains a single species. *Echiopsis curta*, the Bardick is a small (2 feet), smooth scaled heavy bodied snake that is typically a uniformly brown color. Virtually nothing is known of its venom and it is not regarded as deadly to man. Its range is the southern regions of Western and South Australia.

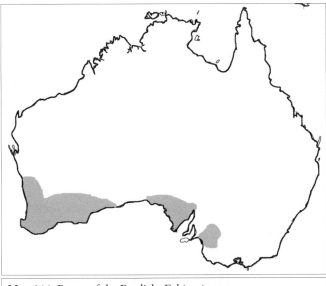

MAP 316. Range of the Bardick, *Echiopsis curta.*

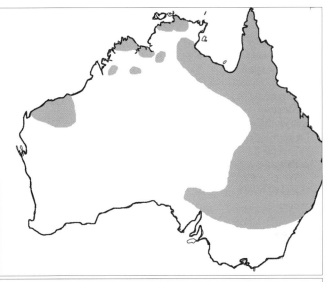

MAP 317. Combined range of the Bandy Bandys, *Vermicilla* species.

Family - Elapidae Genus - Paraplocehalus

Lake Cronin Snake

A single species similar in appearance to the Bardick and listed by some sources in the genus *Echiopsis*. Very limited range in Lake Cronin area of Western Australia. Not dangerous to man.

Family - Elapidae Genus - Vermicella

Bandy Bandys

Five species are recognized. All occur in Australia. None appears to exceed 3 feet in length and they are not considered dangerous.

Definition: Head small and not distinct from neck; no canthus rostralis. Body rather slender and cylindrical; tail very short and obtusely pointed.

Eyes very small; pupils round.

Head scales: The usual 9 scales ordinarily present on the crown; the small internasals sometimes fused to prefrontal, giving 7 scales. Laterally, nasal in contact with preocular and first 2 supralabials.

Body scales: Dorsals smooth, in 15 rows at midbody. Ventrals 126-234; anal plate divided; subcaudals paired, 14-30.

The Bandy Bandys are all similarly colored with distinctive black and white bands.

Family - Elapidae Genus - Toxicocalamus

New Guinea Forest Snakes

In the 1965 edition of *Poisonous Snakes of the World* this genus contained only 2 species. Today at least 9 species are known (some sources list 11). Some of those were formerly contained in the genera *Apisthocalamus* and the *Ultrocalamus.* Both those genera were included in the 1965 edition of *Poisonous Snakes of the World,* but both are now considered synonymous with the genus *Toxicocalamus.*

These are small snakes (from 12 to 24 inches as adults) but one can reach nearly 3 feet. All are endemic to the Island of New Guinea. None are considered dangerous to man.

Species List:
    Buerger's Forest Snake - *T. buergersi*
    Setekwa River Forest Snake - *T. grandis*
    Mt. Rossell Forest Snake - *T. holopelturus*
    Woodlark Island Forest Snake - *T. longissimus*
    Loriae Forest Snake - *T. loriae*
    Misima Forest Snake - *T. misimae*
    Preuss's Forest Snake - *T. preussi*
    Spotted Forest Snake - *T. spiliolepidotus*
    Owen Stanley Range Forest Sn. - *T. stanleyanus*

Family - Elapidae Genus - Cryptophis
Small-eyed Snakes

There are 5 species. Some sources include these snakes in the *Rhinoplocephalus* genus. They are found in coastal areas of northern and eastern Australia and on the island of New Guinea.

Species List:
Carpentaria Snake - *C. boschmai*
Pink Snake - *C. incredibilis*
Eastern Small-eyed Snake - *C. nigrescens*
Northern Small-eyed Snake - *C. pallidiceps*
Black-striped Snake - *C. nigrostriatus*

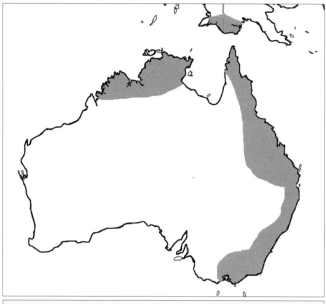

MAP 318. Combined range of the Small-eyed Snakes, *Cryptophis* species.

Family - Elapidae Genus - Furina
Naped Snakes

In 1965 these small snakes were placed in the genus *Glyphodon* and went by the common name Australian Collared Snakes. There are 5 species, all but one restricted to Australia. One species also ranges northward onto New Guinea and small islands off the northern coast of Australia. Collectively they range throughout most of the northern half of Australia. In color they are usually a drab brown, reddish brown, or black without discernible dorsal pattern. The name "Naped Snakes" comes from the presence of a light band across the nape in some species.

Though venomous and members of the cobra family, they are not regarded as dangerous to man and are reportedly reluctant to even bite.

List of Species:
Yellow-naped Snake - *F. barnardi*
Red-naped Snake - *F. diadema*
Dunmall's Snake - *F. dunmalli*
Orange-naped Snake - *F. ornata*
Brown-headed Snake - *F. tristis*

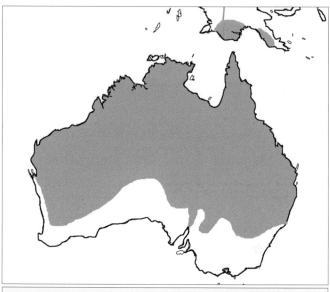

MAP 319. Combined range of the Naped Snakes, *Furina* species.

Family - Elapidae Genus - Brachyurophis
Shovel-nosed Snakes

Known as Girdled Snakes in the 1965 edition of this book. Seven species are currently recognized. They inhabit most of Australia except for the humid southeastern coastal regions. All are small sand dwelling burrowing species and are not believed to be dangerous.

Definition: Head short and not distinct from neck; snout distinctly pointed; no canthus rostralis. Body moderately slender with little taper; tail short.

Eyes small; pupils round.

Head scales: The usual 9 on the crown; rostral shovel-like with sharp anterior edge and with an angulate rear edge that partly divides internasals. Laterally, nasal in contact with preocular.

Body scales: Dorsals smooth;, in 15-17 nonoblique rows at midbody. Ventrals 133-170; anal plate divided; subcaudals paired, 17-27.

Species List:

Northwest Shovel-nosed Snake - *B. approximans*
Australian Coral Snake - *B. australis*
Narrow-banded Shovel-nosed Sn. - *B. fasciolatus*
Unbanded Shovel-nosed Snake - *B. incintus*
Arnhem Shovel-nosed Snake - *B. morrisi*
Northern Shovel-nosed Snake- *B. roperi*
Southern Shovel-nosed Snake - *B. semifaciatus*

Note: Some sources (www.reptile-database.org) place all the above species in the genus *Simoselaps* (below).

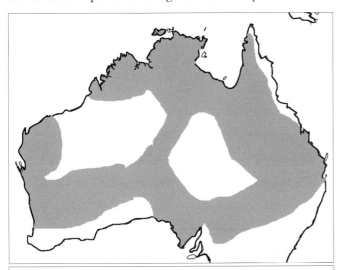

MAP 320. Combined range of the Shovel-nosed Snakes, *Brachyurophis* species.

Family - Elapidae Genus - Simoselaps

Desert Banded Snakes

Some sources regard the genus *Brachyurophis* (pg. 287) as synonymous with this genus. In 1965 only two species of *Simoselaps* were known and they were placed in the genus *Rynchoelaps*. Today at least four species are known. All are endemic to Australia.

These are small snakes that average only about a foot in length. None are dangerous to man. The ground color is orange or greenish gray. Three species are distinctly banded with black bands.

Definition: Head small, flattened above but not distinct from the neck; snout prominent, with obtusely angular edge; canthus rostralis indistinct. Body cylindrical, moderately slender; tail short.

Eyes small; pupils round.

Head scales: The usual 9 on the crown; rostral broad, obtusely angulate posteriorly; frontal long, much broader than superoculars. Laterally, nasal long. In contact with preocular.

Body scales: Dorsals smooth, in 15 nonoblique rows throughout body. Ventrals 122-126; anal plate divided; subcaudals paired, 15-25

Species List:

Desert Banded Snake - *S. anomalus*
Jan's Banded Snake - *S. bertholdi*
West Coast Banded Snake - *S. littoralis*
Dampierland Burrowing Snake- *S. minimus*

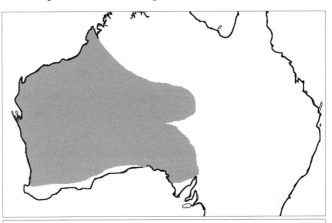

MAP 321. Combined range of the Desert Banded Snakes, *Simoselaps* species.

Family - Elapidae Genus - Ogmodon

Fiji Snake

A singe species, *O. vitianus*, is known from Viti Levu and perhaps other islands of the Fiji group. It is a small burrowing snake; reported lengths are under 20 inches. It is not believed to be a dangerous species.

Definition: Head small and not distinct from neck; no canthus rostralis; snout pointed. Body cylindrical and moderately slender; tail short.

Eyes small; pupils round.

Head scales: The usual 9 on the crown; internasal very small, prefrontals very large and in contact with eye. Laterally, nasal fused to upper labial; small preocular elongate, not in contact with nasal, commonly fused with third upper labial.

Body scales: Dorsals smooth, in 17 rows throughout body. Ventrals 139-152; anal plate divided; subcaudals paired, 27-38.

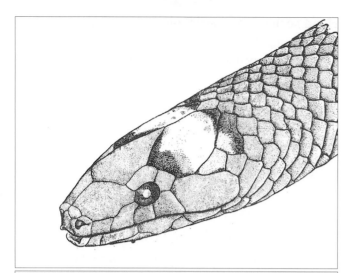

FIGURE 9. Head scales of Fiji Snake, *Ogmodon vitianus*. The top ot the third upper labial is often separated as a preocular. Drawing by Samuel B. McDowell.

Family - Elapidae

Genera - Drysdalia, Antaioserpens, Neelaps, Parasuta, Suta, Hemiaspis, Cacophis

Miscelleneous Small Australian Elapids

The following group of snakes represent a "catch all" listing of the remaining species of small elapid snakes found in Australia. These snakes, although technically venomous, are not a threat to man.

Species List:

Note: The first three species are listed by some sources as members of the genus *Simoselaps*.

Antioserpens:

White-lipped Snake - *A. warrio*

Neelaps:

Black Naped Snake - *N. bimaculata*
Black Striped Snake - *N. calanotus*

Drysdalia:

White-lipped Snake - *D. coronoides*
Master's Snake - *D. mastersii*
Mustard-bellied Snake - *D. rhodogaster*

Parasuta:

Dwyer's Snake - *P. dwyeri*
Little Whip Snake - *P. flagellum*
Gould's Hooded Snake - *P. gouldii*
Monk Snake - *P. monachus*
Mitchell's Short-tailed Snake - *P. nigriceps*
Mallee Black-headed Snake - *P. spectabilis*

Suta:

Rosen's Snake - *S. fasciata*
Ord Curl Snake - *S. ordensis*
Little Spotted Snake - *S. punctata*
Curl Snake - *S. suta*

Hemiaspis:

Marsh Snake - *H. signata*
Grey Snake - *H. damellii*

Cacophis:

Northern Dwarf Crowned Snake - *C. churchilli*
White Crowned Snake - *C. harriettae*
Southern Dwarf Crowned Snake - *C. krefftii*
Golden Crowned Snake - *C. squamulosus*

Current References

Books

Dowling, Herndon G., Sherman A. Minton, and Findlay E. Russell. 1965. *Poisonous Snakes of the World.* Department of the Navy Bureau of Medicine and Surgery. Washington, DC.

Mirtschin, Peter and Richard Davis. 1992. *Dangerous Snakes of Australia.* New Holland Ltd. London, England.

O'Shea, Mark. 2005. *Venomous Snakes of the World.* Princeton University Press. Princeton, NJ.

Williams, David, Dr. Simon Jensen, & Dr. Keith D. Winkel. 2004. *Clinical Management of Snakebite in Papua New Guinea.* Independent Publishing. Port Moresby, New Guinea.

Journals

Raymond Hoser. 1998. "Death Adders (Genus *Acanthophis*): An overview, including descriptions of five new species and one subspecies". Monitor 9 (2), 20-41.

Marcon, Francesca and Graham M. Nicholson. 2011. "Identification of presynaptic neurotoxin complexes in the venoms of three Australian copperheads (*Austrelaps* ssp.) and the efficacy of tiger snake antivenom to prevent or reverse neurotoxicity". Toxicon 58 (5), 439-452.

Websites

University of Adelaide, Clinical Toxinology Resources Wesbsite (2012) - www.toxinology.com

World Health Organization - www.who.int/bloodproducts/snakeantivenoms/database

The Reptile Database - http//www.reptiledata-base.org

Armed Forces Pest Management Board - www.afpmb.org/content/living-hazards-database

Catalogue of Life - www.catalogueoflife.org

iucnredlist.org

Australian Reptile Online Database- www.arod.com.au

Australian Venom Researach Unit - www.avru.org

Original References

BOGERT, Charles M., and Bessie L. MATALAS. 1945. Results of the Archbold Expeditions. No. 53. A Review of the Elapid Genus *Ultrocalamus* of New Guinea. Am. Mus. Novitates 1244: 8 p., 10 figs.

KINGHORN, J. R. 1956. The Snakes of Australia. 2nd ed. Angus & Robertson Ltd., Sydney. 197 p., illustrated in color.

KINGHORN, J. R., and C. H. KELLAWAY. 1943. The Dangerous Snakes of the South-West Pacific Area. Victorian Railways Printing Works, North Melbourne. 43 p., 11 text figs., 3 pls.

LOVERIDGE, Arthur. 1945. Reptiles of the Pacific World. MacMillan Co., New York. 259 p., 7 pls.

LOVERIDGE, Arthur. 1948. New Guinean Reptiles and Amphibians in the Museum of Comparative Zoology and United States National Museum. Bull. Museum Comp. Zool., 101 (2) : 305–430.

ROOIJ, Nelly de. 1917. The Reptiles of the Indo-Australian Archipelago. Vol. II. Ophidia. E. J. Brill Ltd., Leiden. 334 p., 117 text figs.

WERLER, John E., and Hugh L. KEEGAN. 1963. Venomous Snakes of the Pacific Area pp. 217–325, figs. 1–78. *In* H. L. Keegan and W. V. MacFarlane, Venomous and Poisonous Animals and Noxious Plants of the Pacific Region. MacMillan Co., New York.

WILLIAMS, Ernest E., and Fred PARKER. 1964. The Snake Genus *Parapistocalamus* on Bougainville, Solomon Islands (Serpentes, Elapidae). Senckenbergiana-Biol., 45 (3/5) : 543–552, figs. 1–5.

WORRELL, Eric. 1963. Dangerous Snakes of Australia and New Guinea. 5th ed. Angus & Robertson Ltd., Sydney. 68 p., illustrated.

WORRELL, Eric. 1963. Reptiles of Australia : Crocodiles, Turtles, Tortoises, Lizards, Snakes.
Angus & Robertson Ltd., Sydney. 207 p., 64 pls. (some in color).

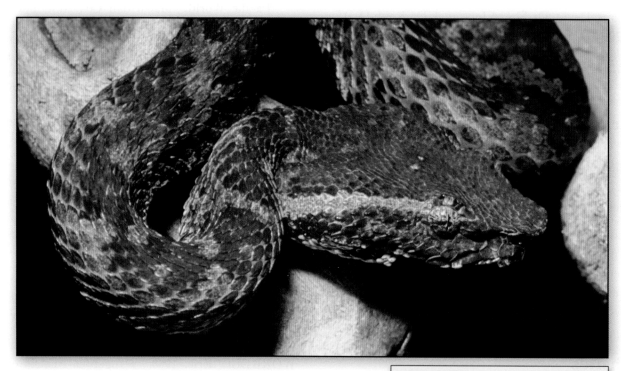

Ashy Pit Viper,
Trimeresurus puniceus

CHAPTER **15**

SEA SNAKES
REGION: GLOBAL

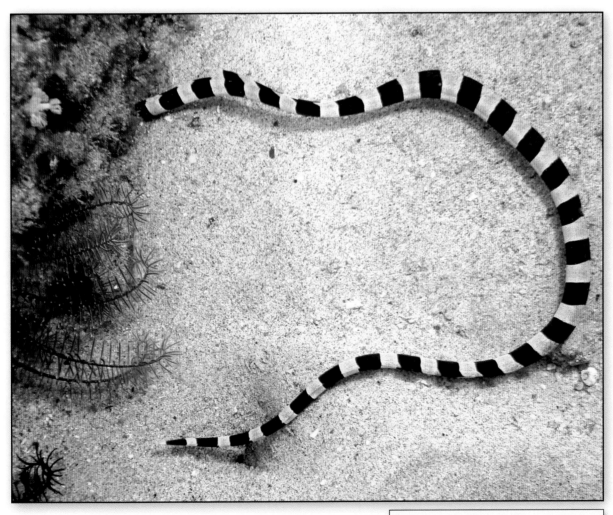

Yellow-lipped Sea Krait,
Laticauda colubrina

Introduction

The sea snakes comprise a group of some 69 species all of which have strongly flattened oar-like tails used as sculls. In addition, most species have nostrils opening on top of the head, a body that is flattened from side to side, and very small ventral scutes that may be difficult to distinguish from the adjoining scales. The scales of several kinds of sea snakes are juxtaposed rather than overlapping as in most land snakes. The only snakes likely to be confused with sea snakes are the elephant-trunk snakes (Acrochordus) and the river snakes (Enhydris and others); these have round or slightly flattened tails, but young elephant-trunk snakes have tails as paddle-shaped as those of some sea snakes. However, all sea snakes have enlarged crown shields and the elephant-trunk snakes have only small juxtaposed scales. Eels are frequently confused with sea snakes; however, no sea snake has fins or gill openings, and none has a smooth skin without scales.

Sea snakes are reptiles essentially of south Asian and Australian coastal waters with a few species found well out into Oceania (Society and Gilbert Islands). One species, the Pelagic Sea Snake (*Pelamis*), occurs far out into the open ocean ranging across the Pacific to the western coasts of Central and South America and south to New Zealand and the Cape of Good Hope. No sea snake is found in the Atlantic, although the Pelagic Sea Snake may eventually find its way through the Panama Canal and become established in the Caribbean. The greatest numbers of both species and individuals are found in warm shallow waters without surf or strong currents. Mouths of rivers, bays, and mangrove swamps are especially favored. Many species of sea snakes enter brackish or fresh water occasionally; two species are restricted to lakes.

The biology of sea snakes is poorly known. There is a general opinion that they can remain submerged for long periods, perhaps a few hours depending upon temperature, degree of activity, and other factors. The depths to which they can dive are also unknown. An observer in the Philippines saw the snakes swim down out of sight in very clear water. Types of bottom dwelling fish found in stomachs indicate the snakes dive at least 20-30 feet to capture food. They are often seen at the surface in calm weather, and some species aggregate there in vast numbers. The reasons for this behavior are unknown, but they may relate to breeding.

There are reports of both nocturnal and diurnal activity. In the Arabian Sea, some species range 10-20 miles off shore during the calm winter months but tend to seek coastal mangrove swamps during the monsoon storms. Their young are born in these swamps. Sea snakes feed largely upon fish. Eels are a favorite food of several species. At least a few species eat prawns and one species feeds on fish eggs.

Sea snakes are generally mild tempered reptiles, although both individual and species variation exists with respect to this trait. In open water they seek to escape or remain almost indifferent to swimmers. Stranded on beaches, some species are almost totally helpless. Others crawl with varying degrees of facility. None can strike on land but most can turn to make an awkward snapping bite. Bites are usually seen when snakes are slapped, kicked, or trodden upon in shallow water or when they are removed from nets, traps, or other fishing gear.

Some kinds of sea snakes are extensively used for human food in China, Japan, and parts of Polynesia.

While some sea snake species can be identified readily by the amateur, many are puzzling even to experienced herpetologists. Color and pattern are extremely deceptive in this family. There are close similarities between remotely related species and marked differences between young and adults of the same species as well as a good deal of variation among adults of the same species.

Sea snakes are members of the family Elapidae (cobra family) and many possess highly potent neurotoxic venom. There are two subfamilies, Hydrophiinae (sea snakes), and Laticaudinae (sea Kraits).

Global Distribution of the Sea Snakes

(family-Elapidae, subfamilies-Hydrophiinae and Laticaudinae)

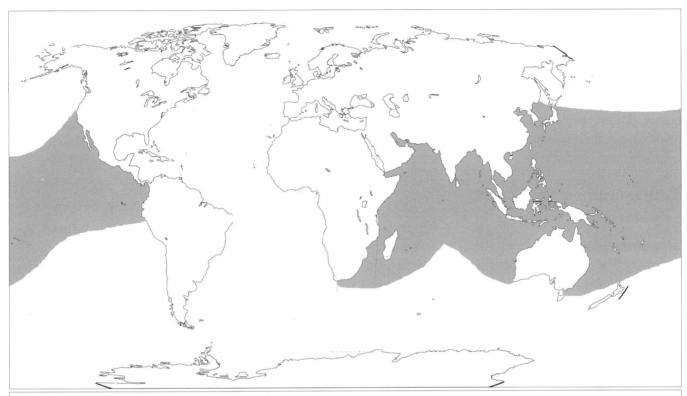

MAP 322. Range of the Pelagic Sea Snake, *Pelamis platurus*

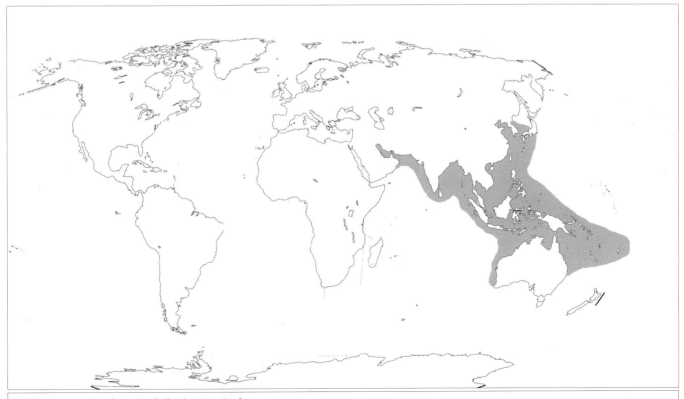

MAP 323. Combined range of all other Sea Snake species.

Sea Kraits

The sea kraits differ from other sea snakes primarily by being less aquatic species that frequently leave the sea and come onto land. They drink fresh water and emerge from their marine environment to sun bath, breed, and lay eggs. Some species occasional travel overland for some distance. This is a small subfamily consisting of a single genus with only 6 species. The snakes of this genus are known to have post-synaptic neurotoxins and myotoxins in their venom. They are quite deadly.

Yellow-lipped Sea Krait,
Laticauda colubrina

Identification: Species of this genus are less flattened and more like conventional land snakes than are other members of the Hydrophiinae (sea snake sub-family). They can be readily identified by the combination of flattened tail, enlarged ventral scutes, and laterally placed nostrils. In this species the pattern consists of black or dark brown bands encircling body and separated by interspaces of pale blue or blue gray ground color; these are about as wide as the bands; snout and upper lip yellow; dark stripes though eye and on lower lip; belly yellow.

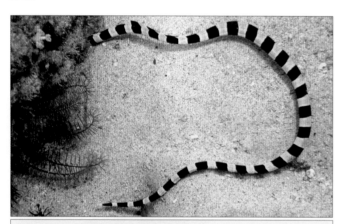

Photo 291. Yellow-lipped Sea Krait, *Laticauda colubrina*

Maximum length about 4.5 feet, average 3-3.5 feet. Females are larger than males.

Remarks: One of the few sea snakes that regularly leaves water to climb onto rocks and pilings. Terrestrial activity usually takes place at night. Eggs are deposited in caves and crevices. Very mild disposition-no report of bite in man although the snakes are freely handled by many natives. Venom of fairly high toxicity bur very small in quantity.

Additional Species: The *Laticauda* are the only genus of the subfamily Laticaudinae (sea kraits). There are a total of 6 known species (some sources list 8). The additional species are listed below:

Crocker's Sea Krait - *L. crockerei*
Vanuatu Sea Krait - *L. frontalis*
Brown-lipped Sea Krait - *L. laticaudata*
L. guineai
L. saintgironsi

The last 2 species have no accepted common name. Antivenom is: Sea Snake Antivenom by Commonwealth Serum Laboratories (CSL Limited) in Australia.

True Sea Snakes

The remaining 63 species of sea snakes are members of the subfamily Hydrophiinae, usually referred to as the "true" sea snakes, these snakes are much more aquatic and never come onto land as do the Laticaudinae (sea kraits). Although totally marine in habits most species associate with shallow waters around reefs, mangroves, mouths of rivers, and shorelines. Several do range many miles from land and one species is totally pelagic.

The venom consists of post-synaptic neurotoxins and myotoxins and in most species it is extremely potent, far surpassing the toxicity of most of the world's deadly land snakes.

Pelagic Sea Snake,
Pelamis platurus

Identification: Head elongate, flat, slightly wider than neck; body of moderate build, very strongly compressed laterally; the entire appearance is very eel-like. Head shields large, symmetrical; body scales small, quadrangular; ventrals not larger than adjacent scales.

The commonest color variety is black or dark brown above, dark yellow to brown below with a pale yellow lateral stripe. Another common variety is yellow with a straight edged brown or black dorsal stripe. In less common forms, the dark stripe may be wavy or broken into transverse bars. The head is usually dark on top and yellow on the sides; the tail is whitish barred or mottled with black.

The average adult length is 25 to 30 inches with a maximum of 44 inches.

Remarks: This is the only truly ocean-going snake; it has repeatedly been seen hundreds of miles from land and has reached many remote pacific islands including Hawaii. It is nonetheless, the most plentiful in the comparatively shallow waters over the continental shelves. Although a graceful, rapid swimmer, it seems to spend much time floating at the surface. It is virtually helpless on land. Great schools of these snakes have been seen in the shallow waters along the west coast of tropical Americas at certain seasons. This is a species that seems to be definitely repelled by fresh or brackish water and does not enter creeks or rivers.

Only minute amounts of venom can be obtained from this species in the laboratory, and the toxicity is about one fourth that of Enhydrina. Only one human fatality has been ascribed to the bite of *Pelamis.*

The Pelagic Sea Snake is the most wide-ranging snake species on earth (see Map 322 on page 289). Although it is quite venomous, it poses little threat to humans because of its adaptation to life in the open sea .

Antivenom: Sea Snake Antivenom by Commonwealth Serum Laboratories (CSL Limited) in Australia.

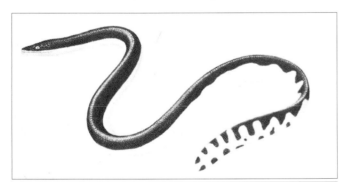

Photo 292. Pelagic Sea Snake, *Pelamis platurus*

Beaked Sea Snake,
Enhydrina schistosa

Identification: The distinctive feature of this sea snake is the form of the lower jaw. The shield at the tip of the chin (the mental) which is comparatively wide and large in most snakes is, in *Enhydra*, reduced to a splinter like shield buried in a cleft between the first pair of lower labials. This gives greater flexibility to the lower jaw and widens the gape thus permitting the snake to seize and swallow large prey. The down curved tip of the rostral is unusually prominent in this snake giving it a characteris-

tic beaked profile. Head shields large, symmetrical; head rather small, very little wider than neck; body moderately stout, strongly compressed; skin especially on neck rather loose; scales keeled; ventrals poorly differentiated, often indistinguishable on anterior part of body.

Adults uniformly dull olive green above or pale greenish gray with dark crossbands that tend to fuse anteriorly; cream to dirty white on sides and belly; head greenish above without marking; tail usually mottled with black. New born young are milk white with crossbands that almost encircle the body; top of head dark olive, tail black.

Remarks: A shallow water snake found over both mud and sand bottom and often very plentiful at the mouths of rivers. In great deltas such as those of the Ganges and Indus, *Enhydra* has been found in channels many miles from the open sea. It has not been reported to leave the water voluntarily and is very awkward although not completely helpless on land. In Indian waters, young are born from March through July. The average brood numbers 4 to 9.

The venom of the Beaked Sea Snake is the most toxic of the better known snake venoms, the lethal dose for experimental mammals being 50-125 micro grams/kilo of body weight. Since the fatal dose for an adult man is estimated to be about 1.5 mg and 10 to 15 mg. can be obtained from a snake of average size, this is clearly a potentially dangerous species, and it does appear to be responsible for more serious and fatal bites than all other sea snakes combined. This may be ascribed partly to its very toxic venom, and partly to its abundance near bathing beaches and fishing villages. It is ordinarily an inoffensive reptile but will bite if restrained.

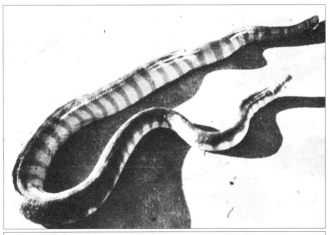

Photo 293. Beaked Sea Snake, *Enhydrina schistosa*

Antivenom: Sea Snake Antivenom manufactured by Commonwealth Serum Laboratories (CSL Limited) in Australia.

Additonal Species: One other species of Enhydrina is known. The Zweifel's Sea Snake, *E. zweifeli.*

Olive Brown Sea Snake,
Aipysurus laevis

Identification: In sea snakes of this genus the nostrils are dorsal in position and the shields on the top of the head are small but regular in arrangement. The ventrals are well developed extending at least one-third of the width of the body. *Aipysurus laevis* is a very heavy bodied snake, often as thick as a man's arm; the body is slightly flattened vertically. The head is large and a little wider than the neck; the end of the tail is usually ragged.

Adults are uniformly olive brown or may have a row of dark spots on the flanks and belly.

Maximum length about 6 feet; average 4.5 to 5 feet.

Remarks: Clumsy on land, it apparently does not leave water voluntarily although it is often found stranded on beaches.

Antivenom: Sea Snake Antivenom by Commonwealth Serum Laboratories (CSL Limited) in Australia.

Additonal Species: There are 8 members of this genus. The remaining seven species are:

    Short-nosed Sea Snake - *A. apraefrontalis*
    Dubois' Sea Snake - *A. duboisii*
    Spine-tailed Sea Snake - *A. eydouxii*
    Leaf-scaled Sea Snake - *A. foliosquama*
    Dusky Sea Snake - *A. fuscus*
    Shark Bay Sea Snake - *A. pooleorum*
    Brown-lined Sea Snake - *A. tenuis*

Hardwicke's Sea Snake,
Lapemis hardwickii

Identification: A rather short, stocky sea snake; head chunky, wider than neck; rostral with 3 stubby downward projections fitting into notches in the chin; ventrals not well differentiated except on neck; irregular rows of enlarged scales low on flanks.

Greenish or yellowish above, with series of dark cross-bands that are much wider than the light areas between them; paler below; head dark with or without lighter mottling; tail barred with black tip.

The average length of adults is 25-30 inches with a maximum of about 35 inches.

Remarks: A very abundant snake in shallow estuaries along coast of Vietnam, Malaya, and the Philippines and often taken in fish nets. It is most abundant during the rainy season (July to November).

Despite its very small venom yield (about 2 mg. from an adult snake) several fatal bites are on record; toxicity of the venom is less than that of the Beaked Sea Snake (pg. 291).

Antivenom: Sea Snake Antivenom by Commonwealth Serum Laboratories (CSL Limited) in Australia.

Additional Species: One other species of *Lapemis* sea snake is known. The Short Sea Snake, *L. curtus.*

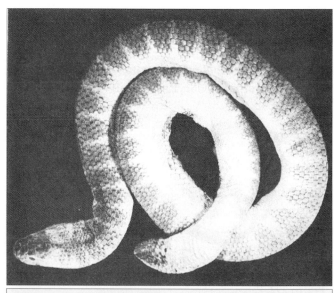

PHOTO 294. Hardwicke's Sea Snake, *Lapemis hardwickii*

Stokes' Sea Snake,
Disteira stokesii

Identification: In 1965 this species was placed in the genus *Astrotia*, and some sources still use that taxonomy. Like the Olive Brown Sea Snake (*Aipysurus laevis*) differs in having ventrals that are fragmented and not well differentiated and larger head shields. The body scales are large, keeled, and strongly imbricate.

Color light brown, yellowish or orange above with broad black rings or bars and spots; belly paler; head olive to yellowish.

Average adult length 4 1/2 to 5 feet; maximum about 6 feet; large specimens are about 10 inches in girth.

Remarks: Although generally an uncommon snake there is a report of a vast aggregation sighted in Malacca Strait on the 4th of May, 1932. The snakes were disposed in a line about 10 feet wide and some 60 miles long. This appears to be a snake of moderately deep open water and is not often taken by native fishermen. There are no reported bites by this species and its venom has never been studied.

Antivenom: Sea Snake Antivenom by Commonwealth Serum Laboratories (CSL Limited) in Australia.

Additonal Species: There are as many as three species of *Disteira*. Those additional two species are:

Spectacled Sea Snake - *Disteira kingii*
Olive-headed Sea Snake - *Disteira major*

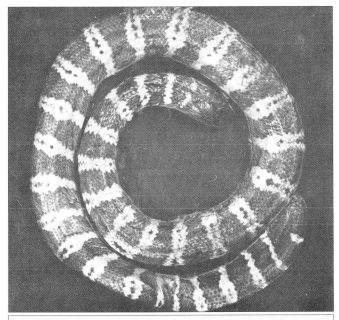

PHOTO 295. Stoke's Sea Snake, *Disteira stokesii*

Annulated Sea Snake,
Leioselasma cyanocincta

In 1965 this snake was placed in the genus *Hydrophis*. Some sources still list it as a member of that genus.

Identification: Head smaller, neck longer and more slender and body more compressed than in the Yellow Sea Snake. Head scales similar to those of the Yellow Sea Snake except that there are usually 2 anterior temporals. Body scales with central keel or row of tubercles. Increase of more than 8 (usually 10-16) scale rows between count at neck and count at midbody.

Color dirty white, pale greenish, yellow or olive with blackish crossbands that may or may not encircle the body, are widest along the vertebral midline and are as wide as or wider than, the interspaces between them. Head in adult olive, reddish or dull yellow; in young blackish with the yellow horseshoe mark seen in some other species.

The adult length averages 4.5 to 5.5 feet with a record specimen of about 6.5 feet.

Remarks: This snake frequents mangrove swamps but has been collected 12 to 20 miles offshore during winter. Although it has not been seen to leave the water voluntarily, it crawls fairly well and can lift its head well free of the ground. It often bites if restrained.

Yellow Sea Snake,
Leioselasma spiralis

In 1965 the original authors of this volume placed this species in the genus *Hydrophis*, and that taxonomic designation is still followed by several sources.

Identification: Head of moderate size and distinct from the neck which is not particularly slender or elongated; body moderately slender, not strongly compressed. Head shields large and symmetrical; the tip of the rostral shows a slight downward prolongation that fits into a notch in the tip of the lower jaw; usually one anterior temporal; body scales smooth or weakly keeled. There is an increase of no more than

8 scale rows between a count made on the neck and one made at the middle of the body.

Color golden yellow to yellowish green shading to a pinkish white below; body encircled by black rings that are widest along the vertebral midline and narrow on the flanks, always much narrower than the interspaces separating them; head uniformly yellow in the adult, dark with a yellow horseshoe shaped mark on the crown in the young.

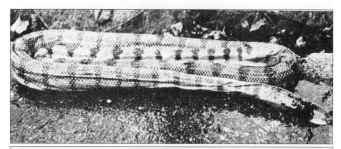

PHOTO 296. Yellow Sea Snake, *Leioselasma spiralis*

This is apparently the longest of the sea snakes.

Adult yellow sea snakes frequently reach a length of 5.5 to 6 feet, and a record length of 9 feet is reported.

Remarks: Very little information is on record concerning the habits and biology of this sea snake. It seems to frequent deep water and often basks at the surface.

Venom yields from this snake are surprisingly small (3 to 10 mg.) and toxicity lower than for most sea snake venoms, nevertheless several fatalities are on record from the bite of this species.

Antivenom: Sea Snake Antivenom by Commonwealth Serum Laboratories (CSL Limited) in Australia.

Additional Species: There are a total of 8 species of *Leioselasma* listed by The Repile Database (www.reptile-database.org - viewed 2012). The additional species not already mentioned are:

Slender-necked Sea Snake - *L. coggeri*
Five-spined Sea Snake - *L. czeblukovi*
Elegant Sea Snake - *L. elegans*
Slender-necked Sea Snake - *L. melanocephala*
Pacific Sea Snake - *L. pacifica*
Lake Taal Snake - *L. semperi*

Reef Sea Snake,
Chitula ornata

In the 1965 edition of Poisonous Snakes of the World this species is listed as *Hydrophis ornatus.*

Some sources still regard this species as a member of the *Hydrophis* genus.

Identification: A large headed, stout bodied sea snake; body scales small, juxtaposed, with a central tubercle that is more strongly developed in the male; increase of 12 to 20 scale rows between count at neck and count at midbody. The combination of regular head shields with

nasals in contact with each other and small, undivided ventrals of almost uniform size the entire length of the body will usually differentiate this species from other sea snakes of similar body build.

The typical form is pale greenish white, olive or yellow with wide dark crossbands or rhomboid spots. The head is olive.

Average length is 28- to 35 inches; maximum about 45 inches.

Remarks: this sea snake has a very wide range extending from the Persian Gulf to the central Pacific and from the Yellow Sea to Australia. It is plentiful in some localities, e.g. Manila Bay, but very rare and apparently a straggler in many others. It evidently frequents shallow water, for dozens have been taken in on haul of a beach seine. At least one fatality is ascribed to its bite.

Additional Species: There are a total of 11 species of *Chitula* listed by The Repile Database (www.reptile-database.org - viewed 2012). The additional 10 species are:

Plain Sea Snake - *C. inornata*
New Caledonia Sea Snake - *C. laboutei*
Lambert's Sea Snake - *C. lamberti*
Persian Gulf Sea Snake - *C. lapemoides*
Bombay Sea Snake - *C. mamillaris*
Kalimantan Sea Snake - *C. sibauensis*
Collared Sea Snake - *C. stricticollis*
West Coast Black-headed Sea Snake- *C. torquata*
Faint-banded Sea Snake - *C. belcheri*
Peter's Sea Snake - *C. bituberculatus*

Banded Small-headed Sea Snake,
Hydrophis fasciatus

In 1965 this species was placed in the genus *Microcephalus*.

Identification: Certain species of the genus *Hydrophis* are remarkable for their tiny heads and long, slender necks. This peculiar body form is most evident in the adult; young are not strikingly different from other sea snakes. Recognition of the young and differentiation of the various species of small-headed sea snakes is difficult. In this species the ventrals are distinctly wider than the adjacent scales throughout the length of the body and the total ventral count is high, usually 400 or more.

Thick part of body gray to dirty yellow crossed by dark bands that are widest in the middle of the back, but taper to points laterally; neck dark olive to black with yellow spots or crossbars; head uniformly dark.

The maximum length does not exceed 4 feet; average specimens are about 3 feet.

Remarks: The heavy body gives stability in floating while the small head and long slender neck permit the snake to explore holes and crevices in search of food. In swimming free, the head and neck are held straight and almost motionless. This species is reported to be primarily nocturnal in the Philippines.

Small-headed Sea Snakes are among the least prolific of snakes, females giving birth to only 1 or 2 young in a season.

Although it is difficult to imagine these snakes biting effectively, there is at least one fatality ascribed to the bite of a small-headed sea snake. Venom yields are minute (less than 1mg. per snake), but their venom is extremely toxic, being about equal to that Enhydrin.

Other widely distributed small-heads of the genus *Hydrophis* include *H. belcheri* of Australian and Pacific seas and *H. brookei, H. caerulescens,* and *H. klossi* of Indo-Malaysian waters.

Antivenom: Sea Snake Antivenom by Commonwealth Serum Laboratories (CSL Limited) in Australia.

Graceful Small-headed Sea Snake,
Hydrophis gracilis

Identification: In 1965 this species was placed in the genus *Microcephalus*. This snake differs from the Banded Small-headed Sea Snake in certain features of the skull and in the type of ventrals which are distinctly wider than the adjacent scales on the slender part of the body but become smaller and fragmented posteriorly; the ventral count does not exceed 300.

Anterior part of body including head black to dark olive with white or yellow spots or bands; posterior part pale yellow to greenish with darker crossbands or uniform gray above and light laterally and ventrally.

Most adults of this species measure 30-35 inches; maximum length is about 42 inches.

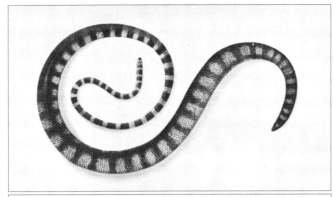

Photo 297. Graceful Small Headed Sea Snake, *Hydrophis gracilis*

Antivenom: Sea Snake Antivenom by Commonwealth Serum Laboratories (CSL Limited) in Australia.

Additional Species: When the original edition of this book was published there were over 25 species placed in this genus. The *Hydrophis* genus is still the largest genus of sea snakes with 15 species currently recognized. Those other 13 species are listed below.

Note that some species have no common name:
Black-headed Sea Snake - *H. atriceps*
Sea Snake - *H. brooki*
Sea Snake - *H. cantoris*
Sea Snake - *H. donaldi*
Sea Snake - *H. hendersoni*
Klossi Sea Snake - *H. klossi*
McDowell's Sea Snake - *H. macdowelli*
Black-banded Sea Snake - *H. melanosoma*
Sea Snake - *H. nigrocinctus*
Russel's Sea Snake - *H. obscurus*
Sea Snake - *H. pachyceros*
Sea Snake - *H. parviceps*
Esturine Sea Snake - *H. vorisi*

The sea snake subfamily Hydrophiinae has undergone many taxonomic changes since the 1965 edition of *Poisonous Snakes of the World*. Many new genera are still placed in the genus *Hydrophis* by some experts. Some genera that were in use in 1965 are no longer regarded as valid and there are several new genera now recognized by some sources that may not be regarded as valid by others. For the sea snakes this author has adopted the taxonomy used by the The Reptile Database (www.reptiledatabase.org-viewed 2012). It should be noted that this arrangement is not adhered to by many other sources. The list below shows the remaining species of sea snakes not already mentioned previously in this book, in alphabetical order.

Genus Acalyptus:

  A. peronii - Spiny-headed Sea Snake

Genus Emydocephalus:

  E. annulatus - Turtle-headed Sea Snake

  E. ijimae - Turtlehead Sea Snake

  E. szczerbaki - Sea Snake

Genus Ephalophis

  E. greyae - Northwestern Mangrove Sea Snake

Genus Hydrelaps:

  H. darwiniensi - Port Darwin Seasnake

Genus Kerilia:

  K. jerdonii - Jerdon's Sea Snake

Genus Kolpophis:

  K. annandalei - Bighead Sea Snake

Genus Parahydrophis:

  P. mertoni - Northern Mangrove Sea Snake

Genus Polyodontognathus:

  P. caerulescens - Dwarf Sea Snake

Genus Praescutata:

  P. viperina - Viperine Sea Snake

Genus Pseudolaticauda:

  P. schistorhynchus - Flat-tailed Sea Snake

  P. semifasciata - Chinese Sea Snake

Genus Thalassophis:

  T. anomalus - Anomalous Sea Snake

References

Books

Dowling, Herndon G., Sherman A. Minton, and Findlay E. Russell. 1965. *Poisonous Snakes of the World.* Department of the Navy Bureau of Medicine and Surgery. Washington, DC.

O'Shea, Mark. 2005. *Venomous Snakes of the World.* Princeton University Press. Princeton, NJ.

Websites

University of Adelaide, Clinical Toxinology Resources Wesbsite (2012) - www.toxinology.com

The Reptile Database - http//www.reptiledata-base.org

Armed Forces Pest Management Board - www.afpmb.org/content/living-hazards-database

Catalogue of Life - www.catalogueoflife.org

Australian Reptile Online Database- www.arod.com.au

Original References

BARME, Michel. 1963. Venomous Sea Snakes of Viet Nam and Their Venoms. *In* Venomous and Poisonous Animals and Noxious Plants of the Pacific World (H. L. Keegan and W. V. MacFarlane, eds.). Pergamon Press: Oxford, pp. 373–378, figs. 1–5.

HERRE, Albert. 1942. Notes on Philippine Sea-snakes. Copeia, no. 1, pp. 7–9. 1949. Notes on Philippine Sea Snakes of the Genus *Laticauda*. *Ibid.*, no. 4, pp. 282–284.

SMITH, Malcolm A. 1926. A Monograph of the Sea-snakes. Taylor and Francis: London, pp. i–xvii + 1–130, figs. 1–35, pls. 1–2.

VOLSØE, Helge. 1939. The Sea Snakes of the Iranian Gulf. *In* Danish Scientific Investigations in Iran (Knud Jessen and Ragnar Sparck, eds.) Copenhagen, Part 1, pp. 9–45.

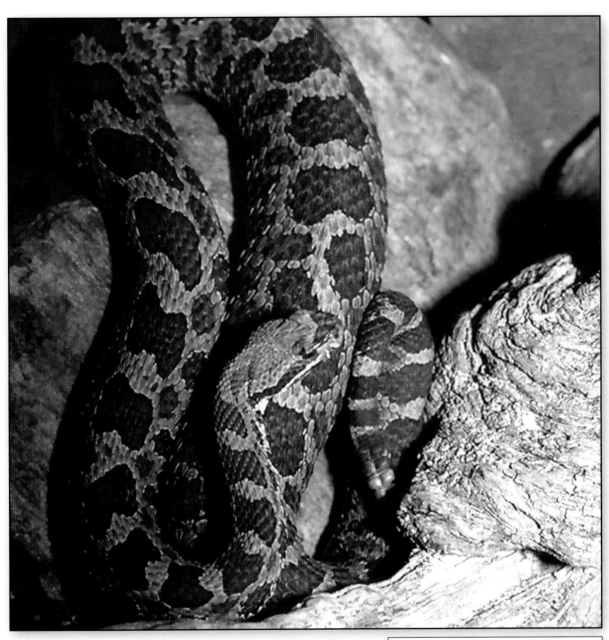

Eastern Massassauga,
Sistrurus catenatus catenatus

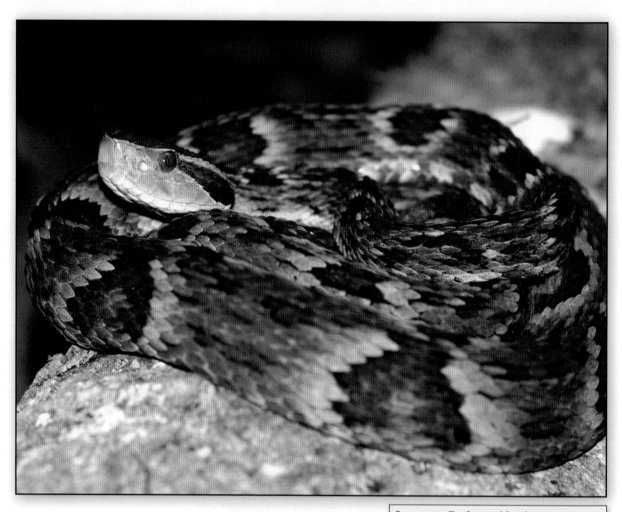

Jararaca, *Bothropoides jararaca*

Acknowledgments

The author would like to thank the following individuals whose support and contributions helped to make this book possible.

Dr. Harold Harlan, Director, Armed Forces Pest Management Board, Silver Springs, Maryland (USA), for his general support of the idea of revising and updating this book; and especially for providing a list of references used in the construction of the AFPMB Living Hazards Database, along with permission to use data found on the AFPMB Living Hazards Database. Dr. David Bates, Toxinology Department, Womens and Childrens Hospital, North Adelaide (Australia) for permission to access the Clinical Toxinology Resources website. From the Kentucky Reptile Zoo and Venom Laboratory in Slade, Kentucky (USA), Jim Harrison and Kristin Wiley assisted with photographing that facilities venomous snake collection and provided valuable advice, support, and encouragement throughout this project. In addition these two individuals were a valuable source of information and advice in the writing of chapters 4 and 5 which deal with snakebite first aid and treatment of venomous bites. Other staff members from the Kentucky Reptile Zoo who contributed to this effort were Taylor Tevis, Mike Lee, Peter Lindsey, Rachel Beasley, and Jackie Swapp. Tony Phelps of the Cape Reptile Institute in South Africa for suppling photos of most of the African snakes in this book and for suppling photos of additional Viperidae species. Dr. Pedro Barnardo of the Royal Ontario Museum (Canada) for suppling reference material and photos. Dr. Anita Mulhotra of Bangor University in the United Kingdom for forwarding papers on the *Trimeresurus* and *Ovophis* genus, and for advice on the current taxonomy of the *Trimeresurus* genus, as well as for providing photos of Asian Viperidae. From the Reptile Discovery Center in Deland, Florida (USA), Carl Barden and Tom Chesley for permission and assistance in photographing specimens at that facility. Dr. Gernot Vogel of Germany for advice on the taxonomy of some Asian pit vipers and for bringing to my attention a number of useful reference materials. Herm Mayes of the Cincinnati Museum (USA) for helping locate photographs.

Other important contributions in the form of photographs were made by David Hegner of the Czech Republic; Daniel Jablonski of Herpetolgie a cestovani; from Reptile Gardens in Rapid City, SD (USA), Joe Maierhouser; Ed Cassano of Clermont, Florida (USA); Sameer Ghodke, Maharashtra, India, and the Andaman Nicobar Islands Environmental Team; Ann Devon-Song, School of Biological Sciences, University of Hong Kong; Michael Cota from the Natural History Museum/National Science Museum of Thailand; Dr. Bruno Gattolin of St. Marcellin, France; Rob Schell from Richmond, California (USA); Roger S. Thorpe, United Kingdom; Raman Upadye, Maharashtra, India; Chris Carille Photography, Bailey McKay, Dick Bartlett, and Nancy-Smith Jones.

Finally, a sincere thanks is due to those at Skyhorse Publishing who helped make this book possible. Thanks to my editor, Jason Katzman, for his patience and counsel during the writing of this book, and to Nick Grant, whose hard work on the layout and design of *Venomous Snakes of the World* made it look better than I could have ever imagined.

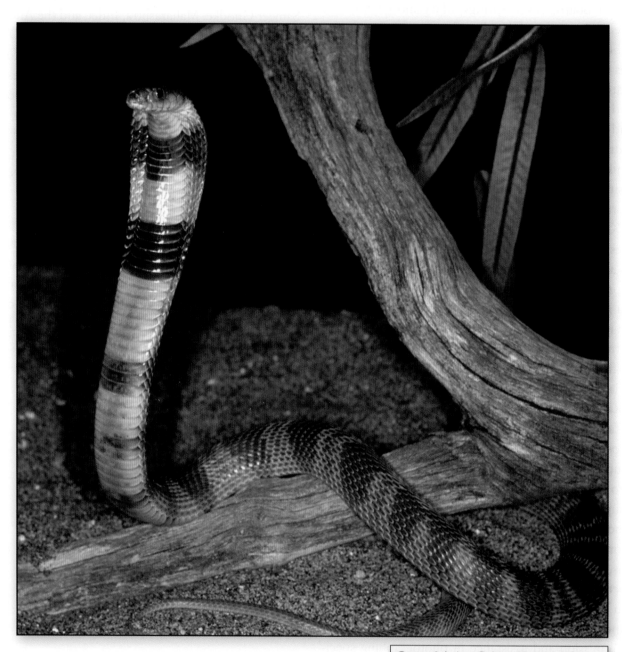

Central Asian Cobra, *Naja oxiana*

Glossary of Terms

Anal plate / Anal scute - the belly scale (scute) associated with the cloaca (anus) of a snake.

Anaphylaxis - a severe allergic reaction that may cause respiratory, circulatory, and neurological symptoms. Often fatal if untreated.

Anterior- towards the front.

Anticoagulant - agent (or toxin) that inhibits the ability of the blood to clot.

Antivenom - an antitoxin serum that neutralizes a venom.

Anuran - frog or toad.

Apical pits - tiny indentations on the apex of the dorsal scales in some snakes.

Arboreal - lives in trees or bushes.

Caniculated - traversed by small tubular passage or channel. Here applied to the fangs of a snake.

Canthals - head scales located between the snout and the eye of a snake.

Canthus rostralis - the angle of the head from the tip of a snakes snout to the front of the eye.

Cardiotoxin - toxin that attacks (or inhibits the function of) the heart.

Caudal luring - a behavior in which a snake wriggles the tip of its tail to mimic a worm, grub, or other prey.

Caudal scales - scales located on the tail of a snake.

Chin shields - scales on the chin of a snake.

Convergent Evolution - the tendency of unrelated animals to acquire similar adaptive morphologies.

Crepuscular - active at dawn or dusk.

Crotalid - refers to a snake of the subfamily Crotalinae (Pit Vipers).

Crown - the top of the head.

Cytotoxic - a toxin that destroys cells (usually by breaking down cell walls).

Disjunct - not connected.

Distal, Distally - away from the central part of the body, towards extremities.

Diurnal - active by day.

Dorsal scales - the scales on the top of a snake's body (the back and sides).

Ecchymosis - discoloration of the skin caused by blood leaking into surrounding tissues.

Edema - swelling caused by excessive fluid in the intercellular spaces.

Elapid - a snake belonging to the family Elapidae (Cobra family).

Elliptical - a shape that is more oval, as in the pupil of the eye of viperid snakes.

Endemic - native to a particular area and found nowhere else.

Equine - pertaining to horses.

Fasciotomy - an incision opening the fascia of the muscles.

Fossorial - burrowing.

Frontal Scale - a large scale located between the eyes on the top of a snake's head.

Fynbos - Mediterranean-like heathland type habitat unique to the Cape provinces of South Africa.

Gular - the throat region.

Haemorragin - agent that induces hemorraging.

Haemotoxic / Hemotoxic - toxic to the blood and/or circulatory system.

Hemipene - the male sexual organ of a snake.

Herpetology / Herpetologist - pertaining to the study of reptiles and amphibians.

Hypotension - abnormally low blood pressure.

Labial scales - scales along the lips of a snake.

LD50 - the amount of venom needed to kill 50% of a group of test animals (usually lab mice) within a 24 hour period.

Live bearing - gives birth to fully formed young.

Infralabial scales - scales of the lower lip of a snake.

Insular - dwelling or situated on an island.

Internasal scales - scales situated between the nostrils on the top of a snake's snout.

Interstitial - the space (skin) between the scales of a snake.

Imbricate scales - scales that overlap.

Keeled scale - a scale with a raised keel.

Loreal scale - a scale on the side of a snake's snout that is located between the preocular and the post-nasal.

Loreal Pit- the deep depressions on the sides of the face of pit vipers.

Maxillary teeth - teeth on the upper jaw of a snake.

Mental scale - anterior-most scale on the chin of a snake.

Monovalent - effective against the venom of a single snake species.

Morphology - pertaining to an organism's body, as in structures, shape, form, coloration, pattern, etc.

Myotoxin - A muscle destroying toxin.

Nasal scale - scales in immediate contact with the snake's nostril.

Necrosis, necrotic - refers to the death of tissues.

Necrotoxin - a toxin that causes necrosis (death of tissues).

Nephrotoxin - a toxin with a destructive effect on kidney tissues.

Neurotoxic / Neurotoxin - a toxin that attacks the nervous system.

Nocturnal - active at night.

Oblique - slanting, at an angle.

Occipital scales - paired enlarged scales that lie immediately behind the parietals in a few snakes such as the King Cobra.

Ontogenic variation - a change in the morphology (usually color or pattern) associated with age.

Ovine - related to sheep.

Oviparous - egg layer.

Parietal scale - large scale located on the back of the head of a snake (there are two).

Phylogeny - the relationship between organisms based on their evolutionary lines of descent.

Pit - see loreal pit.

Polymorphic - occurring in more than one color or pattern.

Polyvalent - refers to antivenom that can effectively neutralize the venom of more than one species of snake.

Posteriorly - towards the tail.
Postocular stripe - a stripe that runs from the eye to the angle of the jaw in a snake.

Postsynaptic neurotoxins - toxins that inhibit the transmission of nerve impulses by blocking the acetylcholine receptors of the nerves.

Prefrontal scale - scale which appears in some species that is located anterior to the frontal scale.

Preocular scale - small scale(s) on the side of the head of a snake located immediately anterior.

Pre-synaptic neurotoxins - a toxin that inhibits the transmission of nerve impulses by disrupting the release of neurotransmitters from the terminal axion.

Procoagulant - An agent that promotes the coagulation of the blood. In snakebite situations procoagulants can ultimately lead to blood incoagulability by exhausting the coagulating elements in the blood.

Proteolytic - breaks down proteins.

Proximal - towards the heart.

Rostral scale - the scale on the anterior tip of the snout of a snake.

Savannah - a habitat type characterized by grasslands having widely spaced trees.

Scute - a type of scale on a snake as in the scales across the ventral surface of a snake (belly scales) or scales on the head.

Sexual dimorphism - sexually related morphological differences within a steppe - a grassland habitat type that is widespread across much of north-central Asia.

Subterranean - living underground.

Supralabial scales - the scales of the upper lip of a snake.

Supraocular scales - scales on the top of the head of a snake immediately above the eye.

Sympatric / Sympatry - occurring together in the same locale / habitat / area.

Synonym / Synonymous - a different name for the same species of organism.

Terrestrial - living on land.

Tubercles - raised, dome-like projection.

Tuberculate - scales having tubercles.

Ventral scales - scales on the belly of a snake.

Ventro-lateral - at the junction of the side and the belly.

Vertebral - having to do with the backbone, as in vertebral blotches (i.e., blotches along the top of the back).

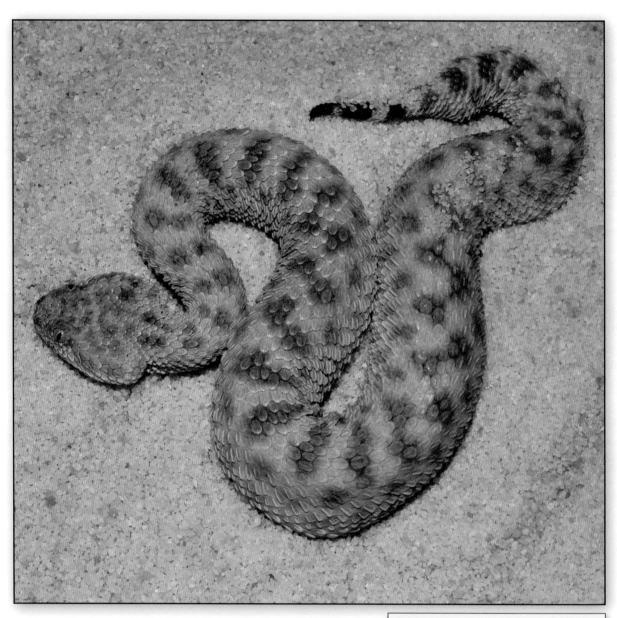

Cottonmouth,
Agkistrodon piscivorous

Index

Throughout this index, names in bold refer to the names as previously listed in the 1965 edition of this book.

Contributing Photograpers

Photographer	Number	Name	Extra Courtesy
Dick Bartlett	1	Sonoran Coral Snake	
Scott Shupe	2	Eastern Coral Snake	St. Augustine Alligator Farm
Scott Shupe	3	Texas Coral Snake	Kentucky Reptile Zoo
Rob Schell	4	West Mexican Coral Snake	
David Hegner	5	Brown's Coral Snake	
Scott Shupe	6	Copperhead	
Scott Shupe	7	Copperhead	
Scott Shupe	8	Cottonmouth	
Scott Shupe	9	Cottonmouth	
Scott Shupe	10	Taylor's Cantil	Kentucky Reptile Zoo
Scott Shupe	11	Common Cantil	Kentucky Reptile Zoo
Scott Shupe	12	Mexican Jumping Viper	Kentucky Reptile Zoo
Scott Shupe	13	Yellow-blotched Palm Viper	
David Hegner	14	Yellow-blotched Palm Viper	
Pedro Bernardo	15	Eyelash Viper	
Scott Shupe	16	Godman's Mountain Pit Viper	Kentucky Reptile Zoo
Scott Shupe	17	Terciopelo	Kentucky Reptile Zoo
Scott Shupe	18	Dunn's Hognosed Pit Viper	
Scott Shupe	19	Yucatan Hognosed Pit Viper	
Scott Shupe	20	Eastern Diamondback Rattlesnake	Kentucky Reptile Zoo
Scott Shupe	21	Western Diamondback Rattlesnake	
Scott Shupe	22	Red Diamond Rattlesnake	
Scott Shupe	23	Mohave Rattlesnake	
Scott Shupe	24	Prairie Rattlesnake	
Nancy Smith-Jones	25	Hopi Rattlesnake	
Scott Shupe	26	Great Basin Rattlesnake	
Scott Shupe	27	Northern Pacific Rattlesnake	
Scott Shupe	28	Southern Pacific Rattlesnake	
Scott Shupe	29	Arizona Black Rattlesnake	Kentucky Reptile Zoo
Scott Shupe	30	Grand Canyon Rattlesnake	Kentucky Reptile Zoo
Ed Cassano	31	Midget Faded Rattlesnake	
Scott Shupe	32	Timber Rattlesnake	
Scott Shupe	33	Timber Rattlesnake	
Scott Shupe	34	Panamint Rattlesnake	
Scott Shupe	35	Speckled Rattlesnake	Kentucky Reptile Zoo
Scott Shupe	36	Sidewinder Rattlesnake	
Scott Shupe	37	Sidewinder Rattlesnake	Birmingham Zoo
Scott Shupe	38	Sidewinder Rattlesnake	
Scott Shupe	39	Mexican West Coast Rattlesnake	Kentucky Reptile Zoo
Ed Cassano	40	Middle American Rattlesnake	
Scott Shupe	41	Tiger Rattlesnake	
Scott Shupe	42	Black-tailed Rattlesnake	
Scott Shupe	43	Mexican Lance-headed Rattlesnake	Kentucky Reptile Zoo
Ed Cassano	44	Baja California Rattlesnake	
Scott Shupe	45	Rock Rattlesnake	
Scott Shupe	46	Rock Rattlesnake	
Ed Cassano	47	Mexican Pygmy Rattlesnake	
Scott Shupe	48	Twin-spotted Rattlesnake	Kentucky Reptile Zoo

Rob Schell	49	Santa Catalina Rattlesnake	
Scott Shupe	50	Massassauga Rattlesnake	
Scott Shupe	51	Massassauga Rattlesnake	
Scott Shupe	52	Dusky Pygmy Rattlesnake	
Scott Shupe	53	Western Pygmy Rattlesnake	
Scott Shupe	54	Carolina Pygmy Rattlesnake	
Chris Carille Photography	55	Central American Coral Snake	
Pedro Bernardo	56	Southern Coral Snake	
Pedro Bernardo	57	Amazonian Coral Snake	
Roy Santa Cruz Farfan	58	Aquatic Coral Snake	National University of San Augustin
Pedro Bernardo	59	Painted Coral Snake	
Pedro Bernardo	60	South American Coral Snake	
Pedro Bernardo	61	Brazilian Coral Snake	
Scott Shupe	62	Central American Jumping Viper	Kentucky Reptile Zoo
Ed Cassano	63	Coffee Palm Viper	
David Hegner	64	Black-speckled Palm Viper	
David Hegner	65	Yellow-blotched Palm Viper	
Scott Shupe	66	Eyelash Viper	
Ed Cassano	67	Eyelash Viper	
Pedro Bernardo	68	Eyelash Viper	
Bruno Gattolin	69	Two Striped Forest Pit Viper	
Scott Shupe	70	Speckled Forest Pit Viper	
Scott Shupe	71	Terciopelo	Kentucky Reptile Zoo
Scott Shupe	72	Common Lancehead	Kentucky Reptile Zoo
Scott Shupe	73	Brazilian Lancehead	Kentucky Reptile Zoo
Scott Shupe	74	St. Lucia Lancehead	Kentucky Reptile Zoo
Pedro Bernardo	75	Jararacussu	
New York Zoological Society	76	Fer-de-Lance	
Pedro Bernardo	77	Whitetail Lancehead	
Pedro Bernardo	78	Barnett's Lancehead	
Scott Shupe	79	Venezuelan Lancehead	Kentucky Reptile Zoo
Pedro Bernardo	80	Jararaca	
Scott Shupe	81	Caatinga Lancehead	Kentucky Reptile Zoo
Scott Shupe	82	Mato Grosso Lancehead	Kentucky Reptile Zoo
Pedro Bernardo	83	Jararaca Pintada	
Scott Shupe	84	Chaco Lancehead	Central Florida Zoo
David Hegner	85	Pampas Lancehead	
David Hegner	86	Golden Lancehead	
Scott Shupe	87	Urutu	Kentucky Reptile Zoo
Pedro Bernardo	88	Fonseca's Lancehead	
David Hegner	89	Rainforest Hognosed Viper	
David Hegner	90	Lansberg's Hognosed Viper	
Scott Shupe	91	Slender Hognosed Viper	Kentucky Reptile Zoo
Chris Carille Photography	92	Central American Bushmaster	
Scott Shupe	93	South American Bushmaster	
Scott Shupe	94	South American Rattlesnake	Kentucky Reptile Zoo
Scott Shupe	95	South American Rattlesnake	Kentucky Reptile Zoo
Scott Shupe	96	South American Rattlesnake	Kentucky Reptile Zoo
Tony Phelps	97	South American Rattlesnake	
Ed Cassano	98	Middle American Rattlesnake	
Daniel Jablonski	99	European Viper	
Daniel Jablonski	100	European Viper	

Daniel Jablonski	101	Portugeuse Viper	
Daniel Jablonski	102	Asp Viper	
Daniel Jablonski	103	Snub-nosed Viper	
Scott Shupe	104	Long-nosed Viper	Kentucky Reptile Zoo
Scott Shupe	105	Long-nosed Viper	Kentucky Reptile Zoo
Daniel Jablonski	106	Transcaucasian Viper	
Daniel Jablonski	107	Meadow Viper	
David Hegner	108	Caucasus Viper	
Joe Maierhauser	109	Caucasus Subalpine Viper	Reptile Gardens
Daniel Jablonski	110	Nikolsky's Viper	
Daniel Jablonski	111	Steppe Viper	
Joe Maierhauser	112	Orlov's Viper	Reptile Gardens
Scott Shupe	113	Otoman Viper	Kentucky Reptile Zoo
Scott Shupe	114	Armenian Viper	Kentucky Reptile Zoo
Scott Shupe	115	Central Turkish Mountain Viper	Kentucky Reptile Zoo
Daniel Jablonski	116	Wagner's Viper	
Scott Shupe	117	Levantine Viper	Kentucky Reptile Zoo
David Hegner	118	Blunt-nosed Viper	
Daniel Jablonski	119	Haly's Pit Viper	
Bruno Gattolin	120	Haly's Pit Viper	
Daniel Jablonski	121	European Viper	
Daniel Jablonski	122	Steppe Viper	
Scott Shupe	123	Levantine Viper	Kentucky Reptile Zoo
Scott Shupe	124	Puff Adder	
Scott Shupe	125	Palestine Viper	Kentucky Reptile Zoo
Scott Shupe	126	Western Russell's Viper	Kentucky Reptile Zoo
Daniel Jablonski	127	MacMahon's Desert Viper	
Scott Shupe	128	Sochurek's Saw-scaled Viper	Kentucky Reptile Zoo
David Hegner	129	Painted Saw-scaled Viper	
Tony Phelps	130	Oman Saw-scaled Viper	
Tony Phelps	131	Arabian Horney Viper	
David Hegner	132	Sahara Horned Viper	
David Hegner	133	Western False Horned Viper (light)	
David Hegner	134	Western False Horned Viper (dark)	
Joe Maierhauser	135	Black Desert Cobra	Reptile Gardens
Joe Maierhauser	136	Central Asian Cobra	Reptile Gardens
Scott Shupe	137	Egyptian Cobra	
Scott Shupe	138	Common Cobra	Kentucky Reptile Zoo
Joe Maierhauser	139	Common Krait	Reptile Gardens
Scott Shupe	140	Puff Adder	
Tony Phelps	141	East African Gaboon Viper	
Scott Shupe	142	West African Gaboon Viper	Kentucky Reptile Zoo
Scott Shupe	143	Nose-horned Viper	Kentucky Reptile Zoo
Scott Shupe	144	Ethiopian Mountain Viper	Kentucky Reptile Zoo
Tony Phelps	145	Horned Adder	
Tony Phelps	146	Berg Adder	
Tony Phelps	147	Southern Adder	
Tony Phelps	148	Many-horned Adder	
Tony Phelps	149	Red Adder	
Scott Shupe	150	Moorish Viper	Kentucky Reptile Zoo
David Hegner	151	Blunt-nosed Desert Viper	
Daniel Jablonski	152	Snub-nosed Viper	

Scott Shupe	153	Western Bush Viper	Kentucky Reptile Zoo
Tony Phelps	154	Green Bush Viper	
Tony Phelps	155	Sedge Bush Viper	
David Hegner	156	Mount Kenya Bush Viper	
Tony Phelps	157	Swamp Viper	
David Hegner	158	White-bellied Saw scaled Viper	
Scott Shupe	159	Egyptian Saw-scaled Viper	Kentucky Reptile Zoo
Tony Phelps	160	West African Saw-scaled Viper	
Joe Maierhauser	161	Sahara Horned Viper	Reptile Gardens
Daniel Jablonski	162	Sahara Sand Viper	
Tony Phelps	163	Common Night Adder	
Scott Shupe	164	Egyptian Cobra	
Tony Phelps	165	Snouted Cobra	
Tony Phelps	166	Snouted Cobra	
Ed Cassano	167	Cape Cobra	
Tony Phelps	168	Cape Cobra	
Scott Shupe	169	Forest Cobra	Kentucky Reptile Zoo
Zoological Society of San Diego	170	Banded Water Cobra	
Tony Phelps	171	Red Spitting Cobra	
David Hegner	172	Nubian Spitting Cobra	
David Hegner	173	Black-necked Spitting Cobra	
Joe Maierhauser	174	Western Barred Spitting Cobra	Reptile Gardens
Tony Phelps	175	Western Barred Spitting Cobra	
Tony Phelps	176	Mossambique Spitting Cobra	
Tony Phelps	177	Rinkhals	
Joe Maierhauser	178	Gold's Tree Cobra	Reptile Gardens
Scott Shupe	179	Black Mamba	Reptile Discovery Center
Scott Shupe	180	East African Green Mamba	
Scott Shupe	181	West African Green Mamba	
Scott Shupe	182	Jameson's Mamba	Kentucky Reptile Zoo
Tony Phelps	183	Shield-nosed Snake	
Tony Phelps	184	Western Coral Snake	
Tony Phelps	185	Boomslang (female)	
Tony Phelps	186	Boomslang (male)	
Zoological Society of San Diego	187	Forest Vine Snake	
Scott Shupe	188	Small-scaled Mole Viper	Kentucky Reptile Zoo
Scott Shupe	189	Common Cobra	Kentucky Reptile Zoo
Scott Shupe	190	Monocle Cobra	Kentucky Reptile Zoo
Sameer Ghodke	191	Andaman Cobra	Andaman/Nicobar Environmental Team
Ann Devon-Song	192	Chinese Cobra	
Joe Maierhauser	193	Peter's Cobra	Reptile Gardens
Nick Baker	194	Sumatran Spitting Cobra (black phase)	ecologyasia.com
Scott Shupe	195	Indo-Chinese Spitting Cobra	Reptile Gardens
Tony Phelps	196	King Cobra	
Joe Maierhauser	197	Common Krait	Reptile Gardens
Joe Maierhauser	198	Banded Krait	Reptile Gardens
Michael Cota	199	Malayan Krait	
Sameer Ghodke	200	Andaman Krait	
Scott Shupe	201	Many-banded Krait	Kentucky Reptile Zoo
Michael Cota	202	Red-headed Krait	
David Hegner	203	Speckled Coral Snake	
Raman Upadhye	204	Indian Coral Snake	

Nick Baker	205	Striped Coral Snake	
David Hegner	206	McClelland's Coral Snake	
Anita Mulhotra	207	Fea's Viper	
Scott Shupe	208	Western Russell's Viper	Kentucky Reptile Zoo
David Hegner	209	Eastern Russell's Viper	
Scott Shupe	210	Saw-scaled Viper	Kentucky Reptile Zoo
Scott Shupe	211	Malayan Pit Viper	Kentucky Reptile Zoo
David Hegner	212	Hump-nosed Viper	
Scott Shupe	213	Snarp-nosed Pit Viper	Kentucky Reptile Zoo
David Hegner	214	Ussurian Mamushi	
Anita Mulhotra	215	Short-tailed Mamushi	
David Hegner	216	Rock Mamushi	
Anita Mulhotra	217	Snake Island Mamushi	
Scott Shupe	218	Hhemihabu	Kentucky Reptile Zoo
Joe Maierhauser	219	Tonkin Mountain Pit Viper	Reptile Gardens
David Hegner	220	Oriental Mountain Pit Viper	
David Hegner	221	Indo-Malayan Mountain Pit Viper	
Anita Mulhotra	222	Taiwan Mountain Pit Viper	
Roger S. Thorpe	223	Mount Kimbalu Pit Viper	
Scott Shupe	224	Chinese Habu	Ross Allen Reptile Institute
David Hegner	225	Elegant Pit Viper	
Bailey McKay	226	Okinawa Habu	
Scott Shupe	227	Takara Habu	Kentucky Reptile Zoo
Scott Shupe	228	Red-spotted Pit Viper	Kentucky Reptile Zoo
Joe Maierhauser	229	Horned Pit Viper	Reptile Gardens
Joe Maierhauser	230	Mangshan Pit Viper	Reptile Gardens
Scott Shupe	231	White-lipped Pit Viper	
David Hegner	232	White-lipped Island Pit Viper	
David Hegner	233	White-lipped Island Pit Viper (yellow morph)	
Ann Devon-Song	234	Kramer's Pit Viper	
Roger S. Thorpe	235	Cardomom Mountains Bamboo Pit Viper	
David Hegner	236	Pope's Bamboo Pit Viper (male)	
David Hegner	237	Pope's Bamboo Pit Viper (female)	
David Hegner	238	Sabah Bamboo Pit Viper (female)	
David Hegner	239	Cameron Highlands Bamboo Pit Viper (female)	
David Hegner	240	Cameron Highlands Bamboo Pit Viper (male)	
David Hegner	241	Siamese Peninsula Bamboo Pit Viper (female)	
David Hegner	242	Siamese Peninsula Bamboo Pit Viper (male)	
David Hegner	243	Vogel's Green Tree Pit Viper (female)	
David Hegner	244	Vogel's Green Tree Pit Viper (male)	
Daniel Jablonski	245	Chinese Green Tree Pit Viper	
David Hegner	246	Gumprecht's Green Tree Viper (female)	
Anita Mulhotra	247	Gumprecht's Green Tree Viper (male)	
Raman Upadhye	248	Indian (Common) Bamboo Viper	
David Hegner	249	Banded Pit Viper (male)	
David Hegner	250	Banded Pit Viper (female)	
Roy Santa Cruz Farfan	251	Ashy Pit Viper (female)	National University of San Augustin

David Hegner	252	Ashy Pit Viper (male)	
Anita Mulhotra	253	Ashy Pit Viper	
David Hegner	254	Wirot's Pit Viper (male)	
David Hegner	255	Wirot's Pit Viper (female)	
Sameer Ghodke	256	Nicobar Island Pit Viper	
Sameer Ghodke	257	Cantor's Pit Viper	
Sameer Ghodke	258	Anderson's Pit Viper	
Scott Shupe	259	Beautiful Pit Viper	
Pedro Bernardo	260	Kanburi Pit Viper	
Tony Phelps	261	Mangrove Viper (dark morph)	
Scott Shupe	262	Mangrove Viper	Ross Allen Reptile Institute
Ann Devon-Song	263	Phillipine Pit Viper	
David Hegner	264	Sumatran Bamboo Pit Viper	
David Hegner	265	Indonesian Bamboo Pit Viper	
Anita Mulhotra	266	Indonesian Bamboo Pit Viper	
Scott Shupe	267	McGregor's Pit Viper	
Anita Mulhotra	268	Schultze's Pit Viper	
Scott Shupe	269	Sri Lankan Bamboo Pit Viper	
Anita Mulhotra	270	Malabarian Pit Viper	
David Hegner	271	Wagler's Temple Viper	
David Hegner	272	Borneo Temple Viper (adult female)	
David Hegner	273	Borneo Temple Viper (immature)	
Joe Maierhauser	274	Common Death Adder	Reptile Gardens
Joe Maierhauser	275	Desert Death Adder	Reptile Gardens
Joe Maierhauser	276	New Guinea Death Adder	Reptile Gardens
Scott Shupe	277	Rough-scaled Death Adder	Kentucky Reptile Zoo
Daniel Jablonski	278	Northern Death Adder	
Joe Maierhauser	279	Eastern Tiger Snake	Reptile Gardens
Joe Maierhauser	280	Western Tiger Snake	Reptile Gardens
Joe Maierhauser	281	Western Tiger Snake	Reptile Gardens
Joe Maierhauser	282	Eastern Brown Snake	Reptile Gardens
Joe Maierhauser	283	Western Brown Snake	Reptile Gardens
Scott Shupe	284	Coastal Taipan	Kentucky Reptile Zoo
Joe Maierhauser	285	Inland Taipan	Reptile Gardens
Joe Maierhauser	286	Papuan Blacksnake	Reptile Gardens
Joe Maierhauser	287	King Brown Snake	Reptile Gardens
Joe Maierhauser	288	King Brown Snake	Reptile Gardens
Joe Maierhauser	289	Red-bellied Blacksnake	Reptile Gardens
Joe Maierhauser	290	Collett's Blacksnake	Reptile Gardens
Shooter Stock	291	Yellow-lipped Sea Krait	
U.S. Navy	292	Pelagic Sea Snake	
Sherman Minton	293	Beaked Sea Snake	
Edward H. Taylor	294	Hardwicke's Sea Snake	
Edward H. Taylor	295	Stoke's Sea Snake	
Serman A. Minton	296	Yellow Sea Snake	
U.S. Navy	297	Graceful Small Headed Sea Snake	

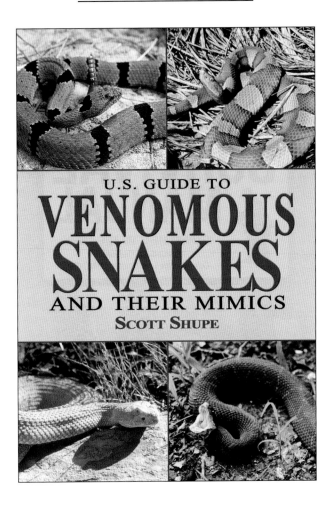

U.S. Guide to Venomous Snakes and Their Mimics

by Scott Shupe

This easy-to-use guide is the most comprehensive resource for snake admirers in the United States. Full-color photographs for almost every snake in the country make for easy reference, and dividing the snakes based on their regional habitats makes finding the right snake a breeze. Whether you are trying to identify a western coral snake or its mimic, the Sonoran shovel-nosed snake, Scott Shupe's guide is the extensive handbook for which all snake aficionados have been waiting. With full-color maps and a thorough glossary of terms, you'll be able to identify Arizona black rattlesnakes, eastern cottonmouths, and more in no time!

Unlike other snake books, Shupe's guide covers the snake population of the entire United States. His expertise and knowledge of snakes are apparent in the thoughtful descriptions and handy hints on how to tell poisonous snakes from their harmless imitators. He also includes an informative natural history of the reptiles and the scientific terms by which they are referred. As a gift for a young naturalist, a reference book for your library, or a handy tool in a sticky situation, this guide is practical, useful, and fun!

$14.95 Hardcover • ISBN: 978-1-61608-182-9

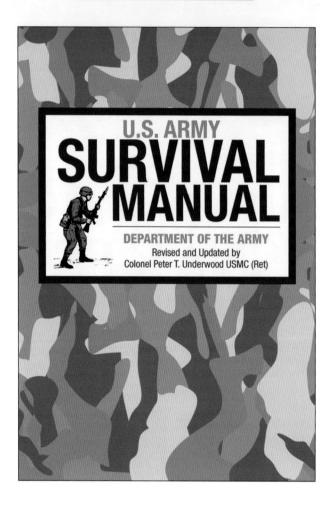
U.S. Army Survival Manual

by the Department of the Army,
Revised and Updated by Colonel Peter T. Underwood USMC (Ret)

Whether you're gearing up for a backcountry trek, preparing for the worst that nature or man can offer, or just want to have a great resource at your fingertips, you need this comprehensive, full-color new edition of the *U.S. Army Survival Manual*, thoroughly revised by Colonel Peter T. Underwood USMC (Ret). Ideal for military personnel, outdoors enthusiasts, and anyone who wants to be ready for anything, this is a thorough road map for all areas of wilderness survival, including:

- Erecting shelters
- Making weapons and utensils
- Fashioning traps for wildlife wrangling
- Preparing food from wild plants
- Identifying poisonous snakes and lizards

From basic first aid to in-depth, step-by-step instructions on overcoming major obstacles and handling emergencies, this guide clarifies all aspects of survival using tactics derived from those whose lives depend on it.

$12.95 Paperback • ISBN: 978-1-62636-158-4

ALSO AVAILABLE

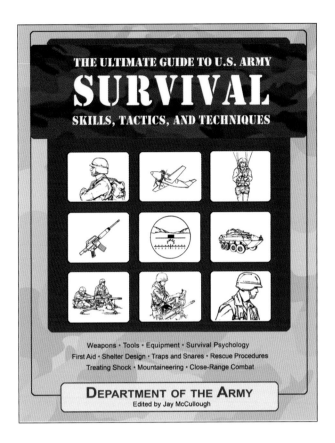

The Ultimate Guide to U.S. Army Survival Skills, Tactics, and Techniques

by the Department of the Army
Edited by Jay McCullough

Drawing from dozens of the U.S. Army's official field manuals, editor Jay McCullough has culled a thousand pages of the most useful and curious tidbits for the would-be soldier, historian, movie-maker, writer, or survivalist—including techniques on first aid; survival in the hottest or coldest of climates; finding or building life-saving shelters; surviving nuclear, biological, and chemical attacks; physical and mental fitness, and how to find food and water anywhere, anytime. With hundreds of photographs and illustrations showing everything from edible plants to rare skin diseases of the jungle, every page reveals how useful Army knowledge can be.

$24.95 Paperback • ISBN: 978-1-60239-050-8